HUMAN DEVELOPMENT

HUMAN DEVELOPMENT

A
TRANSACTIONAL
PERSPECTIVE

IRA J. GORDON
Institute for Development of Human Resources
University of Florida
Gainesville

Harper & Row, Publishers
New York, Evanston, San Francisco, London

To My Wife, Esther,
and Our Children, Gary and Bonnie

Sponsoring Editor: Michael E. Brown
Project Editor: Alice M. Solomon
Designer: Michel Craig
Production Supervisor: Will C. Jomarron
Portions of this book appeared in HUMAN DEVELOPMENT From Birth Through Adolescence, Copyright © 1962, 1969 by Ira J. Gordon
HUMAN DEVELOPMENT A Transactional Perspective

Library of Congress Cataloging in Publication Data

Gordon, Ira J
    Human development.

    Includes bibliographies and index.
      1. Child study. 2. Adolescent psychology.
I. Title.
BF721.G643   155.4   74–14492
ISBN 0–06–042392–7

CONTENTS

PREFACE

In the preface to the first edition, the author suggested that there was a need for a *rapprochement* between self-psychology and general behavior theory. Developmental psychologists in the past decade and a half have moved considerably toward such an establishment of relations through their concern for the educational applications of knowledge of child development and learning. Further, the lines between maturational developmental psychology and experimental child psychology continue to be erased. The concern for individuality represented in self-psychology is presently also found in studies utilizing behavior modification approaches to the disadvantaged child, the child with learning disabilities, and the child with emotional problems. Although there are still three broad divisions of research—cognitive, behavioral, and perceptual-self—barriers and boundaries that formerly existed are somewhat diminished. We find experimentalists utilizing Piagetian concepts, self-psychologists using Skinnerian approaches, and cognitive psychologists borrowing from both. Although this is a healthy sign, harmony is not complete, and we are still a long way from a unified theory. The author of a general text has the obligation to attempt some personal synthesis among these somewhat diverse and still quarrelsome positions.

This book, therefore, attempts to use the self of the child as the integrative theme around which studies of factors both outside him and within his own makeup influence his development and learning. The major unifying concept is that of transaction, in which the developing child is both being influenced and influences his world, and in which his own past experiences and development influence his present development. The developing person represents a synthesis of all influences, internal and external, at any one moment.

In any effort to bridge diverse viewpoints it must be recognized that the author takes certain liberties in interpretation of the findings from individual researches. This book is selective rather than encyclopedic. What is presented here is, therefore, not simply a description of empirical findings about children at different ages but an attempt to organize these findings. The aim for the student of human development is to understand the individual child, who represents his own organization of external and internal forces that have acted and are acting upon him as he grows. With this background as a student, the practitioner may be more effective in helping children and youth to learn and develop, both through direct dealings with children and through changing the social and learning environment in which they are growing up.

Ira J. Gordon

ACKNOWLEDGMENTS

No book is the product of a single person. Although only one author's name may appear, he is indebted to numerous others, both known and unknown to him, for their contributions to his thinking. First, I am indebted to the many researchers and theorists whom I have quoted throughout the book. Each one has contributed either information or an idea without which my attempts would have been futile. The index of names, in effect, forms part of this acknowledgment. I am also indebted to colleagues and students both at the University of Florida and in other institutions who, over the years, have made suggestions toward revision or have read portions of this manuscript and offered constructive help. In particular, I am indebted to R. Emile Jester and Robert S. Soar for specific editorial comments about earlier portions of the manuscript and to Helen Bee for her critical and helpful appraisal of the second edition. My thanks go to Mrs. Denise Stevens, who performed the typing chores, and to Mrs. Ginger Braune for her numerous forms of administrative assistance that smoothed the way for writing.

I owe a debt to the parents, parent educators, teachers, and coordinators, and to my colleagues in the Institute involved in the Florida Follow Through approach. They have all influenced my thinking about the roles of school and home and the needs for partnership that I hope are reflected in many of the chapters. I feel a special debt to my family. Without the support, patience, love, and understanding of my wife, Esther, and the interest of Gary and Bonnie, I could not have written this book. Beyond this, I owe to my wife many of the ideas that have influenced my thought. There are references in the text to the Parent Education Project: Her concern for infancy and her awareness, long before some of the research data were present, of the pliability and learnability of the infant and the importance of the mother as teacher led to the development of that project. Our children, now both finishing university, have really demonstrated the concept of transaction; they have taught us, and they continue to teach us as we strive to help them. Their thoughts, though indirectly, are represented, especially in the chapters on adolescence: Bonnie's because of her interest and work in adolescent self-concept, Gary's in the poem heading Chapter 18, and both in the social background. This book is affectionately dedicated to my family in grateful acknowledgment of their special contributions.

Ira J. Gordon

ONE

A POINT OF VIEW

CHAPTER 1

AN OVERVIEW

In this book we will consider the development of the newborn infant into an adult. The story is one of change, continuous change. The focus is on the child as an individual and on the ways in which he relates to various environments as he grows.

There are various possible ways to study the development of the human being. One approach is to try to see him always as a whole and to look at this whole being in various stages of development. This method has the advantage of maintaining the individual's integrity. Its disadvantage is that we are likely to think of his age or stage of development as the most important factor and to talk as though all children of a given age are alike. We deal with age 6 and age 7, rather than live, whole children.

A second approach is to look at specific processes or areas of development, such as physical growth, social development, and mental growth. The advantage here is that we can learn a great deal about these particular areas through studying them piecemeal. A disadvantage is that we have the child so fragmented that we cannot put him back together again.

Both the above approaches have been supported over the years by considerable longitudinal and cross-sectional research of children at different ages. A third approach, labeled experimental child psychology concerns itself with manipulating the situation in which the child finds himself in order to see in what ways development is influenced by learning.

This book offers the point of view that we can learn from all the above approaches, but that we need to keep the child as an individual continually in focus, correlating our understanding about his environment and biological organism into one system. Behavior and development is a continuous process of transaction between the child's biological organism and his sociophysical environment. Any study that does not look at both elements presents a somewhat distorted picture of the child. In effect, we will attempt to combine an "external" approach of looking at the child's home, his peer group, his school, his society, and his responses to experi-

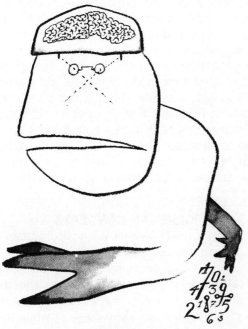

FIGURE 1.1

From Sir P. Medawar, What's human about man is his technology. Copyright 1973 Smithsonian Institution from *SMITHSONIAN Magazine,* May 1973. Illustration by R. Osborn. Used by permission.

mental situations with an "internal" approach of looking at his perception of these various situational forces and of his own body and growth.

The child creates a world of meanings for himself from his experience with his own body and his social milieu. Our basic assumption is that the human being is a meaning-seeking animal. He finds clues in his environment and develops an assigned meaning on the basis of the feedback he gets when he responds to both bodily and external sensations. A simple way of talking about this world of meanings is to label those meanings the child assigns to himself as his *self.* Therefore, an organizing construct throughout this book will be the child's *self-system.* Although it is possible to organize the data in the field of human development in other theoretical terms, the concept of self is a useful organizing one. This concept makes it possible to see the child as a goal-oriented and purposive being who influences the world around him as much as he is influenced by it, rather than as a passive receptacle of data from the outside world or as a simple respondent to external pressure. We will elaborate on this concept later in the chapter and offer some operational definitions.

With the knowledge explosion, particularly in the field of child development, a book cannot be encyclopedic. Each author places his own framework upon the available data. He selects those data that strike him as significant as carefully and objectively as he can from the journal articles, monographs, and books that pour across his desk. He uses them to build his own organization of thought. There is danger that he will select only data that fit his preconceptions or that he will develop his organization free from any attention to data. There is also danger that he will distort the research worker's original intent or interpret his findings in an unacceptable way. Although this book is data-based, the interpretations are the author's. In order to decrease the risk of being influenced by the perceptual bias of the author, the reader is urged to read the originals as much as possible; it is not feasible to describe the research in detail.

GENERAL CONCEPTS

In order to focus on the child, we must acquire certain essential broad concepts about human development and behavior. We need to understand the nature of individual development as it is reflected in the ideas listed below; these serve as the theoretical framework for this book.

In other publications (Gordon, 1965, 1966a, 1966b), a concept of changing views of childhood was developed in which older views were classed as Newtonian and newer views as Einsteinian. These newer views,* which reflect our current social system, technology, and sciences, are:

1. Development is a process of transaction between organism and environment. Therefore, outputs (intelligence, socioemotional behavior, concepts, motor skills) are modifiable by experience.
2. The individual is a functioning whole. A person can be considered a self-organizing system, so that parts must be considered in relation to the whole and behavior understood in context.
3. The individual is an "open-energy" system. The child is characterized by activity. Instead of seeking tension-reduction, the organism seeks energy balance and information.
4. Development and organization are synonymous. From a systems approach, the system develops as it gets more complex and more integrated. Living systems follow this rule.
5. The individual is unique. Uniqueness is continuously evolving from organism-environment transactions. It is both *geno-* and *phenotypical;* that is, behavior is made up of both a contribution from the genes and the impact of the world.

* For a profound, poetical expression of these ideas, see R. Buckminster Fuller, "Now and Then," *Harper's,* April 1972, pp. 58–66.

6. The individual develops a self-system. This idea is not as generally accepted as some of those above. It represents a particular view in psychology and education. It is a basic postulate in the author's system of thought.

DEVELOPMENT AS A PROCESS

When we look at the developing child, it is easy for us to see the continuous activity, but it is not always possible to see this activity as having direction toward maturity. We sometimes think in static terms and take our measurements at a particular point as though what we see at that point were going to stay the same. We often think of stages of development as having sharp demarcation lines between them, rather than seeing development as a gradual, almost imperceptible movement from stage to stage. Birthdays are an example. We gear our expectations to dates—when a child is 5, he should be "acting like a 5-year-old," even though he was 4 only yesterday. When he reaches 18, he is ready to vote, as if this day possessed magical power.

Development, like any process, is influenced by what has gone before. It is not, however, simply a process of adding on, such as increase in height and weight or mental age. It is a process of change in which the child develops by absorbing everything that is happening to him, biologically and mentally, while combining these experiences with previous ones. What emerges is a new organization, a new creation from the blending of these ingredients.

There is a constant interaction between what is biologically given (genotype) and the psychological developments that take place as a result of experience (phenotype). The phenotype of a child is thus not a direct reflection of the genotype but rather a reflection of all that he has experienced up to that particular moment.

Development, then, is the entire series of anatomic, physiological, and psychological changes that represents growth, maturation, and learning. Both increase in size and increase in complexity are developmental processes. Although the increase in size stops, increase in complexity and organization of the person continues throughout his life.

THE INDIVIDUAL AS A FUNCTIONING WHOLE

In the process of developing, different parts and tissue systems of the body grow at different rates of speed. Some tissue systems finish their growth ahead of others, yet they are interrelated in such a fashion that they work as an integrated team.

Therefore, the behaving child must be perceived as he acts—as a whole. Just as in everyday experience the functioning whole is greater than the sum of its parts, so in human development the person is more than the sum of his parts. What does "more than" mean? It refers to the arrangement, or order, or organization of these various parts into a going system. Organization is not static; the person is always in the process of organizing, a process that stops only at death.

Let us look at one example of this organizing process: the interrelatedness of structure and function. These are not discrete, with structure determining function. We will discover in this book that the child's experiences help determine the further development of his bodily structure; thus, sometimes experience influences structure. For example, girls in certain cultures mature later than those in others; children in Samoa can handle their bodies differently than children in New Haven; an American learning French as an adult cannot quite make the language sound the same as a Parisian.

This relationship is reciprocal not only in bodily terms, but in psychological and cultural terms as well. The person's structure, or organization, might be defined as the developed and organized processes at any given moment. This means that what will be developed is a function of the interaction of what is already there and current experience. To some degree, internal and external are one and inseparable, both uniting the body system, both becoming organized into a single system that determines behavior and development.

Projecting the individual in this way resolves the *heredity-environment* conflict. Viewed from our position, there can be no dichotomy between the two. At a given moment, a person's behavior is a product of all his heredity and all his environment wedded within a single organization. Just as the grass is influenced not only by the seed we plant but also by soil conditions, shade, rainfall, insects, and the like, so the growing child is a product not only of his genetic inheritance but also of all that he has experienced from the moment of conception.

A child is not solely a product of his culture, born blank and reflecting only what his society teaches. Yet, he is not purely a product of his genetic inheritance, because what he inherits are only certain potentialities. All of us are distinct and unique individuals who make our own complex of arrangements from the factors that contribute to our self-development.

Similarly, an attempt to split the individual along the lines of a *mind-body* dichotomy is equally false. All tissue systems of the body work with each other, are influenced by each other, and are mutually supportive. We cannot extract the child's "mind" and treat it as an entity removed from his body; the modern physician does not treat even an appendix without recognizing it as a part of a whole person.

Intelligence, too, must be considered with the child as a whole in view. People formerly assumed intelligence to be an isolable trait, fixed by inheritance and consistently measurable. But it is not so simple as that. Intelligence is a form of behavior and, like all behavior and development, reflects the total organization of the person. It is influenced by his biological makeup, by the life experiences of the individual, the type of opportunities he has had, the nature of the culture in which he lives, and the human relationships in which he has engaged. This view will be expanded throughout the book. A continuing argument among scholars is not whether this is so, but rather how much each element contributes. Although some say 80 percent of what we measure as intelligence is inherited, geneticists such as Caspari (1968) and Hirsh (1969) stress that there is no way to use such a dichotomy (genes vs. experience) when dealing with an individual child. His behavior is not divisible in this way.

THE LIFE PROCESS AS AN ORDERING, ORGANIZING PROCESS

Life can be maintained only as long as the body organizes and integrates its world into an orderly arrangement. This organization is a basic activity of the growing person; he must do this for survival. Arranging one's world is not only an internal physiological process but also a psychological process, "making sense" of one's environment. The child, as he grows, needs to feel that there is a constancy about his world. If he does not find it, he invents it. Indeed, there are some data to indicate that the nature of the human brain is such that it finds order satisfying and reinforcing.

The individual is always active; he acts in such a way that he orders himself and his environment. Order and predictability are essential to him and are a necessary basic part of his feelings of security. This need for order means that a person in any given situation will choose that behavior which, from where he stands, preserves and increases his already ordered world. The direction of his behavior is always, in normal development, toward increased complexity. For all of us, behavior is functional and serves to maintain order and organization. This does not mean that growth is completely orderly, or just a matter of unfolding, and that one can sit back and let children grow. It does mean that, even though the surrounding world may be chaotic, each of us takes information in and organizes it within ourselves to make some sense of it and to make our lives orderly. Piaget and Inhelder have expressed this organizational quality of man, this unification of cognition and affect, biology and society, in a single sentence: "The formation of personality is dominated by the search for coherence." (Piaget and Inhelder, 1969, p. 158)

The complex process of organization depends on growth and experi-

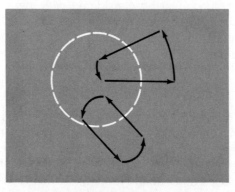

FIGURE 1.2

The child as an open-energy system. The arrows indicate exchange of energy (information) between child and world, modifying both. This can also be seen as a feedback loop.

ence, and on those biological determinants that give the person both his common human inheritance and his unique characteristics.

THE OPEN-ENERGY SYSTEM

All living organisms can be defined as open-energy systems. The openness of a system depends upon the amount of interchange between it and what is outside it. An open system means that the person is continually being influenced by and is influencing his environment.

The person is thus greatly affected by his environment and cannot be considered or understood apart from it. We cannot look at the person in isolation; we cannot understand the individual apart from the culture that has influenced and is continuing to influence him.

The Steady State

There are several characteristics of such an open-energy system as the human organism. One is that it maintains a *steady state;* that is, it attempts to maintain itself and to balance the forces within itself. This concept is not synonymous with that of *homeostasis* (Cannon, 1939), in which there is self-regulation in order to maintain an optimal state of constancy in the internal tissues. Homeostatic processes have been seen as responses to the environment, psychological as well as physiological. Such a concept places the instigation of behavior "outside" the organism. The steady-state concept postulates the organism as actor rather than merely responder. An open-energy system, such as the organism, is constantly and continuously active; indeed, that is its outstanding characteristic. The steady-state means that the organism does not go back to a previous state of affairs but goes forward into a new organization that keeps it somewhat in balance. This new organization, of course, is derived from its previous condition but incorporates the new information received from the environment. *Feedback* is the process of receiving and making use of information from the environment after one has acted. The feedback may indicate that behavior that was formerly appropriate is no longer received with approval and requires modification. It also may be that some behavior that was virtually chance was well received and may then lead down new pathways which might have been unpredictable to an external observer.

There seems to be an optimum range of energy for each individual. We operate to stay within this range, not to go down to complete stability and the stoppage of activity. From this point of view, tension reduction is not the accurate model. If one does not feel active enough, one may actually seek to raise the level of tension and find this satisfying.

The activity of the growing child is essentially undirectional. He does not go back to a previous balance, but forward toward a new steady-state. The organism develops beyond its original state, becoming more complex and differentiated. While, at a given moment, the individual is acting to maintain this steady-state, the cumulative effect is development. The organism, then, is constantly "becoming." Although the child's surroundings become more complex, he also develops a more complex organization that enables him to cope with them. The child develops as he attempts to organize himself and the environment into some meaningful constancy. Because this is an open system, the nature of the forces in the whole transactional field (organism-environment) will determine the rate and direction of the growth and development of the system.

A whole host of studies indicates that growth and rate of development in the present generation of children are more rapid than they were in generations past. The term *secular trend* is used to indicate the fact that over the years there is a curve showing earlier arrival at certain key maturation points. It is not quite clear just what has caused this earlier maturation, but most of the assumptions and the hypotheses offered are concerned with the changing environmental conditions under which children are reared, the changing social and industrial situation, the provision of better prenatal care, the provision of better child care, and the increased immunization to disease. These hypotheses suggest a mixture of physical, social, and psychological reasons for earlier development. The nature of the experience of the child, when viewed in this light, assumes great significance as a potent force in influencing his development, not only psychologically but also physically. We see again that we cannot separate mind and body, structure and function. They are inextricably interwoven into the system.

DEVELOPMENT AS ORGANIZATION
Development Redefined

We can define individual development as the processes by which a person, from the moment of birth, progresses toward maximum organization and integration. Development is directional. As a way of maintaining organization in a fluid environment, the organism reaches out toward it, incorporates what it learns both physically and psychologically, and develops. In moving toward this maximum organization, human beings order their world in terms of meanings. These meanings change as situations change, both internally and externally. Change in behavior patterns can be understood as reflecting the change in meaning or self-organization. Although patterns do change, the stability of certain behaviors through time, as indicated in longitudinal studies, point out that certain meanings acquired earlier in life tend to govern the way we relate to people.

The first two decades of life are not the end of development. However, since change is most rapid during that time, these changes significantly alter the bodily makeup of the child and require him to develop and elaborate his self-system. As aspects of his body change, his systems of meanings must change to incorporate what he is now becoming. Since his organization is also incomplete in these early years, it is far easier for information to penetrate into the system and shape it than it is later on when his defenses are more potent and his perceptions of himself tend to acquire a certain stability.

The problem of the internal versus the external way of studying the child is reflected in our research methods. Thus, the development of the child can be studied from the observer's viewpoint by gathering data about those aspects of development that are measurable or observable physically, such as height, weight, coordination, energy expenditure, and the appearance of secondary sex characteristics. This development can also be seen in another way: in terms of how the person himself continuously organizes and reorganizes his world. In order to understand behavior, it is necessary not only to observe that the child has reached his preadolescent growth spurt but also to observe and to infer from his behavior the meaning this growth has to the child—to discover as best we can what he is experiencing.

Differentiating-Integrating as a Developmental Process

In the course of this book we will be looking at the activities of the child as he searches for meanings in his environment. A major process in this search is differentiating-integrating. Piaget (1961) has talked in terms of assimilation-accommodation in which the growing child not only assimilates information from the environment and makes it part of him but also is forced to accommodate to the environment and to change himself. This relates to Figure 1.2, which can be seen either as differentiating-integrating or assimilating-accommodating. When the information entering the circle is new and requires change, it can be seen as requiring accommodation, or differentiation. When it fits fairly well with what the child already knows, he can absorb or assimilate it, and he can also use it for integrating. Both processes are going on all the time. This process occurs at the biological level as the child matures. From the moment of conception, cells increase in number and tissue systems with specialized functions emerge. These cells undergo a process of differentiation; they become cells with special functions, such as nerve cells and muscle cells. One group of cells, neurons, have as their special function the establishment and maintenance of communication lines among the various subsystems within the organism. These lines of communication provide a means for integrating all the activities of the organism. Any part of the total system can serve as an instigator of behavior, but the system, because of these nerve pathways, acts as a whole.

This process occurs also in a psychological sense. As the child has experiences, he begins to sort them out and to categorize them. The initial categorizations, of course, are highly primitive because of the state of biological development. These may be simply "pleasant or comfortable" or "unpleasant or uncomfortable" feeling states, or "graspable or non-graspable," "responsive or nonresponsive" actions or digests. Later he differentiates "me" and "not me," "living" and "nonliving," "parent" and "not parent." With development, these categories, or differentiated parts of his experience, become more complex and abstract. At the same time that the child is categorizing, he is incorporating these categories into his organization. He arranges and assembles them into some sort of configuration, so that they "make sense" and become constant enough for him to count on when he needs to deal with them again. This is the integrating activity. The child, as he develops, is breaking up his environment and his experiences with himself into pieces that possess constancy for him and then reassembling and reorganizing these pieces into a new whole that he perceives as his self and his world. In Chapter 4 we will explore the reassembling and reorganizing in more detail.

Differentiating and integrating are not and cannot be purely intellectual processes. We have said that any mind-body dichotomy does not exist; thus the process of assigning meanings to one's experience includes affect, or emotion. There is no behavior or experience without affect. The positive or negative emotional loading influences the meaning of an experience to the child. This first rough differentiation of comfort-discomfort is heavily affect-laden. "Me" and "not me," "mother" and "not mother," and all such differentiations carry with them evaluative feelings of comfort and discomfort, tension increase or decrease.

Emotion, then, is a part of the organizing processes of the growing child. It is not something to be avoided (as if we could do so!) but is an essential, basic part of experiencing. Emotions serve a definite purpose in the striving of the individual toward self-realization. When we discuss, in later chapters, the emotional life of the child, we will need constantly to remember that these emotions are an integral aspect of development. It is not sufficient to say that 5-year-olds fear ghosts. We must be able to see what the fear of ghosts means to a child. Emotions can be understood as arousal tendencies. The more intense, the more personal, the more meaningful the experience, the higher the level of arousal, the more intense the emotion. That is why emotions are not separate entities but are states experienced and given meaning by the child as he copes with his environment.

Organizing and Developing

Organizing and developing are, therefore, virtually synonymous terms. No part of this organization operates in isolation from other parts or in opposition to other parts. The total organization always acts as a unit. It reaches out for experience because experience is just as much food for development as are cereal and milk. Development is more than increment; it is the organization of bodily changes and experience into the single unity we call the individual.

This developing process, this organizing and reorganizing process, is a somewhat orderly one. We know that usually certain stages of organization or structure precede others, that certain behaviors come into existence based upon previous behaviors. This orderliness may really be not so much maturational as a result of transaction. It is now becoming clear that if certain experiences do not occur in the life of a child, what we would expect to occur normally in terms of development just does not take place. We know this from studies of cats, rats, chimps, and children. Experience is as essential an ingredient for development as a gene.

Children growing up within a culture share many experiences in common because they are at roughly the same stage of physical development. Although we are concerned primarily with the individual, we cannot consider him unique in all ways. He follows the general laws for his "class of objects"—in this case, humanity.

In order to understand the child in particular, we must comprehend the general developmental laws that govern all of us. Conversely, knowing the general laws will not help us unless we can also find the way these are at work in the individual. Thus, we know that sooner or later all normal children reach puberty. However, one child can be normal and reach puberty at 13, whereas another normal child may not reach puberty until the age of 18. What a difference this will make in his own individual development: "no two people are alike."

THE UNIQUENESS OF THE INDIVIDUAL

To the person beginning in the field of human development, the concept of uniqueness may be disturbing. Although he grants the truth that each person is different, he views it as presenting a chaotic world in which uniqueness means unpredictability from person to person. He knows that people are different; yet he wishes they were less so. It would be so nice if he could standardize them, like so many other objects in our environment. He has this need for "order." If he could reorganize his thinking to see this concept of individuality as lawful rather than chaotic, then he might come to think of individualism as the most promising idea for the future rather than as a fact he would like to eliminate.

Individuality in development is the rule. By individuality, we mean the unique personal organization of normative variables. Everybody has blood pressure, everybody has a pulse rate, everybody weighs a certain amount, and everybody reaches a certain height, but the particular constellation belongs to one individual. Moreover, a person's pulse rate may be normal for him, but at one or the other end of the extreme of a normal distribution. Whether I have "high" blood pressure depends, to some degree, upon my own usual pressure, not just the norm. Norms may tell us something about what might be expected, but longitudinal research studies have clearly shown that an individual, as he develops, moves at his own pace and does not maintain a steady position in relation to the norm. One of the most comprehensive longitudinal studies that has been done is the California Growth Study. As a result of 25 years of following the same group of individuals, a senior researcher reported: "We have become increasingly aware that the growth of individuals is often unstable. In a given [characteristic], such as height, or intelligence, a child may, over a period of years, shift from high to average, to low, and back to average again, as compared to his age peers. The very frequency of these shifts leads us to assume that, for the most part, they are normal and healthy patterns of growth . . . we find that individual patterns are the rule." (Bayley, 1956, p. 45)

Three major influences in the creation and maintenance of this individuality are the genetic origins, the cultural experiences, and the perceptual processes of the child.

The Biochemical Origin of Uniqueness

Uniqueness begins for the individual child at the moment of conception. When the genetic dice are cast, the odds against repeating the same combination of chromosomes are tremendous. This genetic difference is compounded by experiences, both intra- and extrauterine. As Murphy (1966, p. 31) states: "Every individual is an almost infinitely complex pattern of biochemical tendencies. . . . Biochemical individuality is recognizable

even in the embryo and clearly in the newborn; and upon this early individuality are impressed still further individualities due to the vicissitudes of
the individual life process."

The evidence of the uniqueness of individuals is all around us. We
use fingerprints to establish identity. Manufacturers of fountain pens,
shampoos, and electric shavers build their sales appeals around the allowances their products make for individual differences in hands, hair, and
skin. We can visit a hospital nursery and see wide differences among the
newborn in activity rate and movement, as well as in size. Within the first
five days of life, infants have clearly established patterns of individual differences with respect to hand movements, activity level, and other motor
variables. (Kessen, 1961) Genetic composition establishes the first difference among people; intrauterine life builds on this. At the time of birth,
each child is already unique.

The Role of Cultural Experiences

Not only is uniqueness rooted in the biochemical composition of the individual, but it is also fostered by the nature of his cultural experience. When
the child is born, he comes into contact with an already on-going social
environment that immediately begins to shape his development. For example, two children born into the same family experience different environments. Let us suppose the first-born is a boy and the second, born
two years later, a girl. She has an older brother; he has none. Her parents
are two years older and, if not wiser, at least less energetic and less tense
about her care and feeding than they were about her brother's. In addition,
the values, standards, and secret hopes they hold for her are different
from those held for him. Cultural role expectations—although these may
be rapidly changing—present images and create situations, so that each
child experiences something somewhat different from the other.

In addition to family experiences, the child participates in the life of
the neighborhood, the school, and the community at large. Each of these,
in turn, presents images for him to model himself upon and teach him
what it is he should be. Children growing up in different cultural surroundings experience as reality only that to which they are exposed; their concepts of self and of world are strongly influenced by their cultures and add
to their uniqueness.

The Role of Perceptual Processes

Perceiving is "the process by which a particular person, from his particular behavioral center, attributes significances to his immediate environmental situation." (Ittelson and Cantril, 1954, p. 26) This process of at-
tributing significance, or meaning, we have already encountered in our
discussion of differentiating-integrating. We give immediate meanings to
things on the basis of our previous experience with them, our needs at the

moment, our present level of organization or development, and our language.

To some degree, perceptions of what is present in the environment are functions of the need to organize. Seeing certain parts of the environment as structured appears to be due to the innate organizing processes of the human organism. Perceiving is more than seeing. It is the organizing of what is seen, felt, and sensed into a meaningful arrangement related to the already organized system that is the individual.

Since the individual is unique biochemically, has unique experiences in his culture, and is an open-energy system that has constant transactions between these two, his perceptions must, therefore, be unique. In a certain sense, no two people—since they are unique—can ever experience the same thing. They will perceive differently, that is, assign personal and private meanings to, any situation they have in common.

When the individual finds himself in a situation that would present information to him contrary to his present on-going organization, he perceives it in ways that enable him to maintain himself. The two major ways are through denial and distortion. A whole battery of defense devices can be subsumed under these two headings. We are all familiar with the sour-grapes type of rationalization, the shifting of blame to another, the "forgetting" of assignments, and the daydreaming in which the world is reorganized with the person at the center of a delightful universe.

Throughout the book we will be concerned, therefore, with what the child and adolescent perceives to be the nature of himself and his world. He behaves in accordance with his view of the world. We are not implying any philosophical or metaphysical argument about whether or not there is a real world but are assuming the existence of the world outside the growing child. The issue here is that, from our psychological position, there is no reality for the child except that which he creates as a result of the constant transaction between his organism and his environment. The world for him is as he experiences it.

The Common Aspects of Man

When we go for a walk in the woods, we see many kinds of trees. If we were to examine each tree apart from all the others, we would recognize clearly that no two trees are alike. The differences to the layman are not important—they are all trees. To the forester or the lumberman, these differences are important. So it is when we deal with people. If we were removed from the human race, the differences among people would be less vital to us and the common elements would be more obvious.

Human beings, even though they differ, are still human and possess many common characteristics. There is a "human nature" that we all share. It is not composed of common attitudes, beliefs, and the behavior patterns to which the traditionalist refers when he says, "You can't change human nature." Rather, human nature is the ability to learn, the ability to choose, the ability to use language; it includes flexibility of development and the need for activity, love, belonging, and predictability. Men share the need to see meaning in their world as a common aspect of humanity. We share, also, the urge to explore, to create, to initiate. Man must, for survival and sanity, constantly be in a stimulating relationship with his environment. Man has a "taste for excitement." (Hebb, 1955, p. 250)

Uniqueness of the expression of humanness does not imply that there are not these overall common forces. Commonality and uniqueness are not mutually exclusive terms. All men resemble each other more than any man resembles another species. Yet within the species, there are great ranges of individual differences.

Let us look at some other things that all men share. All men live in societies, and these societies provide for their members various experiences that are essentially common. Although one child's perception of the experience may be slightly different from that of another, all children have experienced "parenting" or infant care of some sort. People within a given society more or less care for their children in a similar way, have similar demands, and enforce similar restraints.

Since man is verbal, people within a given society use the words of their language to communicate. Of course, words are subject to misinterpretation and to varieties of connotation; nevertheless, language systems provide for the sharing of experiences and the organization of perception.

That man is a species implies that there are biological characteristics that differentiate man from other animals. We have mentioned some of these in the above list of needs, drives, and abilities. It might be safe to say that, at the moment of birth, two children anywhere in the world are more alike than they are different. Although they will go through about the same pattern of physical development and maturation, the culture will in many ways modify the activities involved in this developing, and it will play a vital role in determining the meanings the child will assign to his development. Nevertheless, although the "culture can alter, mold or reorganize drives—or rather, it can permit them one form of development or expression rather than another— it can hardly 'create' them out of nothing." (Murphy, 1966, p. 128)

Man's individual development may be seen as the emerging of uniqueness from the transactions between (1) a person's organism (which possesses needs, drives, abilities, and tissue systems in common with all men, but in arrangement and organization that is his alone) and (2) a cultural-physical environment (which he shares in large measure with other members of his society, but which also has personal interpretations and meanings for him alone).

The study of individual development requires, therefore, that we look at the processes of this transaction, seeing always both those aspects that are environmental and those that form a part of an individual's private world.

THE INDIVIDUAL DEVELOPS
A SELF-SYSTEM

One way of seeing and labeling the organizing processes of the individual by which he attempts to structure himself and his world is by using the concept of self. This permits us to use a single term to discuss both the consistency of the individual's organization and its forward movement. We call self-processes *the series of interrelated processes by which the individual organizes himself.* The self-system emerges as a result of the operation of the differentiating-integrating processes, including affect as an essential part, and the perceptual processes.

The Self-System

The self-system is the individual's organized experience, both with himself and his world. It includes all that is organized at any given moment. It becomes possible, then, to pull together under this one term all our earlier discussions of organization and reorganization, open-energy systems, and uniqueness-commonality. The organization of the developing person at any single moment in time is his self-system. It includes not only all the internal biological tissue activities but also those phases of the environment that the person has incorporated.

This self-system attempts to maintain a steady-state, has direction toward increased complexity, possesses some degree of internal consistency, and is in continuous transaction with the environment.

While, from moment to moment, its atomistic ingredients change—cells die and are replaced, behaviors, too, die and are replaced—the system goes on and has a recognizable identity.

Self-Concept

Not all parts of the system are equally differentiated and integrated. Some aspects are more clearly defined than others. Although it is the total system that governs the behavior of the person (and this total system is never to be considered in isolation from its situation), some parts seem to exercise a greater degree of influence on the perceptual and interpretational processes and on the choice of situations (as much as the individual can influence this) in which the person will place himself.

One's self-concepts are those central views the individual has that, to him, represent who he is at all times. It is what, as actor, he calls "I," and as subject, "me." These are the highly differentiated, integral, fairly persistent aspects of one's self. They are, of course, not necessarily clear in the awareness of the person. The existence of a person's self-concept and the nature of it cannot be seen directly. The self-system is a construct. We do not ever really see anybody's self-system. We infer its existence from patterned behavior. It is possible to define the self-concept operationally in several different fashions. Some of the confusion in the literature results from poor operational definition. We can hypothesize what a child's self-organization might be by inference from his behavior. We can examine the organized behavior of the individual, his language, his roles, his cognitive style, his expressive behavior, his approach-avoidance techniques. A second technique, and one widely used, is to equate self-concept with the stated view of a child about himself. In this definition, the self-concept is what a child says he is, on some sort of scale, in an interview or in response to an open-ended question. These two definitions are not mutually exclusive, although generally there is little overlap between them. In this book both definitions will be used. We will try to indicate, in connection with research citations, which one was used. Both definitions, however, assume a personal organization lying behind the behavior.

Self-System and Behavior

One characteristic of any system is the maintenance of its identity. The recognizable identity of the individual, in terms of the patterns of his behavior, is a function of the self-system and, to a great degree, that part of the system we have labeled self-concept.

By analogy, today's members of the First Division still wear the *fouragère* awarded the division by the French in World War I. It would be a safe guess that nobody in the present division was there at the time, but the identity of the "Big Red One" is continuous. It preserved its identity in World War II, in the Korean War, and in Viet Nam. To the individual GI, membership in the First Division becomes a part of his central organization and outlook on the world. Conversely, he becomes a part of the ongoing organization that is the division. Although we cannot predict the behavior of an individual soldier, we might safely predict that the unit as a whole would maintain its organization and its tradition in battle. We might predict the future performance of the organization by knowing its present identity, its present self-system, and its concept of itself as visually displayed on the shoulders of its members. However, even this identity has to be placed in a larger context. The soldier brings his views of life, of war, of nation with him, and these views, if widely shared in the larger culture of his age group, may override the more traditional ones.

What faces us here is the puzzle of behavior: it is never as simple as our explanations from any theoretical viewpoint would make it. One way to understand is to see it as the self-system attempting to enhance or develop itself. Behavior is functional; it serves to preserve the steady-state of the self-system. Each person in our culture develops his self-system out of his own needs for maintenance of organization and further development. The developmental processes are governed by the constant inter-action of maturational and interpersonal forces. The individual selects a part of the self-system, which he perceives as "me." This self-concept, which actually consists of several concepts of self, is unique and personal. A person's choice behavior is greatly influenced by his self-concept, and he develops and behaves to maintain this, just as, at an earlier level of development, he attempted to enhance and maintain his body. Through-out this book, we shall discuss the emergence and development of the self-system.

Self-System and Development

Since this self-system is a function of organism-environment transaction, the self a person develops is his real self. There can be no concept of what he "might have been" if things had been different and no concept of a "real" self that would emerge if only the environment were passive or laissez-faire. Although future experiences may modify the self-system, this self is not a mystical thing with which a person was born and which just has to be left to unfold. Neither is it a little man located somewhere up in the brain directing action. It is a construct invented by the psychologist to make behavior understandable. Only in this sense is it real at all.

A person's self-system is continuously developing toward the goal of enhancing itself. The self continues to develop along the lines of previous development. The child's present self-system has within it the seeds of future behavior in the complete integration of biological processes with psychological aspects such as goals, aspirations, self-concept, values, and attitudes. Future development is determined also by what future experiences the child will have. In this sense, change is always possible.

CONCLUSION

In reading about development, we must realize that individuality is the rule and that there is no simple approach to understanding behavior. Those who wish to know about a child must have knowledge not only about children in general but also about the particular child. With this in mind, we can see that it is meaningless to say "all adolescents feel . . ." or "all children growing up in cities think . . ." or "only children are. . . ." We need to recognize that a unique organization of forces is at play in every child. Knowledge of forces and developmental processes aids us to a great degree, but it must always be tailored to fit the youngster.

The remainder of this book will present a detailed account of the general concepts discussed in this chapter in action in the development of the child into the adult. We shall, even while examining the environmental forces at play, keep our focus on the individual as he interacts with his environment. As we increase our understanding of development and behavior, we shall be in a better position to create the kinds of experiences that enable others to develop their potentialities.

REFERENCES AND ADDITIONAL READINGS

Allport, G. *Pattern and growth in personality.* New York: Holt, Rinehart and Winston, 1961.

Bayley, N. Individual patterns of development. *Child Development,* 1956, *27,* 45–74. Reprinted in I. J. Gordon (Ed.), *Human development: Readings in research.* Glenview, Ill.: Scott, Foresman, 1965.

Cannon, W. B. *The wisdom of the body.* New York: Norton, 1939.

Caspari, E. Genetic endowment and environment in the determination of human behavior: Biological viewpoint. *American Educational Research Journal,* 1968, *5,* 43–55.

Chein, I. *The science of behavior and the image of man.* New York: Basic Books, 1972.

Combs, A. W., & Snygg, D. *Individual behavior.* (Rev. ed.) New York: Harper & Row, 1959.

Glaser, R. Individuals and learning: The new aptitudes. *Educational Researcher,* AERA, 1972, 5–13.

Goldstein, K. On emotions: Considerations from an organismic point of view. *Journal of Psychology,* 1951, *31,* 37–49.

Gordon, I. J. Development and learning. In P. F. Regan & E. Pattishall (Eds.), *Behavioral science concepts in psychiatry.* Boston: Little, Brown, 1965. Pp. 441–468.

Gordon, I. J. New conceptions of children's learning and development. In W. Waetjen (Ed.), *Learning and mental health in the school. 1966 Yearbook, Association for Supervision and Curriculum Development,* Washington, D.C.: NEA, 1966a. Pp. 49–66.

Gordon, I. J. *Studying the child in school.* New York: Wiley, 1966b.

Hebb, D. O. Drives and the C.N.S. (Conceptual Nervous System). *The Psychological Review,* 1955, *62,* 243–254.

Hirsch, J. Behavior-genetic analysis and its biosocial consequences. Reprinted in *IRCD Bulletin,* 1969, *54,* 3–4, 16–20.

Hunt, J. McV. *Intelligence and experience.* New York: Ronald Press, 1961.

Ittelson, W. H., & Cantril, H. *Perception: A transactional approach.* New York: Doubleday, 1954.

Jackson, E. B. Child development patterns in the United States. In K. Soddy (Ed.), *Mental health and infant development.* New York: Basic Books, 1956. Pp. 87–92.

Kagan, J. On the need for relativism. *American Psychologist,* 1967, *22,* 131–142.

Kessen, W., et al. Selection and test of response measures in the study of the human newborn. *Child Development,* 1961, *32,* 7–24.

Miller, J. G. The nature of living systems. *Behavioral Science,* 1971, *16(4),* 277–301.

Miller, J. G. Living systems: The group. *Behavioral Science,* 1971, *16(4),* 302–398.

Murphy, G. *Human potentialities.* New York: Basic Books, 1958.

Murphy, G. *Personality, a biosocial approach.* New York: Basic Books, 1966.

Piaget, J. The genetic approach to the psychology of thought. *Journal of Educational Psychology,* 1961, *52,* 275–281. Reprinted in I. J. Gordon, *Human development: Readings in research.* Glenview, Ill.: Scott, Foresman, 1965.

Piaget, J., & Inhelder, B. *The psychology of the child.* New York: Basic Books, 1969.

Pribram, K. H. Neurological notes on the art of educating. In NSSE, *Theories of learning and instruction.* 63rd Yearbook, Part I. Chicago: University of Chicago Press, 1964.

Scheinfeld, A. *Your heredity and environment.* Philadelphia: Lippincott, 1965.

Stoddard, G. On the meaning of intelligence. *Proceedings, 1966 Invitational Conference on Testing Problems.* Princeton, N.J.: Educational Testing Service, 1966.

Tanner, J. M. *Growth at adolescence, with a general consideration of the effects of hereditary and environmental factors upon growth and maturation from birth to maturity.* (2nd ed.) Oxford: Blackwell Scientific Publications, 1962.

Watson, H., & Lowrey, G. H. *Growth and development of children.* (4th ed.) Chicago: Year Book Publishers, 1962.

TWO

IN THE BEGINNING: FROM BIRTH TO SCHOOL

CHAPTER 2

BIOLOGICAL BASES
FOR DEVELOPMENT

In order to examine the organism-environment field in which the self develops, we shall study each aspect somewhat separately and then attempt to synthesize. In this chapter, the organism is the focus of attention. It is from this basic biochemical organization that all behavior and development stem.

HEREDITARY FACTORS
Physical Appearance

Many an anxious expectant parent asks, "What will my child be like? What will he look like?" Just after birth, when the proud parents and the relatives flock to view the new arrival, the first comments usually include, "He looks just like his Uncle John" (who is also bald). Or a dissection process takes place in which his eyes are his mother's, his nose, his father's, his ears, his grandpa's on his father's side, and so on. Everybody gets into the act of comparing the child to all the branches on the family tree.

How much of our knowledge of heredity is based soundly on scientific research and how much on folklore and myth? Just what does the child have as a part of his makeup that comes to him through the genes of his parents?

It is generally accepted by geneticists that physical characteristics such as hair color, eye color, skin shade, blood type, and the like are genetically determined. Without a discussion of the mechanism of genetics, we can safely state that although these characteristics are governed by the genes of the parents, the actual appearance of the child will not be a mirror image of one parent or even a composite picture of the two. Parents carry and pass on to their children genes that, in their own appearance, took "second place" or were recessive genes. Thus a brown-eyed set of parents may each have possessed a gene for blue eyes that did not operate. Since at conception only half the father's genes unite to produce a blue-eyed baby, it does not take an outsider to give the baby a different appearance from his father—a recessive gene from each parent will do the trick. We assume that the reader is already aware of the general principle of genetics from previous work; here we are concerned only with human genetics, with what is known about specific characteristics.

The gene is a chemical messenger; that is, it acts to influence biochemical activity, such as the work of one enzyme, by the information it carries chemically. Since any observable human trait, such as "intelligence" or "schizophrenia" or "aggression," is made up of many activities, it follows that there is no one gene, operating independently, that carries the trait. While there are, no doubt, genetic factors that influence behavior, genetic theory and research at this time indicate that the relationship is far from simple. You may have studied about dominant and recessive genes, but even in that area, real life differs from a chart. When the 23 male chromosomes unite with the 23 female ones at the moment of conception, many things happen (genetically!) that affect the predicted distribution of an observable trait in the offspring.

Life is a gamble, and the first throw of the dice occurs at conception. We should remember that in all genetic factors, what will be passed on is a matter of odds or probabilities. Although physical characteristics are definitely inherited, just what the individual child will look like is largely a matter of chance within the genetic possibilities represented in the total familial background of both parents. Moreover, even these physical characteristics, as static as they may seem, are influenced to some degree by environmental forces such as diet and geographical region. Further, as McClearn (1964) has indicated, one's definition of environment should include not only one's usual notion of the world outside the skin but also neighboring cells and even neighboring contents within the same cell.

Disease Tendencies

It is true that certain ailments run in families, but what seems to be inherited is a predisposition to develop a disease (given certain precipitating environmental conditions), rather than the disease itself. Susceptibility to diseases is on a sliding scale from those that seem most related to genetic factors to those that seem most related to environmental conditions. Table 2.1 shows physical diseases with definite genetic components. Yet the occurrence of disease is a highly complex situation, and the table should be considered relative rather than absolute. "A person's whole genetic make-up—and not merely a specific gene combination—is important in relation to almost every disease." (Scheinfeld, 1950, p. 154)

It is interesting to note that the male is born inherently weaker, in terms of disease susceptibility, than the female. Color blindness and hemophilia are essentially male disabilities. Baldness, too, although not a disease and not even necessarily a handicap (if we look at the success of

TABLE 2.1 HEREDITARY DISEASES AND DEFECTS

DOMINANT	SEX-LINKED	RECESSIVE	CHROMOSOME ABNORMALITIES
Optic atrophy, birth type	Hemophilia	Diabetes mellitus	Mongoloid idiocy (Down's syndrome)
Huntington's chorea	Color blindness	Phenylketonuria	Klinefelter's syndrome
Nerve deafness (middle age)	Sweat-gland defects	Progressive muscular dystrophy, preadolescent types	Turner's syndrome
	Muscular dystrophy (Duchenne)	Glaucoma	
		Tay-Sachs disease	

Source: Data condensed and selected from A. Scheinfeld, *Your Heredity and Environment,* Lippincott, 1965, and personal correspondence, 1974. Used by permission.

Yul Brynner in the American theater and movies), is essentially a male characteristic. On the whole, perhaps because of the mechanism that determines sex, the female of the species is stronger and healthier.

Rosenthal (1971) described the various methods used to estimate the extent of the likelihood of becoming schizophrenic due to inheritance. Several classic methods are used, such as twin studies, pedigree analyses, and consanguinity studies. Twin studies examine the life histories of identical and fraternal twins, pedigree analyses study the individuals' direct family background, and consanguinity studies include the relatives on the family tree. The results are mixed, but there seems to be an emerging picture that schizophrenia and manic-depressive psychosis, in spite of diagnostic problems, are genetic disorders. This means they have a genetic base, which increases the odds of occurrence in certain families. It does *not* mean automatic illness. Rosenthal's discussion of methodological problems is central to our concern with the transactional relation between genetic and environmental factors. In twin studies (the classic model being identical and fraternal twins reared together and apart), the assumption is made that the design controls for environmental effects. If the twins resemble each other in a particular trait, even though reared apart, the resemblance is assumed to be due to heredity. Rosenthal indicates, however, that "such a design virtually assures that heredity will account for more of the variance regarding a particular phenotype than any environmental variable." (Rosenthal, 1971, p. 155) Since many studies of the hereditability of intelligence use the same model, these findings, too, should be questioned.

If we recall our brief discussion about heredity-environment in Chapter 1, we may state that any disease experience, physical or mental, happens to the whole person and is influenced by both the genetic makeup of the person and the nature of his life experiences. Diseases vary from pure genetic disorders, such as phenylketonuria, to more complex diseases, such as tuberculosis. Phenylketonuria is an enzyme defect that is genetic in origin, but even this is influenced by external factors, such as the amount of a particular amino acid in the diet. In tuberculosis, however, the bacillus must act in concert with a series of factors to produce disease. Only one in a thousand persons infected develops progressive disease. Susceptibility seems to be influenced by psychological factors; social factors; physical factors, such as inhaled silica; and genetic factors, such as family or racial background.

Since we are concerned with helping people develop fully, the recognition that a person is not doomed to suffer a common mental illness unless his life situation shares heavily with any genetic factor in its creation gives us the challenge and the hope for prevention.

Further, there are biochemical environmental controls that aid in the treatment of genetic defects. In cases where a specific enzyme cannot be made by the body, it is possible to supply therapeutically the product of its operation or to avoid the substrate in which it operates if the latter accumulates and is toxic. As more becomes known about the biochemistry of the body, it will be increasingly possible to treat genetic defects. For the individual at least, his health and behavior represent an amalgamation of genetic and environmental influences.

Intelligence

Perhaps no more controversial area existed in the old nature-nurture arguments than in the field of intelligence. People have attempted to assign proportions of relative value to each of the two dimensions of genetics and environment. Of course, we realize now that this is fallacious reasoning. First, intelligence is not a single trait carried in a single gene. Intelligent behavior has many more aspects than the ability to do academic classroom work. Although our intelligence tests may measure academic ability with a fair degree of accuracy at a given moment, they are not measuring all the dimensions of intelligent behavior.

Second, the behavior of a person is not the result of an additive process; it develops from an organizing, integrating process in which a self-system is produced that represents a new integration of all organism-environment forces. As Hunt states, "The assumption that intelligence is fixed and that its development is predetermined by the genes is no longer tenable." (Hunt, 1961, p. 342)

The evidences concerning the self-system—a person's organized responses—suggest the following conclusions relative to the roles of heredity and environment in intelligence: (1) there is an organic genetic base for intelligent behavior; (2) the actual measured intelligence of a particular person at a particular time, since performance on a test is behavior, is a result of the complex transactions between the organism and its environment up to that point; and (3) performance, therefore, on an intelligence test can be modified by the exigencies of one's life experiences. "It is very doubtful if any tests [of IQ] have been devised whose results do not depend to a considerable extent on the environment as well as the heredity of the individual." (Boyd, 1950, p. 104) The current theory and research in the 1970s seems clearly to indicate that environmental factors, acting upon the individual's genetic makeup, play a vital role from the time of birth in influencing intellectual performance. We shall refer to this later in appropriate chapters.

Temperament

To what degree are personality patterns or action patterns such as slow response, excitability, high activity level, a tendency to plunge into events versus one to sit back and analyze or reflect due to genetics? We will call such a genetic disposition *temperament* to contrast it with learned behaviors. We have all labeled people as introverts or extroverts, for example. Is this temperament? As in the case of intelligence and schizophrenia, the answer is not a clear one. Individuality is shown, within a few days of birth, in activity level, motor behavior, sucking, and other observable behavior patterns. Further, there seem to be sex differences that are present at birth or appear very early. Van de Riet (1970) reports that "at birth girls are less active motorically, and more sensitive to stimuli and to a greater variety of stimuli, . . . and are more irritable." (Van de Riet, 1970, p. 5)

If we look beyond surface appearances to the actions of body chemistry in the endocrine system, we may find some clues. We know that there are many relationships between hormonal secretions and behavior. To just the degree that predispositions to endocrine function or dysfunction are inherited, the endocrines will affect temperament. Bardwick (1971), for example, indicates that hormonal secretions influence sex-typing of the brain. In the behavior of children, however, we cannot disentangle cause and effect so clearly. Whether these patterns are genetic is unclear, because environment obviously begins before birth. If these behavior patterns are part of what we call temperament, they will influence further transactions and development, but presence at birth does not necessarily indicate genetic origin.

Again we are forced to arrive at the conclusion that temperament probably has genetic components in determining the efficiency and direction of use of the nervous, muscular, and endocrine systems but that the relationship is of an indirect nature.

Heredity-Environment Restated

Throughout our discussion of this topic of heredity and environment, it has become increasingly clear that these two forces must always be considered as a single organization, with now one and now the other contributing heavily to the development of a person. We can see that the genetic influence, except in the case of certain physical characteristics and diseases, is largely an indirect one. Such things as mental defectiveness are party influenced by cultural pressures. Even such physical characteristics as shape of the head and height have been shown (in studies by Shapiro on Japanese in Hawaii and those by Boas on Europeans in the continental United States) to be affected by environment.

Since we are concerned with the study of the whole person as he develops and organizes his self-system, we are primarily interested in those behaviors that are patterned and reflect this self-system in action.

Newman's study of identical twins who were reared apart provides some essential data and conclusions about the combined operation of heredity and environment. With due recognition of the need for caution about the design problems in twin studies, his conclusions still seem useful today. He concluded: "Physical characteristics are least affected by the environment; intelligence is affected more; educational achievement still more; and personality or temperament . . . the most." (Newman, 1937, p. 353) Newman further stated that no form of behavior, even that largely determined by the original character of the organism, is impervious to influence or is most significant. Those behaviors that are not greatly modified are that way "because they have not as a matter of fact been incorporated into an *organized system of learned behavior.** The forms of behavior which constitute the adjustment of the individual to his environment, on the other hand, are on a higher level of performance, which is the product of both the organism and the environment interacting." (Newman, 1937, p. 334)

In actual practice, in looking at the behavior of the growing child, we shall keep him whole instead of attempting to slice him up for analysis into genetic or environmental components. All behavior is both genetic and environmental.

PRENATAL INFLUENCES

The genetic composition of the infant begins its work at the moment of conception. The environment also begins its work at this time. Of course, there is no social environment, but the mother's womb constitutes a physical environment that influences the developing fetus. In this section, attention will be centered on this environment.

Endocrinal Influences

If you want your child to be a classical musician, there's no point trying to teach him while he is *in utero.* If you are afraid of snakes, he cannot acquire this fear at that stage either. Further, he will not have any birthmarks on him reflecting your fears or experiences during his prenatal period. We can safely reject as unscientific the notion that a mother's fears or hopes are transmitted intact to her child. Biology, particularly endocrinology, just does not work that way. But the child's life in the womb is not a blank as far as environmental forces are concerned. Some events do contribute to the child's development.

First, let us take a brief look at the mechanical arrangements of life in the mother's womb. The child's bloodstream is distinct from his mother's, and he is surrounded by a placenta through which there is a constant passage of nutrients to him and of waste products back to his mother. This is accomplished by a process of diffusion rather than by direct connection.

The primary question that confronts scientists working in this particular area is: What can be diffused? They speak of a placental barrier, which implies that only certain products in the mother's blood supply, such as

---

* Emphasis added.

oxygen and digested foodstuffs, are small enough and of such a nature to "get through." Since this is the only place of interchange between two otherwise independent systems, only those substances that can penetrate the barrier affect the developing child.

In the next section, we shall look at certain diseases that are bacterial or viral and, therefore, present in the mother's bloodstream. Here we are concerned with hormonal secretions, such as thyroxin, adrenin, and the like, which come from the mother's endocrine glands.

We know that during emotional periods, endocrine secretions, particularly of adrenin, are increased. Fear and rage, although demonstrated in behavior in different fashions, are accompanied by secretions of the adrenal glands. A change in secretion of a hormone produces changes in the whole body system, affecting the function of the body. The question centers around whether the emotional state of the mother, through her hormones, plays a role in the development of the child by affecting his hormonal processes. Although we have clearly ruled out that the child is afraid, through prenatal influence, of what his mother is afraid, does the mother's fear, since it changes the hormonal balances in her blood, affect his blood supply and his hormones? Can endocrinal secretions penetrate the placental barrier? There seems to be some evidence that these endocrine secretions can, to some degree, do this. Indeed, the evidence is accumulating that the placental barrier is not much of a barrier after all. When the mother experiences sustained emotional stress and her whole system is thereby out of balance, the chances are that secretions reach the embryo. We do not know just what prolonged effect this may have, but it heightens the activity rate and irritability (Sontag, 1966) of the newborn. Further, there are indications that drugs (Thalidomide, LSD) can penetrate the barrier and mar the development of the baby. There are also data to show that smoking during pregnancy affects the baby. The best current advice to pregnant mothers is to restrict their use of any drugs, even aspirin, except those prescribed by physicians.

The Mother's Health

Congenital deafness is due to genetic factors in one-third of the cases. The term *congenital* does not mean present in the genes, but present at birth. Another cause of congenital deafness is illness of the mother; for example, syphilis, German measles, or vitamin deficiencies. With the increase in the VD rate in the United States in the early 1970s, the chances are good for a corresponding increase in birth defects.

The mother's diet plays a vital role in the prenatal growth of the child. It affects not only the presence or absence of congenital defects, but also the general state of health of the infant. Several research studies have led to the conclusion that "infants born to mothers on excellent or good diets [based on caloric, protein, vitamin, and mineral intake] during pregnancy were superior in general health and vigor to infants born to mothers on poor diets.'' (Watson and Lowrey, 1958, p. 40) Burke and Stuart (1948) studied the effect of prenatal nutrition on the first six months of life. They found that the incidence of infections, such as bronchitis, colds, and pneumonia, were higher in the poorer-diet group. The incidence of anemia was also higher in this group.

Timing plays a role in the effect of a disease upon the developing child. If German measles, for example, occurs when a particular development is going on, chances are there will be a malformation or dysfunction of that particular tissue or tissue system. The most vulnerable period is between the second and tenth week of pregnancy, the time during which arm and leg, vital organ and eye and ear cells are differentiated. (NIH, 1972) Certain orthopedic difficulties also are related to prenatal environment.

Studies of brain development show that the last three months of pregnancy as well as the first two years after birth are the critical times. A number of investigations of maternal and child malnutrition (for a description of the methods used to research this issue, see, for example, Cravioto et al., 1966) found that severe malnutrition, especially protein deficiency during pregnancy, permanently decreased the number of brain cells and resulted in behavior difficulties. (Read, 1972) It has been said we are what we eat. To some degree, the baby's potentials are influenced by what the mother eats, not just during pregnancy but in her own long-term diet before pregnancy. (NIH, 1972)

Although much remains to be discovered about this critical period during which the child is growing rapidly in the mother's womb, we do know that the mother's biochemical situation has a direct bearing on the development and health of the child.

NEEDS AND DRIVES

In our discussion in Chapter 1 of the common aspects of man, we mentioned several needs as being forces that form and influence man's behavior and development. These were activity, love and belonging, predictability, esteem, and the like. Lists pages long have been made; people have attempted to categorize needs into biological and social, into basic and derived, into instinctual and learned. Any such analysis overlooks the unity of the person. All forces that compel man to behave are biosocial. We can label them in a multitude of ways, but they all may be seen as aspects of the urge to develop, mature, and enhance the experiencing organism, and to ''preserve, protect, and defend'' the already developed organization. All life seems to follow these two urges—growth and development—and the accompanying maintenance of organization.

Both these urges (or drives or needs) are unspecific to a great extent in man. The child is born with them, but the actual pathways, the details, the patterned ways of working on and accomplishing these urges, are to a tremendous extent learned and therefore culturally determined. We cannot talk about basic biological needs as distinct and apart from social forces. Certainly the infant has to have nutrition to survive, but even such a thing as sucking has learning aspects to it. Indeed, because of the role of learning in development, some psychologists, notably B. F. Skinner (1966) and his adherents, take the view that such terms are not necessary to explain behavior. In contrast to this position, those who use the concepts see them as useful organizing principles for describing human beings and postulate a hierarchy of development from meeting basic survival needs (Maslow, 1954) through needs for competence, for influencing events, for order and predictability, for mastery and identity (Gordon, 1970), and for self-actualization. (Maslow, 1954)

Although all infants have urges at birth, there is a wide range of individual differences in how these needs are manifested. For example, one way in which infants try to follow these urges is through tactile communication with the mother. "The infant evokes from the mother the tactile stimulation which he 'needs' and to which he responds in his own individual fashion as in sucking; the mother solicits from the infant this touching and sucking, which evokes milk from the breast." (Frank, 1957, p. 225) This is a transactional process, as are all developmental processes. Even though feeding is a universal experience, the manner of feeding is somewhat personal and private in each family. There is a wide range of differences in both the provision of and the response to tactile experience. The parents' provision of experience, their feelings, and their reactions to the infant's behavior are also highly individual.

Even at such a common and low level of operation as infant feeding, we see that each situational field has unique components. Each parent-child relationship is personal and private; each baby and parent respond to one another in total ways, both of them attempting to meet their common needs. The feeding situation, therefore, is a perfect example of the combination of needs—nutritional, tactile, experiential—being worked on by the child in a situation, or "field," in which there is another person or persons who relate to the child.

Needs, drives and urges represent potentialities, pushes, and overall directions. They do not operate in a social vacuum. Meeting these needs requires the interaction process, first with the family and later with society as a whole. The self is developed through these transactions with the environment.

Three ideas can serve to sum up the above discussion:

1. All children are born with certain urges or forces for development, such as nutrition, warmth, adequacy, and comfort. These urges

can all be seen as related to one fundamental drive—the drive toward actualization, development, maximal organization, or integration. As a phase of this fundamental urge, the person also attempts to maintain his already developed organization. Maintenance is a part of the process of development.

Bill, a white, middle class, suburban Atlantan has the same fundamental needs as Joe, a black, lower class resident of the Hough district of Cleveland. These needs are shared by the son of a black university professor at Columbia and the son of a white migrant worker in Florida.

2. Operationally, this fundamental urge is not purely biological. From the moment of birth, it finds its expression through biosocial means. The individual differences that develop among the four boys as they grow are due partly to the differences in the cultural experiences with which they are confronted.

3. Although all newborn infants possess this same fundamental urge, the biochemical makeup of each body differs; each has inherited a different set of genes and has had a different intrauterine experience. The intensity of the urge to grow, particularly in its many facets such as nutritional needs, warmth and cuddling needs, needs for sleep, will differ. Bill and Joe will behave differently toward their parents from birth on, not only because their parents behave differently toward them but also because they possess different internal systems.

READINESS FOR EXPERIENCES

We are now ready to look at the infant at the moment of birth. We know that he will be himself and not a carbon copy or simple composite of his mother and father. We know that he will arrive with this fundamental urge to grow toward maximal organization, even though we cannot predict what it will be. We know that he will be shaped by what he experiences in a biosocial field from now on and that he has already had biological experiences *in utero.*

Because experience will play such a crucial role and because experience is related not only to what we do to the infant but also to what he is able to do, let us examine him as the doctor holds him up by the legs and gives him a whack, his first "hard knock," to get him going. Yes, he is all there—two arms, two legs, two eyes, two ears, etc. But are they all functioning? Are they really "ready to go"? How about the internal organs, the muscles, the nerves? Are they all set?

Responsive Readiness

There are two aspects to readiness. One we call responsive readiness, the readiness to learn through contact with the outside world; the other is the infant's organization capability, his internal environment, which we call adaptive readiness. The distinction is artificial, because they interact and influence each other; nevertheless, research clearly indicates that an infant's senses are functional at birth. He experiences the whack from the doctor. He is sensitive to pressure, to changes in temperature, and to pain, and he responds specifically to these stimuli. He responds as well to his position in the total field; that is, he seeks balance, and he can control muscular movement to find, within limits, a comfortable posture. There is controlled movement. "The proprioceptors in muscles, and tendons, and possibly joints are functional well before birth. By the time of birth these mechanisms have undergone such development that they are among the best-organized receptor fields as far as initiation and control of behavior are concerned. . . . It is certain that tonus adjustments of the body muscles in postural responses . . . are among significant prenatal activities." (Carmichael, 1954, pp. 146, 148) Thus, in respect to skin sensitivity and balance, the infant is ready for experience and can differentiate among stimuli.

How about sight? Research on infants 4 to 8 weeks of age shows that they can see about as well as adults. (Bower, 1965) What he sees does register, and he begins to take in visual information at birth. The infant differs, obviously, from the adult in that his systematic processing of visual information has no history yet of personal experience. He is building his "data bank" at this point, rather than using it for selective perception and interpretation of what he sees. In our closer look at infancy, we have discovered that "infants from birth have the capacity to receive and discriminate patterned stimulation." (Fantz, 1967, p. 218)

The infant will be able to hear as soon as the middle ear has lost the amniotic fluid it collected in birth, and he will respond to a loud noise within the first few days. There is some evidence of discrimination of pitch and direction.

Reactions to temperature are also within his capability. However, there is a "normal" temperature range that does not evoke reaction. Changes outside the individual infant's normal range produce vigorous attempts to alter the situation; for example, both respiration and circulation are stepped up. The infant mobilizes what organization he has in an attempt to maintain a steady-state.

The responses he is able to make are functions of his state of development. A basic principle of growth is that development proceeds in a cephalocaudal, proximodistal fashion; that is, it proceeds from the head region down, and from the center out. As we would expect to find, the infant responds more around the head region, particularly around the mouth, than at any other place. Although there are gross muscular movements of arms and legs, there is little control of them. Reactions are either specific reflexes, such as the grasping movement of the hands, or general reflexes, such as the *Moro response* (general clutching movements) to something startling. This capacity to grasp, even if seen as involuntary (the infant's hand will close and grasp your finger if it is laid in its palm), represents the beginnings of sensorimotor experience. In Piaget's terms, from it the child will develop organized actions of grasping and then the use of these actions in building intelligence. He will distinguish, for example, the "graspable" from the "nongraspable" by what happens. In terms of sex differences, the girl's nervous system is more advanced at birth than the boy's.

In summary, the *neonate* (an infant less than a month old) is sensitive not only to internal but also to external stimuli. He takes in and processes information. In the last fifteen years, we have substantially altered our view of his capabilities. The infant enters the world as a competent organism, ready and able to learn and able to make some specific responses to stimuli. The laboratory work of Lipsitt (1971) on infants' ability to discriminate odors and to learn to respond differentially to them is an example of a learning experiment used to extend our knowledge of infant capabilities. These and other studies support the view of competence. He is certainly not the completely internally controlled, insensitive, passive animal we pictured him to be a decade or so ago.

Adaptive Readiness

There has been considerable controversy over the state of organization of the infant. Much of it has centered around the importance of parenting in the physical survival of the infant. Ribble (1944) has claimed that there is inadequate development of primary functions and that the infant therefore needs psychological mothering to aid in physiological as well as psychological development. Pinneau, on the basis of a careful study of the research, has written a devastating reply to this thesis. In relation to respiration, he states: "One, normally the birth process augments the oxygen supply of the fetus; two, newborn infants appear to reach the adult level of oxygenation in a few hours; three, they appear capable of enduring an extraordinary degree of asphyxia." (Pinneau, 1950, p. 209)

Additional medical research data indicate that the old notion that neonates were immunologically incapable is now in serious doubt. Instead, the newborn seems to be able to deal with most bacterial and viral infections. (Smith and Eitzman, 1964) However, although the infant may have a high degree of organization in some tissue systems, such as heart and lungs, on the whole he is inadequate to face the task of survival on his own. The first function of the family or its surrogate is to keep the child alive.

Survival is one standard; efficient growth is another. There is increasing recognition of the importance of adequate nutrition not only for the maintenance of life but also for psychological and physical growth. For example, malnutrition not only affects direct development of tissue, but also has indirect effects. Cravioto et al. indicate these as (1) loss of learning time because of less responsiveness to the environment, (2) interference with learning which, if it occurs in infancy, cannot be fully recovered, and (3) motivation and personality changes because the apathetic behavior of the malnourished infant "can provoke apathy and so contribute to a cumulative pattern of reduced adult-child interaction." (Cravioto et al., 1966, p. 358)

All research illustrates the tremendous range of individual differences among infants in their degree of organizational maturity. For example, research with neonates at the University of Illinois hospital indicated "that there are qualitative and quantitative individual differences in autonomic function apparent within the first few days of life. These differences are both in terms of autonomic-system endowment and the rate of maturation." (Richmond and Lustman, 1955, p. 274) Not only is there a wide range of individual differences, but the fluctuations within the individual are of a high order. Kessen (1961) has demonstrated stable individual differences evident in the first five days of life in movement and hand-mouth contacting. Further, although ways to investigate and analyze data are difficult and although most of the data concern animals, it seems clear that there are innate, basic biological differences as a function of sex. These must always be considered in both the design of research on children and in the interpretation of results.

The main question is the importance of parenting to the child's total self-development—not merely to his survival as a physical being. No research in the field of child development denies the importance of the parenting process. The question of the mechanisms involved is at issue, but as we shall see in Chapter 3, the role of parenting is a vital one in self-development.

SUMMARY

What can be concluded? (1) The child comes into the world with a highly complex organization, some subsystems of which are able to function at a high level in helping the body maintain itself. Some parts of his body, such as the organs of sight and hearing, and especially the neuromuscular systems of the extremities, are able to perform some efficient operations. (2) The infant is basically still an immature organization, unable to modify its environment to meet its drive for growth and maintenance without help through the parenting process. This process is one of communication, not only of food but of all kinds of stimulation. (3) The infant responds to tactile communication, to changes in temperature, to body position, and to changes in his internal state, such as hunger. The infant can and does learn to respond to systematic changes under experimental conditions. Changes in sucking behavior, for example, can be conditioned. (Lipsitt, 1967) (4) The head region, particularly the mouth, is the vital center for stimulation. (5) The infant can differentiate between comfort and discomfort. (6) There are measurable individual differences in behavior among infants.

This combination of readiness for experience, ability to respond, and individuality lay the groundwork for the development of the child's unique self-system. What he will become is not set, but neither is he a *tabula rasa*.

REFERENCES AND ADDITIONAL READINGS

Bardwick, J. *Psychology of women: A study of biocultural conflicts.* New York: Harper & Row, 1971.

Bower, G. T. The visual world of infants. *Scientific American,* 1965, *215,* 80–92.

Boyd, W. C. *Genetics and the races of man.* Boston: Little, Brown, 1950.

Burke, B. S., & Stuart, H. C. Nutritional requirements during pregnancy and lactation. *Journal of the American Medical Association,* 1948, *137,* 119–128.

Carmichael, L. The onset and early development of behavior. In L. Carmichael (Ed.), *Manual of child psychology.* (2nd ed.) New York: Wiley, 1954. Pp. 60–185.

Coursin, D. Nutrition and brain development in infants. *Merrill-Palmer Quarterly,* 1972, *18,* 177–202.

Cravioto, J., et al. Nutrition, growth and neurointegrative development: An experimental and ecologic study. *Pediatrics,* 1966, *38,* 319–372.

Fantz, R. L. Visual perception and experience in early infancy: A look at the hidden side of behavior development. In H. W. Stevenson, E. H. Hess, & H. Rheingold (Eds.), *Early behavior: Comparative and developmental approaches.* New York: Wiley, 1967. Pp. 181–224.

Fantz, R. L., & Nevis, S. Pattern preferences and perceptual-cognitive development in early infancy. *Merrill-Palmer Quarterly,* 1967, *13(1),* 77–108.

Frank, L. K. Tactile communication. *Genetic Psychology Monographs,* 1957, *56,* 209–255.

Freedman, D. G. An evolutionary approach to research on the life cycle. *Human Development,* 1971, *14(2),* 87–99.

Gordon, I. J. The needs of children and youth. In *Pupil personnel services, working papers.* Buffalo: University Press at Buffalo, SUNY, 1970. Pp. 52–59.

Hunt, J. M. *Intelligence and experience.* New York: Ronald Press, 1961.

Kagan, J., et al. *Change and continuity in infancy.* New York: Wiley, 1971.

Kessen, W. Research in the psychological development of infants: An overview. *Merrill-Palmer Quarterly,* 1963, *9,* 83–94. Reprinted in I. J. Gordon (Ed.), *Human development: Readings in research.* Glenview, Ill.: Scott, Foresman, 1965.

Kessen, W., et al. Selection and test of response measures in the study of the human newborn. *Child Development,* 1961, *32,* 7–24.

Kessen, W., Haith, M., & Salapatek, P. Human infancy: A bibliography and guide. In P. H. Mussen, *Carmichael's manual of child psychology.* (3rd ed.) New York: Wiley, 1970. Pp. 287–445.

Lipsitt, L. Learning processes of human newborns. In I. J. Gordon (Ed.), *Readings in research in developmental psychology.* Glenview, Ill.: Scott, Foresman, 1971. Pp. 114–126.

Lipsitt, L. L. Learning in the human infant. In H. Stevenson, E. Hess & H. Rheingold (Eds.), *Early behavior: Comparative and developmental approaches.* New York: Wiley, 1967. Pp. 225–248.

McClearn, G. E. Genetics and behavior development. In M. L. Hoffman & L. W. Hoffman (Eds.), *Review of child development research.* Vol. 1. New York: Russell Sage Foundation, 1964. Pp. 433–480.

Maccoby, E. (Ed.) *The development of sex differences.* Palo Alto, Calif.: Stanford University Press, 1966.

Maslow, A. H. *Motivation and personality.* New York: Harper & Row, 1954.

Milner, E. *Human neural and behavioral development.* Springfield, Ill.: Charles C Thomas, 1967.

National Institute of Health. *How children grow, clinical research advances in human growth and development.* Washington, D.C.: U.S. Department of Health, Education and Welfare, PHS, NIH, DHEW Publication No. (NIH) 72–166, June 1972.

Newman, J. J. et al. *Twins: A study of heredity and environment.* Chicago: University of Chicago Press, 1937.

Pinneau, S. R. A critique on the articles by Margaret Ribble. *Child Development,* 1950, *21,* 203–227.

Pratt, K. The neonate. In L. Carmichael (Ed.), *Manual of child psychology.* (2nd ed.) New York: Wiley, 1954. Pp. 215–291.

Read, M. S. The biological bases: Malnutrition and behavioral development. In I. J. Gordon (Ed.), *Early childhood education.* NSSE, 71st Yearbook, Part II. Chicago: University of Chicago Press, 1972. Pp. 55–70.

Ribble, M. Infantile experience in relation to personality. In J. McV. Hunt (Ed.), *Personality and the behavior disorders.* Vol 2. New York: Ronald Press, 1944. Pp. 621–651.

Richmond, J. B., & Lustman, S. L. Autonomic function in the neonate: Implications for psychosomatic theory. *Psychosomatic Medicine,* 1955, *17,* 269–275.

Rosenthal, D. *Genetics of psychopathology.* New York: McGraw-Hill, 1971.

Ross, S., Fisher, A., & King, D. Sucking behavior: A review of the literature. *Journal of Genetic Psychology,* 1957, *91,* 63–81.

Schaeffer, D. L. *Sex differences in personality: Readings.* Belmont, Calif.: Brooks/ Cole Publishing Co., 1971.

Scheinfeld, A. *The new you and heredity.* Philadelphia: Lippincott, 1950.

Scheinfeld, A. *Your heredity and environment.* Philadelphia: Lippincott, 1965.

Skinner, B. F. *Beyond freedom and dignity.* New York: Knopf, 1971.

Skinner, B. F. Phylogeny and ontogeny of behavior. *Science,* 1966, *153,* 1205–1213.

Smith, R. T., & Eitzman, D. V. Development of the immune response. *Pediatrics,* 1964, *33,* 163–183.

Sontag, L. W. Implications of fetal behavior and environment for adult personalities. *Annual New York Academy of Sciences,* 1966, *134,* 782–786.

Van de Riet, H. Achieving equity for women. Address presented at the meeting of the American Association for Higher Education, March 1970. (Mimeo) P. 5.

Watson, E. H., & Lowrey, G. H. *Growth and development of children.* (3rd ed.) Chicago: Year Book Publishers, 1958.

Woodworth, R. S. A survey of studies of identical twins reared apart. In W. Dennis (Ed.), *Readings in child psychology.* New York: Prentice-Hall, 1951. Pp. 353–359.

Young, W. C., Goy, R. W., & Phoenix, C. H. Hormones and sexual behavior. *Science,* 1964, *143,* 212–218.

CHAPTER 3
THE FAMILY SETTING

His own parents, he that had father'd him and
she that had conceiv'd him in her womb
and birth'd him,
They gave this child more of themselves than that,
They gave him afterward every day, they became
part of him . . .
The family usages, the language, the company, the
furniture, the yearning and swelling heart,
*Affection that will not be gainsay'd . . .***

THE DUAL ROLE OF THE FAMILY

If a cultural anthropologist from outer space were to drop in on the earth to explore our ways of living, he might first report on the universal phenomenon of the family unit. Family must be defined more broadly than the idealized image of mother, father, two children, and a dog. Alternative life styles have been prevalent throughout the history of man. The idealized American family is late on the scene and rare, and now new patterns are emerging in America. Indeed, a special symposium on alternative life styles was held at the American Psychological Association's convention in 1972, and projects were funded that year to begin the investigation of the effects of various communal and other alternative patterns on children. The 1970 census showed that 10 percent of all families in the United States were headed by women, one-sixth of all children were living with one parent or none, and one-fourth of all wives with husbands present and with children under 6 were in the labor force. Further, 40 percent of all adult women were in the labor market. Divorce rates were high, and many children were living in homes with remarried parents.

* From Walt Whitman, ''There Was a Child Went Forth,'' in *Leaves of Grass.*

The immediate living group constitutes the infant's initial source of experience and shapes what he will become. The family, however defined, provides first an emotional setting, a climate of affection, an interpersonal network in which the growing child can work toward self-enhancement through feeling warm, comfortable, loved, and accepted "at home." Second, the family is a teacher of culture to the child, passing on from its adult members to its children the appropriate behaviors and beliefs to enable the child to "grow out" from home and meet the world face to face, knowing how to behave.

Of course, especially in a complex civilization such as ours, the family is not an isolated unit, and other cultural agencies begin their work early in the game. The family acts as the anchorage point, the mediator, and the interpreter of the culture to the child.

In addition to interpreting the culture through explanation, family members teach by example. The child learns how to behave by the way he is treated and by the way he sees others behave toward the people and objects that surround him. He discovers that "the news" is important, because he has to be quiet at the dinner table "while the news is on." He soon learns that time holds much meaning. Long before he can read the clock, or "tell time," he sees that many aspects of his behavior are regulated by time; for example, he cannot invoke his favorite cartoon program by wishing it there but has to wait until it is the right time.

He sees life on the street and asks for explanations; he sees violence in a variety of forms on the TV screen and also "Sesame Street." He turns to other family members for interpretation and may either receive some or be left to make his own sense out of all the inputs. In either case, he is still receiving a message from inside as well as outside the family unit about values, conditions, ways of behaving. He sees the way family members talk to and treat each other and the pattern of daily life. In all his learning, the interpersonal relationships in the home provide the emotional setting, the backdrop, and the stage.

The Security-Adequacy Constellation

The infant and small child, before the advent of language, begins to organize himself in relation to this family setting. At this early stage of development, he is unable to differentiate outer from inner, self from world, mother from others. He is living almost from moment to moment. He experiences comfort and discomfort, even though he is unable to label his discomfort as "hunger," or "wetness," or "air bubbles," or other physical states. The way he is handled, the way in which his needs are met, initiate the psychological processes of the development of both his intellectual abilities and his attitudes toward himself. A sense of trust and love, or "security," and a sense of competency are influenced by the behavior of adults toward him.

THE FAMILY AS
AN INTERPERSONAL FIELD
The Family Structure

No behavior takes place outside a field, or situation. The organization of this field and the individual's own perception of the field play important roles in determining behavior. The family is such a field for the growing child. Who the members are and his own particular location in the organized pattern influence his own self-development. Of course, we need to recognize that there is no simple one-to-one cause-effect relationship. We cannot say, as we view a child in action as an adult, that he acts this way "because he was an only child," as if this were a sufficient answer; or, in another case, "because his sister was born when he was 2." These may be crucial considerations for some children; they may mean very little in the lives of others.

Ordinal Position.   With this caution as a guide, what are the probabilities that youngsters will develop different facets in terms of the order in which they are born into a family?

Although folklore and some research indicate the significance of *ordinal position*—whether one is oldest, youngest, middle, or only child—the issue is not completely clear-cut. A basic problem in psychological research, especially that which is not experimental, is the establishment of certainty that all possible errors in selecting cases (sampling errors) are ruled out and that any factors that might bias the results are determined and either ruled out by the selection of subjects for the sample or handled by some statistical means. In ordinal position research, a bias favoring the firstborn creeps in. This is because high-income, professional families have few children and send them to college and low-income families have more children and the oldest has to work to send others to school. Therefore we are bound to find more "firstborns" among professionals than among working class people. Schooler (1972), after reviewing the research on ordinal position and carefully analyzing such problems as the one above, concludes that, as of now, research cannot support any definitive statements about the role of birth order, by itself, in psychiatric illness, professional attainment, intelligence test scores, self-concept, and social views. Even our common sense notions that parents treat children differently have not been demonstrated. So, where are we? A nonscientific look at families based on our own experiences and on the swapping of stories suggests that birth order plays some role in parent behavior and in child development; careful studies do not. The question then is, do we abandon the idea or conduct better studies? Do we recognize that any attempt to use a single fact, such as birth order, or sex, or race, or genetics, or social class, or (as we shall see) breast feeding, is doomed because life is complex? The researcher faces the problem of designing his studies to show how all the facts go together and of doing what he can to see just what part each plays. We shall refer to this and to other methodological problems as they turn up throughout the book.

Family Composition.   An increase in the number of family members by one increases the interactional possibilities by many more than one. For example, in a family with 3 members, 4 interrelationships are possible (mother-father, mother-child, father-child, and father-mother-child), but in a family of 4 there are 11 possible interrelationships. All these interrelationships have emotional loadings and, in addition, serve to present to the child many models of possible behaviors that he might emulate. At the present time, research does not clearly indicate any personality patterning typical of the child from a large family as compared to an only child or a child from a small family. Indeed, we probably shouldn't expect to find a typical "large family" or "small family" member.

Another aspect of the family field of forces is the presence or absence of a parent. What does it mean to the child to grow up in a broken home? Since there are many "parents without partners" in the American society, large numbers of children are growing up in father-absent homes. This fact was clearly indicated by the 1970 census. These homes range from those in which a stable father figure was never present (children living with their unwed mothers) to homes split by divorce or a succession of fathers. There are, in addition, the communal living patterns. Again, our beliefs about the effects of this type of group living upon children contain more myth than data.

There seems to be some evidence of negative effects of father absence on boys' sex-role indentification (Biller, 1970; Santrock, 1970; Biller and Bahm, 1971), cognitive development (Landy et al., 1969, Blanchard and Biller, 1971), and emotional and social adjustment (Siegman, 1966; Cortes and Fleming, 1968; Hoffman, 1970). Girls' social adjustment seems also to be negatively influenced by father absence (Biller and Weiss, 1970). However, as we have said before, single-variable (such as father absence) research is usually inconclusive because of the many other variables that need to be taken into account. The age of the child, the length and reason for the parent's absence, the emotional strength of the mother, income level, cultural patterns, and the presence of siblings are all factors that influence the effect of the absence upon the child.

Summary

It is generally agreed, both by scientists and lay people, that such family factors as size, stability, and composition influence child development. The basic scientific issues lie in the development of adequate research strategies and measurement tools to assess just how the situations are translated into child learning and what the actual effects are. The curious student can raise a number of researchable questions, and the field is still wide open.

CHILD REARING AND THE DUAL ROLE

The admonitions of the experts, both those who are qualified by training and those who are self-appointed, are on all sides of the new mother. Suggestions and advice are offered by Gesell and Spock on the one hand and by the neighbors and relatives on the other. The advice, particularly from the self-appointed, is usually arbitrary and heavily laden with "thou shalts" and "thou shalt nots." Everybody, it seems, has an opinion on how to raise children, and often those with no children have the loudest voices. There are two major clusters of experience around which much of the advice and concern are grouped. The first is feeding and weaning; the second is toilet training. Of course, there are other concerns that face the parents as they attempt to bring up the child, but these two seem to be primary.

Feeding and Weaning

To breast feed or bottle feed, which is better for the health and security of the child? Nursing has both cultural and interpersonal aspects, and these exist within a particular family in a special and unique combination. Different segments of our society advocate different practices. Whether the child is bottle fed or breast fed, maternal behavior ranges from permissiveness and its misinterpretation of license to rigidity and the notion that "crying is good for the lungs." These differences stem from ethnic backgrounds, from religious viewpoints, from social class values, and from the personalities of the mother and father. The mass media magazines (such as those given out in store nursery departments, those sold at supermarkets, or full-length ones like *McCalls*) add their voices to the confusion.

What does research establish? First, any direct relationship between a particular approach to feeding and adult personality is not shown by the data. (Orlansky, 1949; Thurston and Mussen, 1951; Caldwell, 1964)

Most of the research of a single-variable nature looks at the technique being studied and overlooks the mother-child interaction. Breast feeding, when the mother desires it and the child responds, seems to enhance the emotional relationship between mother and child as well as give the baby some antibodies in the colostrum that precedes the true milk in the early days. The mother's physiological functioning is such that there is a tie between breast feeding and uterine contraction. The mother who breast feeds and is uninhibited in it helps her organs get back to normal shape; she "not only gives her baby the pleasure of a secure and abundant milk supply, but she, herself, derives pleasurable physical sensations from the act of breast feeding . . . and thus the mother-child relationship starts on the basis of physical desire as well as companionship." (Newton, 1965, p. 137) On the other hand, being breast fed by a rejecting mother or by one who is doing it only because it is expected probably operates to create anxiety rather than security. How the father views the situation is also part of the field. His attitudes and behavior affect the mother's decision and in turn the mother-child relationship. All three— mother, father, child—are bound together and influence each other. If father is upset by breast feeding because of his own immaturity or cultural background, this may prove disruptive.

As Newton and Newton (1971) conclude, there are a variety of factors that seem to account for the decline of breast feeding around the world, such as the psychological ones just discussed and social factors such as the female role in society, industrialization, and cultural patterns (see Chapter 7 for more detail).

If we approach the answer from a transactional point of view, the child will develop and thrive when the feeding situation is constructed in such a way that (1) his biological needs are met and (2) his mother is comfortable and relaxed. This can occur, depending upon the family, under a variety of circumstances. In essence, it doesn't seem to make much difference whether the baby is breast fed or bottle fed, has an essentially demand feeding or a not completely arbitrary routine, as long as the above two conditions are met.

There doesn't seem to be an optimal time for weaning. If we go back to Chapter 2 and recall what was said about the wide range of individual needs for sucking and the wide range of maturation, this conclusion should not surprise us. Some children need mothering longer than others; some cultures impose weaning much sooner than others. When we approach this in terms of individual behavior, we find no clear-cut evidence favoring a particular pattern.

Toilet Training

In the case of toilet training, we are faced with somewhat the same range of demands upon the child, from permissiveness and delayed expectations to harshness and early demands. In a comparison of 20 societies, these expectations ranged from beginning training at 6 months to waiting until the child was 5 years old. The American middle class ranked with one other subgroup at the extreme of early expectation. In harshness of training, the American middle class norm again was at the most severe end of the group. (Whiting and Child, 1953, pp. 74–77) Comparisons have been made within American society between classes and castes, and the picture again shows wide ranges of individual differences. The average middle class parent expects that children should be trained early and that cleanliness is an important attribute to learn. "Clean" and "good" are associated early.

Considerations of the impact of toilet training on self-development differ in one respect from feeding and weaning. In the latter two, the infant is capable of functioning in response to the stimuli of bottle, breast, or cup. Toilet training demands the ability to control. Such control is a function of both maturation and learning, and there is no set time for an individual child. Although the data indicate some relationship between severe demand and child behavior disturbance and between onset of demand and the length of time required to train, we must conclude that there is no single cause-effect relationship between toilet training and general personality development.

Here again, a basically common-sense idea—at least, common sense since Freud—is difficult to substantiate by research. The movement, partially aided by the development of computers, to multivariate studies should help. Such studies combine data on a number of variables, such as age of parent, sex of child, socioeconomic status, home conditions, baby's health, and other factors, in order to examine the patterns of relationships among them and some other variable thought to be dependent on them, such as a child's susceptibility to allergies, aggressive behavior, and the like. As we engage in more of these studies and improve our measurement techniques, our information should become less myth-ridden and more factual. Further, the use of experimental methods, such as certain studies of infant learning (Lipsitt and Eimas, 1972), should enable us to understand better just how a child-rearing pattern, embedded in the host of stimuli that surround the child, influences his development.

Child Rearing as a Complex

What do these results mean? The child-rearing situation must be viewed as a phase of the total family pattern and family value system. Any specific technique reflects both the cultural expectations and the interpersonal climate of the home. An important point is the meaning a pattern has in its own culture. In discussing national differences found in a European study, Hindley et al. state: "It cannot, therefore, be assumed when a Brussels mother weans early, that this has the same connotation as when a Stockholm mother does so. In the latter culture breast-feeding is part of the accepted pattern of life, and failure to breast-feed is the more likely to imply unusual maternal attitudes; whereas in the Brussels culture—it would be likely to have much less significance." (Hindley et al., 1965, p. 198) Further, within a nation, there are subgroups with distinct cultural patterns that influence all aspects of child rearing. (Castaneda, 1971; Coles and Piers, 1969; Grier and Cobbs, 1968; and Rainwater, 1970)

To understand the impact of the experience upon the child, we must include his own organism as a part of the process. Infants are individuals and partly shape their own destinies. They can reject or distort inputs from the environment. (Kagan, 1971) They help create the home environment, and it is the interpersonal climate of the home, in which specific techniques are employed, that seems to be a major contributing factor in development.

LOVING AND THE DUAL ROLE

We have said several times that the network of family relationships is the major force shaping self-development. For example, in the discussion of feeding, the degree of comfort of the parent was stated as a major criterion in determining the best individual procedure. A healthy parent-child relationship that is nonexploitive and provides the child with security seems to be the desirable pattern. We know that a number of homes depart from the so-called ideal pattern. The word *nonexploitive* is a key one. The late 1960s and early 1970s saw in the United States and in other places around the world the emergence of women's liberation. A basic element in the movement is the desire for women to cease being victims of cultural stereotyping and exploitive relationships. In terms of the family, the mother's comfort depends to a considerable extent on whether she perceives herself as valued, loved, and respected for herself and not because she plays particular roles. The husband-wife relationship has been subjected to severe strains as each seeks to come to grips with emerging perceptions of sex roles.

Although different social classes and ethnic groups within American society define the role of wife-mother in different fashion, a basic underlying thread of a valid family relationship must be a perception on the part of each parent of acceptance by the other.

Since so many women are in the labor market, a major question has been the effect of the working wife-mother on her child's development. The data are certainly not complete and are far from unequivocal, but as in the case of other single variables described above, the fact of working is probably not the significant fact. What seems to be significant is the role that work has in the mother's perception of self, the effect that this has on her husband, and the meanings that each assigns to conventional roles. Questions seem to be: How free is the mother to choose? Why does she work? A recent survey (ISR, 1972) indicates that, as with men, women work for major income, not pin money, and are just as concerned as men with self-satisfaction from the job. If the mother can choose between working or staying at home, the choice must be judged in the context of the way in which provision is made for adequate child care and the means by which the family unit carries on its primary functions. Since a primary function is child rearing, many mothers are faced with the necessity of staying home because of the lack of adequate substitutes, such as day-care institutions or family day care. Thus, the mother's choice is not a fully independent one. The question of adequate care remains. What we need is attention to and investigation of the effects of mother absence similar to the studies on father absence cited earlier in the chapter. One might guess that the results would be similar; that is, that mother absence has different meanings when embedded in different social contexts. It probably contributes in some systematic fashion to the intellectual and personality development of children.

Parent-Child Relationships

With our present view of the infant and young child as able to select and respond to inputs from the world around him, we would expect that he would pick up cues about this world from how he is held, how and when he is talked to, the sight and sounds that surround him. Studies of institutionalized children show that mothering is an important variable in development (Dennis and Najarian, 1957; Provence and Lipton, 1962; Tizard and Joseph, 1970; Tizard et al., 1972) and that mothering is far more than feeding and changing the baby. Unfortunately, emotional deprivation exists and leaves its mark in families as well as in institutions.

There have been a great many studies investigating attachment, the bond between parent and child, especially in infancy. (Gewirtz, 1972; Moreno, 1973). As one example, Ainsworth and Bell (1972) reported that the sensitivity of mothers (their responsiveness to the attempts of the children to call attention to their needs) and the provision of freedom to explore were both positively related to children's cognitive and social behaviors in infancy. They stress the importance of a harmonious infant-mother relationship and state that for socioeconomically disadvantaged infants it is "the single most important factor alleviating" such disadvantage. (Ainsworth and Bell, 1972)

The way parents relate to young children and the general climate of the home have been studied in naturalistic field observations; that is, the investigator visits the home for long periods of time, both within a single observation period and over several months or years, and records the pattern of interactions. There are, as with any method, problems. How true is the picture the observer sees? What goes on when an observer is not present? Nevertheless, studies such as those by Escalona (1972) and B. White (1972) within the United States and those by Caudill and Weinstein (1969) in Japan and the United States are examples of a host of literature that supports the idea that the parent-child interaction pattern has measurable effects on the cognitive and social behavior of the young child. Longitudinal research such as that of Kagan and Moss (1962) and the collection of reports stemming from the California Growth studies all indicate relationships to later life.

Parent-child relationships affect physical growth as well as personality and intellectual development. Studies of a small group of hospitalized children led Powell and his colleagues to conclude that growth failure was related to emotional disturbance in the home in the first few years of life. (Powell et al., 1967) This is a landmark study, because we so often assume that growth is not affected by external events.

The "Climate of Feeling" as a Complex

The child begins to develop his sense of competence, his sense of self-worth, from the way he is treated and evaluated by the other members of his family. We have seen that it is not techniques alone that convey to him the attitudes and beliefs his parents hold about him. The presence of love and his perception of being loved is important. This climate is created by the ways all members of the family treat each other, by the tones of voice used, by the kinds of tactile sensations that are denied or offered the child. Both societal expectations and parental attitudes are combined into parental behavior. Further, the child himself is a part of the field of forces. He is not mere passive recipient—he is an active person, contributing his share to the development of the family "climate of feeling."

From the very beginning of his life, the child's sex and appearance are stimuli that evoke parental feelings and responses. His cries, his being a "good baby" who sleeps 20 out of 24 hours, his lack of colic, his reactions to their behavior, all leave their mark upon the parents. The infant has a share in the determination of his own fate. He shapes his parents' behavior toward him. What happens to him is influenced by what he does and how his behavior is perceived by his parents.

Summary

The climate of feeling in the home, mutually created by all members of the family but most strongly influenced by the parents' love and acceptance of each other, provides the original environmental source for the child's development. If this climate is a loving one, he will be more able to develop his competencies and positive notions of self and world.

AGE-SEX STANDARD SETTING AND THE DUAL ROLE

Along with the pattern of relationships within the family, we must consider what parents expect of each other and what they expect of their children as potent forces that shape the behavior and development of the child. We mentioned earlier that there are many ways in which a woman can behave and still perceive herself as female and a good wife and mother. Similarly, there are many roles the man can play—from "breadwinner" to part-time cook, to partner-in-housework—and still perceive of himself as male and a good husband and father.

Expectations are held for the children and rewards and punishments, smiles and frowns, praise and reproof meted out in accordance with the child's attempts to meet these standards. Parents are not necessarily aware of their expectations for their children, although certainly these expectations reflect the parents' own sex and cultural experiences. The injunction that parents should always agree overlooks the perceptual realities of each—each sees life in his own fashion.

Expectations for Infants

Luckily for the infant, both parents usually are more in agreement during this beginning period. They expect him to be helpless, and cuddlesome, and completely dependent. They look forward to his accomplishing such feats as rolling over, or following an object with his eyes, or grabbing his toe. Only the most sophisticated parents realize that these seemingly meaningless activities are the beginnings of intellectual development. Most parents enjoy their infants as spectators or see their "playing with the baby" as amusement only, but these activities are fundamental to adequate development.

The expectation of the parents toward their own roles as teachers of infants helps determine whether a child will be educationally advantaged or disadvantaged. For instance, Smilansky (1968) found that Israeli mothers from Middle Eastern backgrounds did not see themselves as teachers, whereas Israeli mothers from European backgrounds did. The latter broke learning tasks up into small steps and taught the child how to perform. The differences favoring the European children were clearly apparent in the sociodramatic play of preschoolers.

This concept of parent as teacher, even in relating to the infant, seems to be a crucial one in influencing cognitive development. We cited some naturalistic studies above. Such studies, like those of Wachs, Uzgiris, and Hunt (1971), indicate that teaching activities such as direct instruction, spontaneous teaching, and placing objects in the environment are all positively related to intellectual performance in infancy. An experiment in parent education showed that parent-child interaction patterns before age 1 in a teaching situation were predictive of child performance at age 1 on a mental development scale. (Gordon and Jester, 1972; Gordon, 1972) The child's view of self also develops from these expectations and from the responses of parents to child performance. One might speculate that the parent who expects performance but doesn't help the child to master the steps might be communicating to the child in a way that contributes eventually to his diminished self-esteem.

The first expectation is one of dependency. The expectancies are asexual at this point, although we find the beginnings of cultural differentiation in the "blue for boys, pink for girls" gifts that shower upon the new baby. It is enough for the parents if the baby responds, sleeps well and long (especially through the night), and gains in height and weight.

The pressures for movement from dependence to independence vary, of course, from family to family, but in the middle class they begin early and are persistent. There have been two major studies of patterns of child rearing in modern America. Sears and his colleagues at Harvard used interviews with 379 mothers who had children attending public kindergarten in two suburbs of a large metropolitan New England area. They conducted standard open-ended interviews with these mothers and then scaled the responses for comparison. They used the Warner scale for determining social position. In relation to dependence, they report that individual mothers report wide differences in their own feelings regarding the dependent behavior of their children, but most accept it as normal and natural in infancy. They see their task as enabling the small child to broaden his base of attention and affection to include other adults and peers. (Sears, Maccoby, and Levin, 1957, p. 141)

The other major study was made by Miller and Swanson in the Detroit area. In comparison with the other studies to determine child-rearing practices, they attempted to use current concepts about the changing American culture toward increased organization. In effect, they asked if the children of "organization men" were reared differently from those of the older, entrepreneurial family. Their term for the newer type is "bureaucratic," which they defined essentially as working for someone else in a large organization for wage or salary. The entrepreneurial family is engaged in small enterprise of a risk-taking nature. Their results "show only a modest correspondence with those found elsewhere." (Miller and Swanson, 1958, p. 144)

But do we really know much about what goes on in homes? Probably not. Interview techniques, as indicated by Yarrow, Campbell, and Burton (1968), have many flaws. Their study points up the problems of investigating home situations in ways that yield valid data and at the same time meet ethical and cost considerations. They advocate observation, but here too the problem is tremendous. Escalona (1972) and B. White (1972) both mounted major efforts to observe family interaction with infants and developed elaborate coding systems for analyzing the interaction, but they could use their schemes—at great expense—with only a few families. Although all agree on the importance of the issue, we are a long way from answers.

"Children Should Be . . ."

When we move past the first six months or so, particularly when the child is mobile, a number of other expectations combining cultural and individual factors become more evident. Standards for cleanliness and sexual modesty are laid down; areas and objects are placed "off limits" to curious hands; the child's own safety poses limits on mobility, etc. Again, these demands and restrictions, these "dos" and "don'ts," are a function of the age and the sex of the child. They are certainly a function of the culture and class position of the family, and they are related to the personality structure of the adults. Concern for visiting neighbors may dictate that the living room is out-of-bounds, and closing bathroom doors may reflect both the sexual concern of the mother and the particular ethnic or class culture of the parents.

Our culture has many age-graded expectations, and the child learns "his place" in the scheme of things through the ways these are communicated to him. His sense of selfhood, of who and what he is, of what he can and cannot do, is developed partly as a result of his experiencing these demands. They are, of course, never communicated apart from the parental attitudes and feelings that surround them. They are defined in myriad ways, but they all have in common the injunction: this is what children should be. "From a comparative point of view, our culture goes to great extremes in emphasizing contrasts between the child and the adult. The child is sexless, the adult estimates his virility by his sexual activities; the child must be protected from the ugly facts of life, the adult must meet them without psychic catastrophe; the child must obey, the adult must command his obedience. These are all dogmas of our culture. . . ." (Benedict, 1953, p. 466) Although more than twenty years old, the basic statement still holds.

During this period when selfhood is being initiated, what are some of the specific demands and expectations held for children?

First, there are expectations concerning conduct with other children. Here we can see again the type of discontinuity of which Benedict spoke. We expect children to share toys, to play nicely with each other, to take turns, to cooperate; that is, do what the adults want done. ". . . let us consider how often children are expected to share their most cherished possessions, toys, with one another, and how we try to educate them to do that, while at the same time expecting them to succeed in a highly competitive society when they grow up." (Bettelheim, 1952, p. 77)

Second, there are expectations about sexual activity. "The task of the mother in our society . . . involves training the child to inhibit sex impulses toward family members, avoid erotic play with other children, and avoid sexual self-stimulation." (Sears et al., 1957, p. 181)

The Detroit Area Study found the differences in permissiveness to be related to the type rather than the social class of the family. "Entrepreneurial middle-class mothers are more likely than bureaucratic mothers of the same social class to use harsh means to stop a child from sucking his body, to declare that their children did not touch their sex organs, and to say that they took measures to stop a child who touches his sex organs." (Miller and Swanson, 1958, p. 105)

Third, there are the continued expectations about relationships to authority. One of the differences between social classes, which affects language and cognitive learning, is in this area. The middle class child is expected to be obedient, but the adult is expected to have reasons for his requests. Although final authority may rest in the adult because of his physical prowess, rational authority is usually presented to the child as the basis for expectations. While parents will say in exasperation, "Do it because I told you to!" they usually offer reasons to the child when he asks, "Why?" In turn, they expect the child to have reasons for his requests and his behavior. In terms of the development of self, children learn that people (including themselves) are expected to be rational, that authority rests on reason, not force, and that "just because" is usually not an acceptable reason for either a request or behavior. This perception of causality and rationality becomes clarified further as language develops, because our language structure is organized in this fashion.

A variety of studies using survey methods structured "teaching" situations in which the parent is asked to interact with the child, and naturalistic observation in homes all seem to indicate that parental teaching style is intricately interwoven with language usage and expectations of reasoning responses, even in young children. Miller (1971) and Goodacre (1970) in England, Rupp (1969) in Holland, Olmsted and Jester (1972), Hess and Shipman (1965), and Streissguth and Bee (1972) are examples of the spread of this research. Further, there seem to be clear relationships between these home activities, beginning in infancy, and school achievement.

But all the facts are far from known, and social class distinctions are far too simple. We have found that there are poor (income) parents who rate high on effective interaction in a reasoning fashion, and comfortable (income) parents who offer their children a deprived social interactional environment. At the risk of redundancy, think always in multivariate terms! Nothing is as simple as we would like it to be.

The handling of aggression is a fourth area in which expectations are held for the child. In addition to age and sex, social class is a major variable affecting the expectations parents hold. Independent of sex, lower class mothers were less permissive about aggression toward themselves and other children and were more restrictive and punitive toward aggressors. (Sears et al., 1957, p. 254) Although parents expect youngsters to know how to defend themselves physically—even when they are 2 and 3 —social class differences about physical aggression become more evident as children grow. Middle class children are expected to move from physical to verbal means, whereas physical means remain more acceptable to lower class groups.

Along with aggression, the whole area of emotional expression has heavy cultural influences. As in the case of all the above expectations, this is a mixture of cultural and personal pressures. Age and sex are again factors. The younger the child, the more permissive the parent toward "explosions" of negative feelings and the more acceptant of physical affectional demonstrations. As children grow, they are expected to be less demonstrative in middle class families, in terms of both negative and positive feelings. Words become substitutes for actions.

Boys as "Frogs, and Snails, and Puppy-dogs' Tails"

Perhaps one of the areas in greatest ferment as this is written is that of sex-role expectation and identification. How much is biological and how much socialization? If the latter, just how do boys and girls learn these roles? There seems to be evidence suggesting that aggression has some biological overtones that both lead males to be more aggressive than girls and to be expected to be so. Consequently, there is more acceptance of aggression in boys.

A prime problem in the early formative years for boys is that they have not too much contact with male models. Since identification is a major way in which the young child learns about and shapes himself, the lack of father figures during much of this early time poses problems and questions. The boy child learns what is expected of him as a boy largely from his mother, so that he receives feminine perceptions of maleness. Research has shown that mothers have wide varieties of sex-role expectations. The boy, to some degree, receives his instruction "secondhand" and gets images of maleness that not only reflect general cultural images but also, and probably more significantly, reflect his mother's perception of appropriate male behavior. This is compounded of her images of her father, her perceptions of her husband, and her hopes and aspirations. So we have the strange situation in early childhood (as well as in primary school for many children) that boys learn boyness first from the feminine point of view.

Girls as "Sugar and Spice"

Cultural stereotypes for young girls seem to cut across class lines more than those for boys. Except in the area of sexual modesty, where lower class mothers are stricter and more punitive, the individual differences from family to family are greater than the differences between social class groups.

Although it would seem that the girl is presented with a clearer and more persistent image of her sex-role early in life because the primary caretakers are usually female, some research (Rothbart and Maccoby, 1966) suggests this may not be such a simple issue.

Standard Setting as a Complex

It is evident that our concept of individuality permeates what research shows about the standards parents hold for children as boys and girls begin the process of development. While there are broad cultural images that play roles in defining what the child should become, these are highly modified within any given family by the personal views of the parents, particularly the mother's. The child's perception and acceptance of his own sex will be determined by the perceptions held by others in his family. These, in turn, are compounded by the transactions in their personal experiences between person and culture. Each family presents to the child his first image of himself, and this image grows out of the adult's perception of the culture in which he lives.

In addition, as society changes, we need to ask what effects cultural stereotypes have on the ability of the person to adapt to changing roles. Does the child who learns his role too well become ill adapted? Is the child who is presented with many models of appropriate behavior in better shape to develop his own personal pattern? We do not know, and it will take a different kind of research than we have engaged in to answer these questions.

SUMMARY

In this chapter we have looked at the family setting that surrounds the child at birth and along with his organism sets the stage and provides the materials for his self-development. We have seen that the family is not a simple mechanical unit directly reflecting the society. It is a highly dynamic organization with (1) a network of interpersonal relationships that are basically emotional in tone, (2) a set of goals, values, and aspirations, not necessarily known to the parents, that affects the ways in which the infant and child will be treated, and (3) the infant himself, with his rhythm of activity and rest, his needs and urges, his sex and appearance.

As Lipsitt and Eimas express it, "These processes [sensory, learning, etc.] get themselves together in diverse and fascinating ways in different people . . . [This does] honor to the devotees of individual differences in man. . . ." (Lipsitt and Eimas, 1972)

Throughout the chapter, we have indicated what we do not know, as well as what seems to be known, and have referred to methodological problems. It seems clear that we need to make more use of longitudinal studies that are more broadly based than our earlier efforts (Sontag, 1971); we need more sophisticated observational efforts in both naturalistic and semistructured situations; we need to focus on multiple variables in social context; and we need more straight experimentation from a variety of orientations. Rather than being discouraged, we should be challenged to continue to pursue, from as many angles as possible, the principles that explain the impact of family on the developing child.

REFERENCES AND ADDITIONAL READINGS

Ainsworth, M., & Bell, S. Mother-infant interaction and the development of competence. In K. J. Connolly (Ed.), *Development of early competence.* London: Academic Press, 1972.

Benedict, R. Continuities and discontinuities in cultural conditioning. In J. Seidman (Ed.), *The adolescent.* New York: Dryden, 1953. Pp. 465–475. Reprinted by permission of Holt, Rinehart and Winston, Inc.

Bettleheim, B. Mental health and current mores. *American Journal of Orthopsychiatry,* 1952, *22,* 76–78.

Biller, H. B. Father absence and the personality development of the male child. *Developmental Psychology,* 1970, *2,* 181–201.

Biller, H. B. *Father, child and sex role.* Lexington, Mass.: Heath, 1971.

Biller, H., & Bahm, R. Father absence, perceived maternal behavior, and masculinity of self-concept among junior high school boys. *Developmental Psychology,* 1971, *4,* 171–181.

Biller, H., & Weiss, S. The father-daughter relationship and the personality of the female. *Journal of Genetic Psychology,* 1970, *116,* 79–93.

Billingsley, A. *Black families in white America.* Englewood Cliffs, N.J.: Prentice-Hall, 1968.

Blanchard, R., & Biller, H. Father availability and academic performance among third-grade boys. *Developmental Psychology,* 1971, *4,* 301–305.

Bloom, B. *Stability and change in human characteristics.* New York: Wiley, 1964.

Brown, R. Development of the first language in the human species. *American Psychologist,* 1973, *28,* 97–106.

Caldwell, B. M. The effects of infant care. In M. L. Hoffman & L. W. Hoffman (Eds.), *Review of child development research.* Vol. 1. New York: Russell Sage Foundation, 1964. Pp. 9–88.

Castaneda, A. et al. (Eds.) *Mexican-Americans and educational change.* Riverside, Calif.: University of California, 1971.

Caudill, W., & Weinstein, H. Maternal care and infant behavior in Japan and America. *Psychiatry,* 1969, *32,* 12–43.

Clausen, J. A. Family structure, socialization and personality. In M. L. Hoffman & L. W. Hoffman (Eds.), *Review of child development research.* Vol 2. New York: Russell Sage Foundation, 1966. Pp. 1–54.

Coles, R., & Piers, M. *Wages of neglect.* Chicago: Quadrangle, 1969.

Cortes, C., & Fleming, E. The effects of father absence on the adjustment of culturally disadvantaged boys. *Journal of Special Education,* 1968, *2,* 413–420.

Dennis, W., & Najarian, P. Infant development under environmental handicap. *Psychological Monographs,* 1957, *71,* 1–13.

Escalona, S. K. The differential impact of environmental conditions as a function of different reaction patterns in infancy. (Mimeo) Rose F. Kennedy Center for Research in Mental Retardation and Human Development, Albert Einstein College of Medicine of Yeshiva University, N.Y., 1972.

Frank, L. K. Tactile communication. *Genetic Psychology Monograph,* 1957, *56,* 209–255.

Gewirtz, J. (Ed.) *Attachment and dependency.* Washington, D.C.: V. H. Winston, 1972.

Goodacre, E. *School and home.* London: National Foundation for Education Research in England and Wales, 1970.

Gordon, I. J. What do we know about parents as teachers? *Theory Into Practice,* 1972, *11,* 146–149.

Gordon, I. J., & Jester, R. E. Instructional strategies in infant stimulation. *Selected Documents in Psychology,* 1972, *2,* 122.

Grier, W., & Cobbs, P. *Black rage.* New York: Basic Books, 1968.

Hawkes, G. et al. Marital satisfaction, personality characteristics, and parental acceptance of children. *Journal of Counseling Psychology,* 1956, *3,* 216–221.

Henry, J., & Warson, S. Family structure and psychic development. *The American Journal of Orthopsychiatry,* 1951, *21,* 59–73.

Hess, R. D., & Shipman, V. C. Early experience and the socialization of cognitive modes in children. *Child Development,* 1965, *36,* 869–886.

Hindley, C. B. et al. Some differences in infant feeding and elimination training in five European longitudinal samples. *Journal of Child Psychology and Psychiatry,* 1965, *6,* 179–201.

Hoffman, L. W. Effects of maternal employment on the child. *Child Development,* 1961, *23,* 187–197. Reprinted in I. J. Gordon (Ed.), *Human development: Readings in research.* Glenview, Ill.: Scott, Foresman, 1965.

Hoffman, M. Moral development. In P. Mussen (Ed.), *Carmichael's manual of child psychology.* (3rd ed.) Vol. 1. New York: Wiley, 1970, Pp. 261–360.

Hunt, D. *Parents and children in history.* New York: Basic Books, 1970.

Institute for Social Research. Women in work—facts and fictions. *ISR Newsletter,* Autumn 1972, *1(16),* 4–5. Ann Arbor, Mich.: University of Michigan.

Kagan, J. On the need for relativism. In I. J. Gordon (Ed.), *Readings in research in developmental psychology.* Glenview, Ill.: Scott, Foresman, 1971. Pp. 42–53.

Kagan, J., & Moss, H. *Birth to maturity.* New York: Wiley, 1962.

Klatskin, E. et al. The influence of degree of flexibility in maternal child care practices in early child behavior. *American Journal of Orthopsychiatry,* 1956, *26,* 79–93.

Landy, F., Rosenberg, B. G., & Sutton-Smith, B. The effect of limited father absence on cognitive development. *Child Development,* 1969, *40,* 941–944.

Lipsitt, L., & Eimas, P. Developmental psychology. In P. H. Mussen & M. R. Rosenzweig (Eds.), *Annual review of psychology.* Palo Alto, Calif.: Annual Reviews, Inc., 1972. Vol. 23. Pp. 1–50.

Lynn, D. B. Sex-role and parental identification. *Child Development,* 1962, *33,* 555–564. Reprinted in I. J. Gordon (Ed.), *Human development: Readings in research.* Glenview, Ill.: Scott, Foresman, 1965.

Miller, D., & Swanson, G. *The changing American parent.* New York: Wiley, 1958.

Miller, G. W. *Educational opportunity and the home.* London: Longman, 1971.

Mischel, W. Father absence and delay of gratification: Cross-cultural comparisons. *Journal of Abnormal and Social Psychology,* 1961, *63,* 116–124. Reprinted in I. J. Gordon (Ed.), *Human development: Readings in research.* Glenview, Ill.: Scott, Foresman, 1965.

Moreno, P. The assessment of attachment. *Selected Documents in Psychology,* 1973, *3,* 121.

Murphy, L. et al. *The widening world of childhood.* New York: Basic Books, 1962.

Newton, M. The influence of the let-down reflex in breast feeding on the mother-child relationship. In I. J. Gordon (Ed.), *Human development: Readings in research.* Glenview, Ill.: Scott, Foresman, 1965. Pp. 136–138.

Newton, N., & Newton, M. Psychologic aspects of lactation. In I. J. Gordon (Ed.), *Readings in research in developmental psychology.* Glenview, Ill.: Scott, Foresman, 1971. Pp. 133–145.

Olmsted, P., & Jester, R. E. Mother-child interaction in a teaching situation. *Theory Into Practice,* 1972, *11*(3), 163–170.

Orlansky, H. Infant care and personality. *Psychological Bulletin,* 1949, *46,* 1–48.

Powell, G. F. et al. Emotional deprivation and growth retardation simulating idiopathic hypopituitarism. *The New England Journal of Medicine,* 1967, *276,* 1271–1278.

Provence, S., & Lipton, R. *Infants in institutions.* New York: International Universities Press, 1962.

Rainwater, L. *Behind ghetto walls.* Chicago: Aldine, 1970.

Rothbart, M., & Maccoby, E. Parents' differential reactions to sons and daughters. *Journal of Personality and Social Psychology,* 1966, *4,* 237–243.

Rupp, J. C. C. *Opvoeding tot school-weer baarherd (Helping the child to cope with school).* Groninger, Netherlands: Walters-Noordhoff, 1969.

Santrock, J. W. Paternal absence, sex-typing and identification. *Developmental Psychology,* 1970, *2,* 264–272.

Schooler, C. Birth order effects: Not here, not now! *Psychological Bulletin,* 1972, *78,* 161–175.

Sears, R., Maccoby, E., & Levin, H. *Patterns of child rearing.* New York: Harper & Row, 1957.

Sells, S. B., & Roff, M. Peer acceptance-rejection and birth order. A paper presented at the American Psychological Association convention, 1963.

Siegman, A. Father absence during early childhood and antisocial behavior. *Journal of Abnormal Psychology,* 1966, *71,* 71–74.

Smilansky, S. *The effects of sociodramatic play on disadvantaged preschool children.* New York: Wiley, 1968.

Sontag, L. W. The history of longitudinal research: Implications for the future. *Child Development,* 1971, *42,* 987–1000.

Streissguth, A. P., & Bee, H. L. Mother-child interactions and cognitive development in children. *Young Children,* 1972, 154–173.

Stroup, A. Marital adjustment of the mother and the personality of the child. *Marriage and Family Living,* 1956, *18,* 109–113.

Thurston, J., & Mussen, P. Infant feeding gratification and adult personality. *Journal of Personality,* 1951, *19,* 449–458.

Tizard, B. et al. Environmental effects of language development: A study of young children in long-study residential nurseries. *Child Development,* 1972, *43,* 337–358.

Tizard, B., & Joseph, A. Cognitive development of young children in residential care: A study of children aged 24 months. *Journal of Child Psychology and Psychiatry,* 1970, *11,* 177–186.

Wachs, T. D., Uzgiris, J. C., & Hunt, J. McV. Cognitive development in infants of different age levels and from different environmental backgrounds: An exploratory investigation. *Merrill-Palmer Quarterly,* 1971, *17,* 283–317.

Wenar, C., & Wenar, S. The short term prospective model, the illusion of time, and the tabula rasa child. *Child Development,* 1963, *34,* 697–708.

White, B. L. Fundamental early environmental influences on the development of competency. In M. Meyer (Ed.), *Third symposium on learning: Cognitive learning.* Bellingham, Wash.: Western Washington State College, 1972.

Whiting, J., & Child, I. L. *Child training and personality.* New Haven: Yale University Press, 1953.

Wortis, H. et al. Child-rearing practices in a low socioeconomic group. *Pediatrics,* 1963, *32,* 298–307.

Yarrow, M. R., Campbell, J., & Burton, R. *Child rearing: An inquiry into research and methods.* San Francisco: Jossey-Boss, 1968.

CHAPTER 4

THE EMERGENCE OF "I"

THE ORGANIZING PROCESSES AT WORK

In Chapter 1, we said that the development of the self-system depends upon two major processes—differentiating-integrating and perceiving. Both of these are transactional, involving both the organism and the environment. The infant has a drive, or urge, to create order in his world, to assign meanings to events, to create stability, and to push toward higher and higher levels of organization. In this chapter, we will consider these organizing processes at work in the development of the self-system up to the point where the infant conceives of himself, however vaguely, as a person with some stability.

The Development of Motor Control

As we have seen, the infant possesses at birth a certain degree of organization. The process of motor control development illustrates one way in which the infant, through his increasing ability to differentiate and integrate, develops some control over himself and his environment. This development, while having strong biological components, is not purely a matter of maturation or the unfolding of biological development without the influence of experience or learning. We need to keep two factors in focus: (1) the purposiveness of this process of extending control and (2) its transactional nature.

Direction of Development.   The direction of control proceeds along two major axes: cephalocaudal and proximodistal. The infant's head region is more highly developed than his extremities. Coordination proceeds downward from the head and outward from the center line. The head-turning and sucking reflexes are part of the infant's system and are major beginning contributors to infant learning. Both Russian (Papousek, 1967) and Swiss (Piaget, 1963) research are illustrative of the importance of these two organic activities in the transactions between body and world. The oral region is highly sensitive to tactile stimuli at birth, a condition that is essential to meeting hunger needs. The mouth is, thus, a major communication zone for the infant. Everything gets tested, tasted, and experienced orally during this period. Indeed, the infant would take literally the advice of Sir Francis Bacon that "some books are to be tasted, others to be swallowed, and some few to be chewed and digested. . . ." The whole head region is more highly developed than other parts of the body. Even in size, the head is one-fourth the newborn infant's total length.

As we move down the vertical axis of the body, we find that sphincter control is not necessarily established before the child is well into his second year, or even later. And, moving along the horizontal axis, we find the infant making total arm and leg movements before he is able to move or control his feet and hands independently.

Generally, increasing organization means a reduction of extraneous movement, a trend in the direction from grosser to finer movements, a trend from involuntary to voluntary control.

Significance of This Development. We can see that the infant is actively engaged in the process of organizing and controlling himself while, at the same time, he is beginning to create some order in his world. The more organized his motor responses become, the freer the infant is to divert energies into other experiences, widening his horizons. What he is able to see is partly dependent upon how much head control he has; what he is able to get into his mouth depends not only on what his parents leave within his reach but also on how well he can grasp and retain it. The infant's world is constantly and rapidly expanding as he gains control over his own muscles.

Piaget (1963) has labeled the time from birth to approximately two years the *sensori-motor period* and has described in detail the stages through which the child goes as he actively engages in dealing with his environment. In essence, he says that the child uses his already established ability because it exists and extends its use to assimilate, or take in, elements of the environment. This view corresponds to our active view of the infant. He seeks to suck because he can suck; he seeks to look because he can see.

Accompanying this rapid expansion in horizons—a change from virtual helplessness at birth to an ability to walk at approximately 1 to 1½ (see Figure 4.1)—is a wide variety of feeling tones. The beginnings of feelings of adequacy and achievement may be found in the infant's experiences with his own body, his efforts to make it do what he wishes. Along with this, the parents' provision of experiences and opportunities—from toys to space—and their words of praise and encouragement may be significant factors not only in the development of control but also, and more

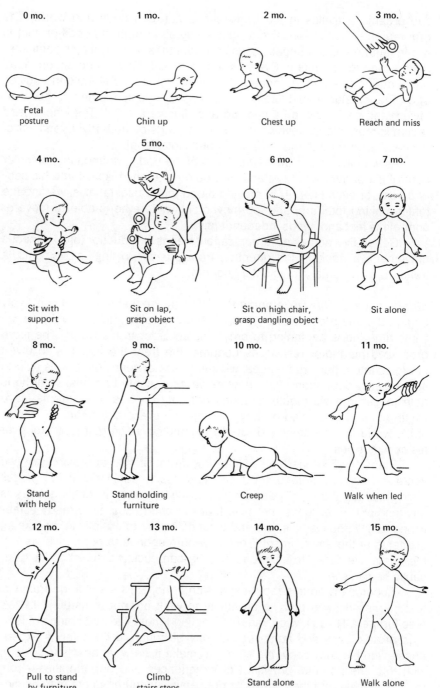

FIGURE 4.1

significantly, in the beginnings of the child's feelings about himself. Self-awareness begins during this time, as the infant moves from an objectless world in which all objects are part of him and magically subject to his control (he cries, and is fed) to the point, somewhere about his first birthday, when objects are seen as separate from him.

The Development of "Meanings"

Accompanying the increasing neuromuscular control of the infant is the process of assigning "meanings" to events. A "meaning" is defined here as a cue to action or a response accompanied by a feeling tone, ranging from comfort and satisfaction to discomfort and heightened tension; that is, the child begins to recognize that some act is symbolic of a coming event that affects him. He may see his mother approaching with a bottle; he may be lifted up into the bathinette; he may experience wetness. In each case, he learns that another event, either pleasant or unpleasant, will follow. This does not and should not imply any high level of thought, but it does suggest the beginnings of cognition. The child assigns meanings by establishing a relationship between himself and the objects and people in his world. This involves a sorting-out process, a differentiating process, a movement from a blooming, buzzing world of isolated, unconnected sensations toward an organized, stabilized, limitedly predictable world.

The developing degree of control over his own body permits the infant to begin the exploration of himself and his world through which he acquires meanings.

Exploring the Physical World.   One of the most important ways in which the infant explores his environment is through tactile communication. This begins at birth and is concentrated for some time around the mouth. The abilities to grasp, to hold, and to let go are not fully functioning until about the eighth month. The infant learns that some objects are hard, some soft; some too large, some small; some satisfy hunger, others soothe aching gums. Gradually, the objects begin to assume a quality of permanence to him. The bottle or breast is differentiated fairly early in the sequence. We can tell that these objects are stable, because the infant makes consistent responses to them.

The motor sequence. Age in months should be seen as approximate; the sequence of development corresponds closely with other research findings. Many American children today would tend to exceed these age norms. It must be noted that this diagram does not reflect cultural experience and should not be seen as purely maturational. Reprinted from M. M. Shirley, *The first two years, a study of twenty-five babies,* Vol. II. The University of Minnesota Press, Minneapolis, © Copyright 1933 by the University of Minnesota. Used by permission.

Obviously, a child learns to make these differentiations, and he can only learn if he is presented with opportunities from his environment which require that he make different responses to different objects and people. During the first year of life, as Hunt (1966) has indicated, the infant seeks the familiar when presented with both familiar and unfamiliar objects, but gradually he seeks out the novel, the different, the unusual aspect. He enjoys both the familiar and the unfamiliar. If his world does not provide him with a variety of familiar and novel cues, development is retarded. Provision of experience during the last few months of the first year of life seems to be able to make up the gap. (Sayegh and Dennis, 1965) Just how to provide such experience and how much and in what order stimulation is desirable is a focus of current research on infancy. (Ambrose, 1969; Gordon, 1973; B. White, 1972; Levenstein, 1971; and Fein and Clarke-Stewart, 1973)

For example, researchers ask such questions as how and when does a child learn that an object has permanence; that is, that it exists even when unseen? Such a concept is basic not only to the development of scientific concepts but also to the development of stable interpersonal concepts.

Indeed, current research offers much evidence of the close ties between affect or feelings and cognition in early life and strong evidence of the close relationships between the mother-child interpersonal transactions and the child's arrival at object permanence. (Ainsworth and Bell, 1972) Our basic understanding of object permanence stems from Piaget, and investigators have now developed procedures for observing the child's development along this dimension. (Uzgiris and Hunt, 1966; Escalona and Corman, 1968; Yarrow, 1971)

The sample items from Escalona and Corman's Object Permanence Scale shown below indicate how such a phenomenon is measured. The first item is the earliest and demonstrates that the child can seek an object when he has observed where it has been hidden. The second item reflects the ability of the child to follow the path of an object and to predict where it will be even though he has not seen its final location.

ITEM (1)   OBSTACLE TO VISUAL PERCEPTION

> *Administration:* Using a pillow or cloth, E. holds screen directly in in front of child's face, so as to block the child's entire field of vision; or, alternatively, a cloth may be draped over child's head and face.

> *Response:* Child removes pillow or cloth; or child alters his position so as to peer above or look out beneath the obstruction on at least two occasions. In any case, he must manipulate the obstacle or his own body so as to restore unimpeded vision.

ITEM (14) *SERIAL INVISIBLE DISPLACEMENT—TWO SCREENS*

Administration: Two screens are in the field. Having secured child's attention, E. conceals an object in his hand (or in rectangular box) and brings his closed hand first beneath Screen A and then beneath Screen B, where he invisibly releases the object. (One slow sweeping motion from A to B.) Then exhibits empty hand or box. If child goes directly to B, E. must repeat the item, moving his hand in the reverse (BA) sequence.

Response: Child first checks hand or box, then searches under A and thereafter goes to B.

Response: Child goes directly to screen visited last by E's hand, on two successive trials in opposite direction (AB and BA).

Source: Adapted from S. K. Escalona and H. H. Corman, Albert Einstein Scales of Sensorimotor Development, Object Permanence Scale, 1968. Mimeo. Used by permission.

Decarie (1965) attempted to relate the modern psychoanalytic position concerning the processes by which a child develops a stable image of his mother to the Piagetian concept of object permanence; she found they have much in common. As Piaget and Inhelder say, "There is no behavior pattern, however intellectual, which does not involve affective factors as motives; but, reciprocally, there can be no affective states without the intervention of perceptions or comprehensions which constitute their cognitive structure. Behavior is therefore of a piece. . . . the two aspects, affective and cognitive, are at the same time inseparable and irreducible." (Piaget and Inhelder, 1969) So we cannot separate the sensorimotor development of the child from the family context in which it occurs, even though much of the development has a maturational base. Examples of efforts to bring these in harmony are depicted in Figures 4.2 and 4.3.

As the infant gains control over his arms and hands, he explores the world of his crib. He reaches out and touches the dangling cradle gym and finds it moves to his touch. As he attempts to do it again and again, he is able gradually to grasp it at will and to produce the effect that came at first by chance. Through tactile communication and increased motor control, the infant begins to establish order in his world. He develops the ability to make certain events occur; he knows that the appearance of certain objects means increased comfort; he learns that certain tactile sensations—such as a satiny blanket, warm bath water, mother's arms around him—are highly pleasurable. He learns, further, that some of these events occur with regularity, and he can begin to predict them.

This predictability and the ability to make things happen come about not only because of the development of the central nervous system but

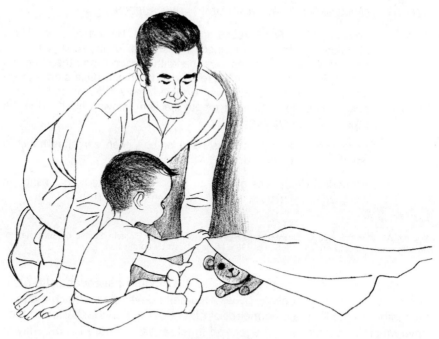

FIGURE 4.2
From I. J. Gordon, *Baby learning through baby play,* St. Martin's Press, New York, 1970, p. 35. Used by permission.

also through experience. Watson (1972) describes "the Game" as the process by which the infant, seeing connections between familiar stimuli (bottle, face) and his behavior (smiling and cooing) engages in the former in order to elicit the latter. Piaget (1963) describes the discovery by his daughter of the fact that bouncing in the buggy made the fringe move—a phenomenon similar to the game. Kagan (1972) links this to the development of thought and suggests that 9-month-olds hypothesize in the sense that they attempt to make the unfamiliar fit into the familiar. All these views are incomplete. We have much to learn, but they do indicate that psychologists from diverse points of view are applying observational and experimental techniques that yield common information. Although the explanations are different, they tend to agree on the observed behavior.

The boundaries of the infant's world increase when creeping and crawling begin. He enters his individual "space age," analogous in his development to the leap man took when the New World was discovered or Sputnik launched.

He is no longer confined to objects that come to him; he can now go to his world. This is not an unmixed blessing. Previously, his experiences with his environment, through mouth and hands and body surfaces, have

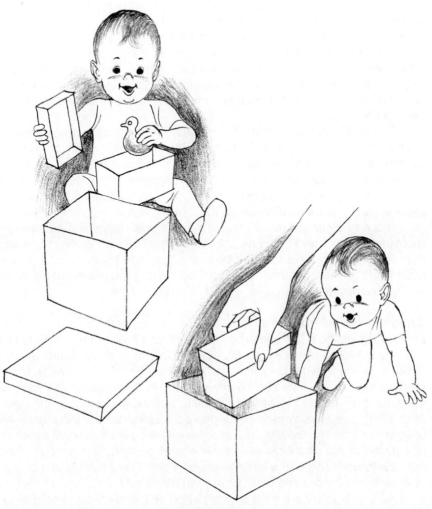

FIGURE 4.3

From I. J. Gordon, *Baby learning through baby play,* St. Martin's Press, New York, 1970, p. 49. Used by permission.

been controlled without his knowledge. The censorship of materials was accomplished before they reached his vicinity. Mother, in trying to protect him, didn't place him near electrical outlets or give him toys that could hurt him. In terms of the appearance of her home, a child in a crib could hardly damage furniture or bric-a-brac.

Now the house gets "child-proofed." The child's discovery of the physical world—and of himself in relation to it—is influenced by his parents' attitudes toward safety and property and by their notions of what and how children at this stage learn. In one house, all dangerous, breakable, or precious objects are placed out of reach, and the crawling child is given free movement to explore. In another house, he is placed for long hours in a playpen, which offers very restricted movement at a time when movement has so much meaning. In a third house, he is met with a barrage of "don't touch!" and similar commands, or with hand slapping, or with sudden pickups and relocation. In a fourth, once he begins to be mobile, he is ignored.

These, of course, represent extremes. Probably each house offers a mixture of all four. The child's concepts of himself, his feelings of satisfaction and adequacy, his developing notions of mother and father, his sense of the world as safe and interesting, his cognitive competence—all are related to the way he experiences and is encouraged or permitted to experience this growing physical world.

It seems clear that infants must have the opportunity and encouragement to explore. They should be able, within the limits of safety, to see and handle objects, to have experience in reaching, grasping, touching, manipulating. To deny or restrict most likely has a negative influence on intellectual development.

Exploring the Interpersonal World.   Concurrent with the expansion of physical limits, the infant's interpersonal horizons broaden. During the first year, he develops from being influenced mainly by internal stimuli at birth through seeing parents as objects meeting his psychological needs, to the point where he responds and becomes social in his behavior. Throughout this time the infant is establishing a basic orientation toward people—an orientation that Erikson calls "basic trust." (Erikson, 1951) We have already seen how the feeding situation, viewed as a transactional process, is a phase in the establishment of feelings of comfort. The control situation, described above in relation to exploration of the physical world, also plays a role in the development of the child's attitudes.

All of the infant's contacts with people influence these attitudes toward self and others. Sullivan has coined the phrase "significant others" (Sullivan, 1953) to describe the people who are crucial in the child's early development. Before he is able to walk, before he has language, the infant has developed a crude differentiation of his own limits and is able to perceive others as being distinct from him. Of course, he is a long way from any awareness of personality of others or of the motivations and separate lives of others, but he is able to respond to different people in different ways.

The concept of *attachment* (Bowly, 1969) has been used as a way of conceptualizing the tie between parent and child. Attachment in the young is defined as seeking proximity to a special adult, usually the mother. Investigators have used a number of laboratory designs to measure and describe attachment, such as Lewis and Ban's (1971) procedure of placing mother and child in a room and recording the distance the child wanders, the amount of physical contact, etc., or Ainsworth's (1969) use of strange situations in which mother and stranger approach and handle the baby. Home observations (Escalona, 1973, and Maccoby and Masters, 1970) have also been widely used. Moreno's (1973) review of the techniques used illustrates the problem of defining in agreed-upon terms the phenomenon we can all easily see, the special link between mother and child. By about 6 months, the child responds differently to familiar and unfamiliar people; at about 9 months or so, he's usually unhappy if quickly picked up by a stranger (even a previously unseen grandma needs to remember the child does not know she is grandma!); but by about 15 months, he is at ease with others when mother is around.

If we look at this through the child's eyes, it makes sense. He has just come to some crude differentiation between himself and others; he is keenly aware that people, and the way they treat him, strongly affect his feelings of comfort and happiness; he is still establishing his basic trust with his parents. This is enough to do without being faced with new people who suddenly overwhelm him with unsought attention and affection.

Exploration of his interpersonal world is rooted in his needs for the familiar and the predictable and only gradually extends beyond the immediate family. Within the family he develops meanings about people and self through the channels mentioned earlier: tactile communication and motor control. As he becomes more social, he responds to affection by giving affection; as his motor control increases, he can play social games, such as pat-a-cake. Peekaboo and hide-and-seek delight him, and delight the adult too, who soon discovers the child's fascinating concepts of space and body. The adult sees that if the child cannot see the adult, he thinks the adult cannot see him (although all but his face may be in full view). "I see you" means to the child "I see your face." This mutual and reciprocal delight in games, in the giving and receiving of affection, and in the accomplishment of new things serves to strengthen the emotional ties between the parents and the child and to aid him in the establishment of concepts of himself as lovable and adequate. These simple games also contribute to cognitive development, to the child's concepts of object permanence, to his ability to anticipate cues.

Studies of parent education designed to help parents engage in a more stimulating relationship with their infants and toddlers have revealed, as we would expect, wide ranges in parenting skill, attitudes toward babies, and attitudes toward self as teacher and mother. (Gordon, 1972, 1973)

Home conditions contribute to difficulties; as one paraprofessional described it: Sometimes they have too many children, they work, and when they come in they have to cook, clean up, feed the children, and in the afternoons they're tired after they've done all that, and they just don't have time. And so some of them have problems that make it hard for them to concentrate on solving their problems and getting these things done with the baby. (Gordon, 1967, p. 73) But this is not all there is to it; there are parents who effectively surmount these difficulties and relate beautifully to their children; there are parents who, materialistically, have it made, who don't relate at all. Ainsworth and Bell describe infant competence as resting on "The cooperation of his mother figure. . . . This definition implies a competent mother-infant pair—an infant who is competent in his preadapted function and a mother who is competent in the reciprocal role to which the infant's behavior is preadapted. The infant in such a competent pair is effective in getting what he wants at least in part because he can influence the behavior of a responsive mother. Furthermore, one facet of competence, important throughout the entire life span, is social competence—the ability of the person to elicit the cooperation of others. . . . maternal responsiveness provides the conditions for a normally functioning infant to influence what happens to him by influencing the behavior of his mother. This, we believe, fosters a general 'sense of competence' . . . and a sense of competence—or confidence—influences the development of increased competence in other realms, whether viewed in age-relevant or absolute terms." (Ainsworth and Bell, 1972, pp. 2, 3–4)

Maternal behavior is a critical variable. During infancy and early childhood, there is a positive relationship between mother love and the happy, calm, positive behavior of the child. (Schaefer and Bayley, 1963) But not all mothers are loving, nor do all mothers understand the need to transact and to play with their infants, nor do all of them have the time.

Exploring the Body.   Anyone watching babies sticking their fingers into their mouths and, a little later, putting their feet (one at a time, of course) into their mouths, is aware of the great pleasure the infant receives from these experiences. Throughout this first development period, the infant is experiencing what is him and what is not him through the process of feeling, handling, and tasting. The thumb in the mouth is a classical example of the body experiencing itself, or what Sullivan calls "self-sentience." "The mouth feels the thumb and the thumb feels the mouth; that is self-sentience. This is the point of departure for an enormous development." (Sullivan, 1953, p. 141) When one part of the infant's body touches another and the infant experiences both feeling and being felt, we have self-sentience. Knowledge about the self-sentient is elaborated into the child's conception of his body.

The infant experiences "me" and "not me" in a bodily sense from as early as birth on. Since, at least in middle class America, he is diapered except when in a bath, his experiences in handling genital and anal areas are limited and occur mostly when being changed or bathed. Again, the transactional, interpersonal nature of this experience becomes significant. The child is not alone to enjoy himself in his exploration, to know kinesthetic satisfaction. His mother is not a mere onlooker, a passive observer, but a participant in the situation. Her attitudes about sex, about bodily processes, about elimination and waste, are part of the situational field in which the infant comes to learn about his body. The meanings he assigns to fondling his penis or seeing it erect grow out of the transaction between the kinesthetic satisfactions he receives and the behavior of his mother. If she permits the exploration, accepting it as a normal part of the development of her child, the meanings he connects with his body and its functions will probably be healthy; that is, he will conceive of his body as good, of all parts of his body as good, of bodily processes as normal and natural activities. He will have no guilt or shame at this level of development.

If, on the other hand, he is prevented or stopped when he attempts to fondle himself or is treated with harsh words and facial expressions that convey shock and rejection, the infant will develop unhealthy views about his body. Free of his diapers as he grows, he is bound to discover that the genital zone is pleasure-producing. We mentioned in the previous chapter that, according to the Sears study, the mother saw her role in the sexual domain as preventing stimulation in infancy and early childhood. Faced with bodily satisfaction on the one hand and the condemnation on the other, the child is placed in a situation in which he develops concepts of his body (or at least of part of his body) as being somehow evil. Further, if this part of him is evil but enjoyable, what is he to make of this? His experiences with himself and his mother do not seem to equip him (according to Sears) with the labels (culturally-accepted meanings) for handling this confusion. The origins of guilt, of shame, of unhealthy sexual attitudes may possibly be attributed to this initial period of bodily exploration and the parent-child situation in which it occurs. Certainly, clinical evidence suggests that this is so.

Bodily exploration not only leads to the development of the differentiation of "me" from "not me" and the meanings attached to "me" in the area of the goodness or badness of the body, but this exploration also aids the infant in determining the things he can do with his body—the effect his body has on the "not me" that surrounds him. We see infants and young children repeating a performance again and again. The mere act of repetition seems to be rewarding to them. This is what Piaget calls "exercise play"—"repeating for the pleasure of causing an effect and confirming his newly acquired skill." (Piaget and Inhelder, 1969, p. 59)

Why is this so? We may infer that it is related to their attempts to handle their world, to arrange, order, and predict their environment. If I (the infant) can do this act at will and it "feels good" to do (and brings appropriate adult approval), why then I'll keep trying it. When we turn to language, we can see this as a part of the process by which language is learned.

Of course, there is the danger of reading adult thoughts into infants' minds. We must recognize that these are not intellectual, rational activities of the infant but only inferences from his behavior.

Exploration of the body, then, contributes to the development of meanings about its value as an agent in producing satisfaction in relation both to itself and to the world. Acceptance of the body as part of "me," and particularly as a "good" part of "me," is determined by the way in which the infant's behavior is experienced by himself (self-sentience) and the way in which he perceives others reacting to his explorations.

Developing "Anchorage Points."   Just as the navigator at sea uses his instruments to find his location, the child, too, needs to establish his location in his field. He develops what would correspond to a map of the area in which he lives. His map is not limited to a representation of geography; it is a representation of the interpersonal field as well. This map of the infant we can call his perceptual field. It is personal, and it provides him with the sense of stability and order he needs.

Anchorage points are to the self as the stars are to the navigator; they orient him in his world. They are essential to normal self-development. Hebb and his colleagues have reported many interesting findings about what happens to people when they are deprived of normal perceptual stimulation. Although this is not the place to describe Hebb's position, his finding, in a study of brainwashing, that "merely taking away the usual sights, sounds, and bodily contacts from a healthy university student for a few days can shake him, right down to the base: can disturb his personal identity. . . ." (Hebb, 1958, p. 111) can be utilized here. It seems to suggest that throughout life one has to keep himself oriented to his world and that perceptual stimulation is a basic part of this orientation process. The adult has a whole host of orientations that depend upon continuous perceptual information from his environment. The open-energy concept may help us to understand that the person is always immersed in his surroundings and that his self-orientation is related to his orientation in the real world. The perceptual anchorage points provide the adult with the stable world he needs. The child, too, needs a stable environment, and the process of establishing anchorage points begins early.

What are the primary anchorage points of the infant by which he orients himself? They are threefold: first, his body; second, the caretaking ones or "significant others"; and third, his physical environment. Each is value- and feeling-laden. The value of the anchorage point is derived from the degree of satisfaction, comfort, and predictability the infant has received in relation to it. The anchorage point of caretaking ones, for example, may be "good mother" or "bad mother"; it is not just "mother."

By the end of the first year, both his body and his parents have become fairly stable elements in his perceptual field. His physical world begins a rapid expansion at this time. This does not mean that his image, knowledge, or acceptance of his body and his parents are crystallized and complete. His basic orientations, however, his knowing that this is "me" and that is "my parent," along with the emotions that are a part of knowing, are somewhat stable. His notions, we may assume, are primitive and vague. What takes place after this is elaboration, further differentiation and integration, and modification.

The development of additional anchorage points continues throughout life. People and objects become differentiated out of the welter of stimuli and are assigned fairly stable places on the growing child's map as a result of the meanings they and their behavior have for him. He learns patterns of behavior and action in relation to them. These initial anchorage points always remain central to the self, and the new ones that are acquired through life are, to a large degree, selected and evaluated in relation to these early ones.

Meanings are learned through the transactional process of exploring the interpersonal and the physical world, and one's own body. In time, the infant learns that certain objects and people are associated with certain experiences. Through learning, these people and objects become known and take on meaning to the child. Certain people, and the child himself, acquire so many meanings for him that they form a constellation, or cluster. For example, parent is perceived as cuddler, feeder, soft voice, etc. Gradually, parent as a totality is conceptualized. The infant learns to predict and expect certain behaviors and feelings in relation to this person who becomes an anchorage point he uses to establish himself in his world.

One mother's observations of her infant (Debbie, at 7½ months) illustrate how a mother acts as an anchorage point:

> She [Debbie] also has begun to take toys with her as she creeps about the house, either carrying a soft squeaky-toy in her mouth as she goes, or clompety-clomping around with a block or rattle in one hand making an odd sound pattern as she travels. She plays well for 10 or 15 minutes in another room without any direct supervision, returning to home base to crawl up Mama's leg and be greeted for a moment or be offered a sip of liquid. Then off again about her business. [Church, 1966, pp. 25–26]

The infant's perceptual field is composed of those aspects of his total environment to which he has assigned meanings. It is organized around the various anchorage points he has extracted from his experiences. The word "meaning," used earlier, was defined as a clue to action.

The infant's perceptual field, then, is action oriented. It enables him to know what to do, how to respond, what to expect. He perceives his world along two major dimensions: (1) what it can do to *him* and, later, (2) what he can do to *it*. On both dimensions, the orientation is toward action.

The actions he takes have results, and these results are incorporated into new meanings, leading him to modify and enlarge his perceptual field. As this process continues, accompanied by the internal maturational process, he reaches the next breakthrough on his road to maturity, the breakthrough that enables him to extend his meaning system widely. This is the development of language.

The Development of Language

One of the great mysteries of human development is how the child acquires language. Although various theories have been advanced and argued, the best we can say today is what Ervin-Tripp said in 1966: "The basis for the child's most important and complex achievement still remains unknown." (Ervin-Tripp, 1966, p. 81) Although learning explanations are popular among psychologists who assume that either operant or classical conditioning are explanations, McNeill, after an extensive review, states in relation to the learning of syntax (the rules of sentence structure and grammar) that "Theories of learning based on S-R principles are inappropriate to the task." (McNeill, 1970, p. 1063) On the other hand, the linguists led by Chomsky (1965) have had to create fictions, such as a Language Acquisition Device, to explain the facts. This LAD acts to translate the raw data of words heard into the regularities of the language. But there is still no explanation of how this occurs, of how the brain is organized to do this. What we do know is that by the time they are 5, somehow children have learned the rules of grammar and apply them in their speech. This does not mean they can recite the rules but rather that their speech shows they know them. Syntax, then, is acquired early.

A second aspect of language is semantics, that is, what we would commonly call word meanings. This goes beyond just vocabulary and has been likened to the compiling of a word dictionary. "Semantic development is at once the most pervasive and least understood aspect of language acquisition." (McNeill, 1970, p. 1119) For our purposes, the syntactic and semantic aspects are seen as related to both the acquisition of meanings and their expression by the child. The third aspect of language acquisition is phonemic development; that is, sound production and differentiation. Friedlander (1970) indicates that even this begins early in the child's hearing of sounds before he reproduces them. Elkonin (1971) indicates that the infant responds to the rhythm and melody of speech before he attends to the content. This leads to attention to the sound of the word, and he stresses the acoustic quality. Elkonin links phonetic development

to syntactic and semantic by emphasizing the importance of verbal transactions and the child's own independent practice.

All three aspects—syntactic, semantic, and phonetic—rest not only
upon maturation of the organism but also upon the family environment.
Indeed, in studying the content of a child's language, the latter is perhaps
more significant. We need to understand something about the order in
which language activity emerges, but we need to see this as functional in
the life of the child, as a development that contributes heavily to the communication process between him and his family and thus affects his development. We need to ask ourselves how language develops and how this
development serves the child.

It is generally agreed that language learning begins at birth and that
it is in the prelinguistic period that the child begins to acquire the passive
understandings that words have meanings. (Ervin-Tripp, 1966)

Table 4.1 summarizes the findings of eight research studies dealing
with the order of emergence of language activity. It has been arranged
so that one can see the progressive level of complexity in language activity up to the personal pronoun, but more than that, it makes it possible to
see how language serves the infant's developing self. We can see that his
first essential communication is of feeling and that discomfort seems to be
expressed before pleasure. Expression of discomfort brings activity on the
part of those who care for the child and enables the organism to maintain
its steady-state. Whereas this is not true speech, it is communication.

Perceptual transactions, awareness of vocal stimuli and response to
them (item 4 in Table 4.1), also begin very early and establish still another
link between parent and child. As the child responds, the parent feels
closer to him, and this, in turn, elicits more attempts on the part of the
parent to talk to, play with, and relate to the child. The child, then, is not a
mere recipient; he is an active participant, contributing to the development of the climate of feeling that surrounds him.

The next higher level of communication, which occurs roughly in the
last quarter of the year, has been labeled in Table 4.1 as conceptual transactions, because it is clear that the child's response is in relation to the
meaning of the words being used. It shows an understanding of the symbol itself, which is a higher order of differentiation than repetition of
sounds or expression of feelings. This might be said to be the real beginning of language—when it is being used as a symbolic process. Words do
not have dictionary definitions to the child; their meanings grow out of
their usages in the family. Words are said in a tone of voice and are accompanied by gestures and actions. Meanings are derived from the total
context. Further, words are learned or not learned, depending upon the
family atmosphere and the provision of verbal experiences.

Young children respond to the paralinguistic (tone, sound) as much

TABLE 4.1 THE DEVELOPMENT OF LANGUAGE ACTIVITY BY AGE LEVELS

ACTIVITY	AGE RANGE (IN MONTHS) AT WHICH ITEM FIRST IS REPORTED TO OCCUR*	
	FROM	TO
1. Vocalization	0.25	4
2. Cooing	2	6
3. Vocalization of feelings		
a. Discomfort	1	5.9
b. Pleasure	3	5.9
c. Eagerness	5	5.6
d. Satisfaction	6.5	7
e. Recognition	7.4	8
4. Perceptual transactions		
a. Response to another's voice	1.3	4
b. Vocalizes to social stimulus	3.1	4
c. "Talks" to a person	6	
d. Imitates sounds	6	10
e. Imitates syllables (mamma)	11	11.7
5. Conceptual transactions I		
a. Understands gestures (for example, bye-bye)	9	12
b. Listens with *selective* interest to familiar words	8.5	9
c. Differentiates words	9.8	10
d. Adjusts to and understands simple commands	10	15
e. Understands a demand and gesture	15	23
f. Responds to inhibitory words	12	20
6. Conceptual transactions II		
a. Names objects	17.4	22.5
b. Asks with words	17	18
c. Simple sentences	23	23
7. Self-reference		
a. Points to nose, eye, hair	18	
b. First pronoun	23	
c. Uses pronouns past and plural	36	

* The age in months should be used merely as a guide to the order of occurrence rather than as a figure to be viewed as having any intrinsic merit as a yardstick. The *from* column indicates only that a researcher observed this behavior at the age cited, the *to* column indicates the *first* time another researcher observed this behavior. Other researchers found a particular behavior emerging any time between these two ages.
Source: Adapted from Dorothea McCarthy, "Language Development in Children," in L. Carmichael (Ed.), *Manual of Child Psychology,* Wiley, 1954, pp. 499–502. Used by permission.

as to the linguistic. They also deduce word meanings from the variety of ways in which a word is used rather than from the number of examples shown. For instance, the word "doll" is learned from the contexts of commands or instructions (such as "Look at the doll" or "Bring me the doll") rather than from seeing a variety of dolls. (Razran, 1961)

In level 5, it is *receptive language* that is being assessed; that is, we infer that the child understands from his response to the verbal stimuli of others, not by his own production of language. All three aspects are required; he has to understand not only individual words but also their grammatical arrangement and the rhythm of the sentence so that "Bring me the doll" and "Bring the doll to me" both carry the same message. Bzoch and League (1970; League, 1973) have developed an assessment tool for receptive language called the Receptive-Expressive Emergent Language Scale. Such a device is possible because there is orderly development.

Expressive language is found at levels 6 and 7. It is here that the linguists begin; but language development, as we have indicated, begins earlier in the first sounds and vocal transactions within the family.

Language as a Means of Clarifying Meanings.   "Every individual speech performance is understandable only from the aspect of its relation to the function of the total organism in its endeavor to realize itself." (Goldstein, 1948, p. 21) How does the use of speech for this purpose operate in the infant? The infant's behavior is rooted in the present. He is moving from a world of hazy perception and unconnected stimuli toward an organized, somewhat more integrated environment we call his perceptual field. As he assigns meanings to events and as he learns name words that have a constancy to him in terms of their action potential, he becomes more able to put things and people into place. The speech performance thus enhances his ability to differentiate and integrate. It enables him to do this not only spatially but also temporally; that is, he can now use words to project himself forward into the future. As he develops, his language will enable him to speak of past events and to recall and label past events as well.

When his world is a world only of images—and nonsymbolic—the degree of perceptual distortion and inaccurate communication is high. As he acquires meanings and assigns words to these meanings, the degree of this distortion is decreased. "Dog" represents all dogs—and all things he might do to dogs or that dogs might do to him; it embodies all his wants, hopes, and fears. Still, it is a classification word, and it enables him to convey more clearly his perceptions of "dog" to mother, who can then respond to him. The use of words, combined with the parental response to them, clarifies meanings for the child and gives his world more integration.

We need to reiterate that meanings of words are not "intellectual" in the sense of being dictionary definitions. They are cues to action and heavily tinged with feelings. The infant responds, as we all do, with all of himself, not just a part of himself. Each word he learns is thus colored by the emotional context in which it was experienced. Words are not neutral; they are symbols of events, objects, and people and call forth in the child his total previous response to the situation. What does "dog" mean? Depending upon the tone of voice, the gestures, and bodily movements, it may mean, "I'm scared, get me away, hold me and comfort me," or "I want to pet the dog, I like dogs, come here, dog." With the use of a word, the child conveys his total impression of dogs. He can then begin to reflect upon this impression; his parents can then aid him in the modification of his impression. He moves forward into a world of thought and concepts. This phenomenon, in which the word carries with it a concept and an emotion, in which it stands for an idea, is called *holophrastic speech,* and it occurs in the second six months of life (levels 3 and 4 on Table 4.1). It is syntactic and semantic—it conveys meaning.

Semantically, the child engages in two forms of categorization, what Church (1961) calls upward and downward. "Dog" becomes broken down into types of dogs and also becomes part of the class "animal." This process, which is begun in the second year, continues throughout life. Syntactically, he will begin to add words, such as "dog go" or "good dog"; by age 3 he can ask "where those dogs goed?" This development of language, this sharpening of his perceptions through the acquisition of both the word meanings and the grammar that enable him to describe, place, and recall enables the child to move toward self-realization. As other objects become more constant and can be symbolized, moving beyond the immediate, he himself becomes more constant and can become more clearly an object that can be symbolized to himself. His self-identity grows as the identity of others grows.

He first calls himself "Tommie," because this is the name that has been applied to him; next, he moves to self as object, "me do this"; and finally, perceiving of self as doer, "I do this." At each stage in this process, he has sharpened his meanings about self. His language both reflects this sharpening and provides him with the sharpening tool.

Language and New Interpersonal Horizons.   Another major function of speech in the infant is to provide him with the means for the establishment of interpersonal relations. Here, in particular, the nature of the interpersonal, transactional field of the family plays a decisive role in the determination of his development. The behavior of his parents toward his attempts to use language will either promote or retard his speech development. If they encourage him, speak often to him, and, most important of all, *listen* to him, his ability to express, to communicate, to symbolize and categorize will be enhanced.

The relationship between parents' language and child language development within a disadvantaged population was clearly shown by the high positive relationship between aspects of the mother's language in a free-play situation with her two-year old and the child's performance on the Bayley Scales at 2, on the Stanford-Binet at 3 (Resnick, 1972), and three years later at age 5, on the Stanford-Binet. (Gordon, 1973)

Language activity grows as the infant finds a warm, accepting emotional climate in the home. Again we have the cyclical pattern repeated: With acceptance, the child takes over the sounds of speech, then the understandings of the meanings of words, then the use of the words themselves; as he does this, and thus becomes more like his parents, he gains further acceptance, support, and encouragement from them. The initial impetus for growth is within the child, but the impetus needs a nourishing environment in order for normal speech development to occur. "The average infant must be exposed to spoken language for about eight months before he begins to comprehend the speech of others . . . unless the child continues to identify with the talking human, unless he finds language enjoyable instead of threatening and anxiety-producing, he might reject the world of talking." (Myklebust, 1956, p. 164)

Further, if the child grows up in an essentially nonverbal environment (home or institution), his store of words, and thus concepts, is reduced. He lacks the particular symbol, and he also loses out on the use of language as a tool for understanding, expression, and communication. He gets locked into a narrow, restricted world.

As the infant uses vocalizations and then words to express first his feelings and then his needs, as he responds to the voices of others, he feels more related to those around him. He strengthens the bridge that already exists between him and his parents, and he begins to reinforce it from his side of the transactional field. As he learns to say "Mama," "Dada," and the like, he makes a tremendous emotional impact upon his parents and reaps the rewards in joy and affection. He, of course, finds this satisfying, so he repeats not only these words but also other words he hears and finds that language is a highly satisfying experience. This is quite apart from understanding the words; here we are concerned mainly with the feeling tones, the subtle connections that exist between people when they speak, apart from the words they use.

When the infant meets new adults, he uses this delightful new thing he has discovered and finds out, on the whole, that these other adults respond favorably to his efforts too. They talk back to him, making the sounds he makes, using (by dictionary standards) nonsense syllables that are communicative to the infant because they express feelings of delight, of interest, of rapport, or are rhythmically interesting.

These two major functions of language, the clarification of meanings and the expansion of interpersonal horizons, continue as long as we live.

What occurs in further development is increased complexity and higher levels of organization, but the dynamics remain the same.

The development of language in infancy is closely related to and, to some degree, dependent upon another phase of development, the process of identification.

THE IDENTIFICATION PROCESS

The behavior and development of the infant is many-faceted and can be approached from several directions. Just as we turn a precious stone around and around in our hands, holding it up to the light and admiring the beauty reflected from its many surfaces, so it is with understanding the developing self. We have approached this understanding from several sides: organic and genetic contributions, transactional relationships, and the role of language. We have seen that each of these is only one facet, a contributing variable in the total picture. We turn now to still another facet, but one which perhaps serves to unite and organize, to act as a catalyst, and to provide a framework upon which all these other processes, in varying degrees, depend. This is the process of identification.

The Nature and Functions of Identification

Identification has been defined as that process by which a person views himself as being like another and then behaves accordingly. (G. Murphy, 1966, p. 989) It has been variously viewed as behaving like another (Bronfenbrenner, 1960), as a disposition to be like another (Kohlberg, 1966), or as a belief that one is like another (Kagan, 1963). Mischel (1970) indicates that it has also been seen as the process by means of which the above behaviors, dispositions, and beliefs come about. Like so many other psychological terms, identification is a construct; that is, it is a shorthand device for both describing and explaining the many behaviors we all see about us. In this case, it covers sex-role—"boys will be boys"—and more specific resemblances—"she's just like her mother." As such, it is hard to test and verify through research. Mischel's (1970) review indicates little support for the original Freudian notion of the processes by which the boy tends to identify with father and the girl with mother, but the observed behavior is a reality.

Although there is lack of agreement about how it comes about (and again there is much opportunity for further research), our view is that the beginnings of identification behaviors, beliefs, and dispositions lie in the infancy period. Identification is the major way in which the infant tackles the task of self-definition. He perceives or views himself as a variety of others, takes on their behaviors as he sees them, tries them out, selects aspects of their roles as meaningful to him, and incorporates them into his own image. The child becomes "mother," or "father," or "other" to himself, emulates them in so far as he is able, and develops a common ground with them.

How does this begin? We mentioned in our discussion of language development the idea of dialogue. The same applies here; pat-a-cake, clap hands, vocal interaction all demonstrate that the infant models his behavior on the interesting adult. Direct imitation and the pleasure it leads to is one activity. But as any acute observer can see, the infant learns a good deal by hearing and seeing what goes on around him, even when he is not central to it and even when he is not "behaving." Modeling and imitating, then, have cognitive aspects that emerge in later behavior, such as the child playing by himself or talking to himself in the absence of the person he is imitating. The infant is learning what it is to be human by observing human behavior. Research findings do not support the notion that specific reinforcement is a useful explanation for something as complex as identification. Indeed, as Mischel indicates, "On the contrary, . . . children may rapidly learn large and complex sequences through cognitive-perceptual processes that hinge on their observing events rather than on their being reinforced for specific acts." (Mischel, 1970, p. 31)

But the child sees a number of models and, especially in these early years, has little history to aid him in either selecting or interpreting the events and behavior he sees. In reference to his parents, the child does not literally assume a facet of a parent; he incorporates *his* perception and *his* understanding of the parent's behavior. If we look back at how meanings are developed and anchorage points derived, we can see that identification does not mean being like, in any exact sense, another person. One parent, viewing the misbehavior of a child, may say to the other, "That's because he's just like you!" This is not quite correct. No one is "just like" another person, and no child is a mirror image, either bodily or in his behavior, of his parents. He sees himself as being like another, but he does not become the other. He becomes, for the time in which he plays the particular role, the other *as he perceives the other.*

The child's behavior, as Bandura, Ross, and Ross (1963) have shown, is a synthesis of his own that he has drawn from models, and we still do not understand this selection process very well. No doubt attachment plays a strong role, as does the child's own sex, which he is able to identify early (see Chapter 6), the nature and variety of models he has seen, and so forth. But this begs the question. We know it is not simple reinforcement; we know that some combination of cognitive and perceptual processes are involved, but we cannot at this point describe or explain how it takes place.

Sullivan, writing from a psychoanalytic viewpoint, indicates the difficulty of the simplified notion of taking over another's personality. He indicates that between the other's behavior and the mind of the one taking it over "is a group of processes—the act of perceiving, understanding, and what not—which is intercalated, which is highly subject to past experience and increasingly subject to foresight of the neighboring future. Therefore, it would in fact be one of the great miracles of all time if our perception of another person were, in any greatly significant number of respects, accurate or exact." (Sullivan, 1953, p. 167)

At this point, then, we can say that the process of identification probably can be understood as consisting of both direct imitation, modeling, some reinforcement (including self-reinforcement) and also the particular way in which the infant puts this all together and builds his own organization.

Piaget describes the infant's and young child's thought as egocentric, or as he now prefers, "symbolism centering on the self" (Piaget and Inhelder, 1969, p. 61) in which the child, through symbolic play, handles the conflicting reality situation and makes reality over to suit himself. He also implies the inability of the infant to be aware of the fact that the thoughts and feelings of others may differ from his own. In this sense, the child has not yet recognized that different people hold different beliefs (some adults have not yet accepted the notion that beliefs other than their own are not inferior!). The process of identification needs to take into account the growing awareness of the young child of the fact that he is a distinct individual, and therefore cognitive development is closely interwoven with identification. At the same time that the infant separates himself from others, he also models himself on aspects of others that he observes.

Like all the other facets we have discussed, this too is a transactional situation. (Rheingold, 1969) The infant identifies with the parents, and the parents identify with him. They too do not necessarily see him as fully differentiated from them. They often see him as an extension of themselves, as part of their selves, and they invest their feelings, hopes, and aspirations in him. They shift their unfulfilled dreams to him and glow in his accomplishments as though they were their own. There is, then, a mutual identification.

The process of identification contributes to the development of self by (1) enabling the child to develop a sense of identity with others, (2) enabling the parents to feel closer to the child, (3) providing the child with models of behavior (that is, parents) upon which to build his own, and (4) providing him with information from the responses of others to his behavior that he can experience as being his own feelings. Later on, he no longer needs the behavior of others as a cue—he is able to feel how they would feel without their presence. The latter point can be understood as the beginnings of conscience, or what Freud labeled the "superego." It is the valuing process by which the child experiences behavior as good or bad on the basis of the feelings he perceives others as having. Since how *others* feel is inextricably interwoven with how *he* feels and since self and other are not clearly differentiated at this time, his perception of their feelings *are also his feelings.* In this sense, he incorporates them into him.

Identification with the Mothering One

The infant's primary identification is with the mother or those who serve in place of the mother. The process begins probably about the middle of the first year, when mother is becoming an anchorage point, when her existence in the child's eyes is not merely related to her presence, and when he knows he can bring her into being through his behavior.

We, of course, cannot know what the infant really perceives, but it is possible that the child's earliest notions of mother are of her as a part of himself. With the exploration and establishment of bodily limits through self-sentience, the mother becomes a more or less fixed object in the field —not part of his body, but still not separate and distinct from him, still not a person in her own right. The mother affects his bodily state—of comfort and discomfort—and, to some degree, he can predict what she will do or when she will appear. Gradually, he perceives her, although still crudely, as another person, and here begins the process of imitating her behavior because it is her behavior. Before this, imitation is indiscriminate; now it becomes more focused. We see this imitation in making sounds, in attempting to feed himself, in smiling, and in many areas of behavior.

The child also identifies with other family members, but his strongest emotional ties during this period are with the mother.

In Chapter 6 we will look further at identification and see how its direction and operation are modified as the child moves out of infancy and into and through the preschool years.

THE EMERGENCE OF SELF-AWARENESS

The culmination of all the child's previous experiences during infancy is the emergence of expressed awareness of self. This might be considered the demarcation point between infancy and childhood. It is an emergent— a new thing created out of social experience. It is epigenetic.

What particular experiences shape the formation of the self-system? What contributes to the child's sense of self? Primarily, it develops from the transactional process, in particular the evaluational interactions between the infant and the people who surround him, and his own evaluation of his body and his behavior. The child's awareness of himself emerges from the total experience of the infant with himself, with his physical surroundings, and with his interpersonal world. He seeks to enhance his feelings of comfort and stability and to avoid those periods of discomfort and strain that occur in his daily life.

A deprived environment not only retards language development but also affects the essential orientation of the child. A whole host of objects develop meanings. When we examine the child's langauge, we find him referring to himself by name (as object) before referring to himself as "I" (as subject). Although he achieves a sense of personal identity before he is able to handle the complexities of "I," it is this shift in language that indicates that he has become more precise in his self-definition.

Through exploring, identifying, talking, and feeling, each child develops a crude sense of selfhood sometime during the second year of life. By this time, self and other have been differentiated. The infant now seeks not only to maintain his organic existence but also to enhance and preserve this self, which is both more than and less than his body. As G. H. Mead states: "The self has a character which is different from the physiological organism proper. The self is something which has a development; it is not initially there at birth, but arises in the process of social experience and activity."(Mead, 1940, p. 135)

The Measurement of Self-acceptance

What kind of self-picture will the child possess? According to the viewpoint of this book, this will depend upon the nature of his previous experiences with his body and his world. If, on the whole, life has been a satisfying experience for him, he will develop a picture of self that will be one of adequacy and security. He will perceive and conceive of himself as being loved and being lovable, as being able to do what his parents expect of him and what he expects of himself. We may then postulate that his basic orientation toward self and the world will be one of basic trust.

If, on the other hand, his background of experience has been harsh, deprived, inconsistent, or cold, he may develop either a confused, conflicted view or a negative view. It may be difficult to conceive of a very young child as possessing negative feelings, but clinical evidence is full of examples of even so extreme a nature as autistic children who did not respond to human beings as people and lived in a completely private world without much communication with people.

We can see the gross manifestations of the effect of life on the young child. We can recognize the extremes—the happy, outgoing, responsive, curious youngster, and the autistic one. But we lack considerable precision in measuring what we've labeled as self-concept in the young child. What behaviors indicate competence and a sense of competence, a feeling of being loved and valued? How do these relate to other measures, such as those of cognitive development? Our procedures are crude, and our understandings are weak. For example, a two-year-old child is busy playing with a toy in a day-care center. Another two-year-old grabs it away. The first child can do a variety of things: he can cry, grab it back, sit stunned, go to the teacher, get another toy, go over and hit another child, etc. Which of these is indicative of a positive self-concept? Since this author grew up in New York City, hitting the other child back and hanging on to the toy might be seen as positive. In other cultures or groups, it is not so.

We can make some inferences from behavior, provided we are aware of the above problem. There are ways to assess attachment, responsiveness to others, and exploratory activities, but at this point the gap between our measurement capabilities and self-concept theory is still very wide. As we shall see in subsequent chapters, the problem is not easily solved as the person grows older.

The Openness of the Self-System

Sometime during his second or third year, the child calls himself "I," has a rudimentary sense of identity, and a constellation of attitudes about this "I." Does this mean that his self is a well-organized, well-integrated system, essentially fixed and not subject to change? Or is this self still essentially a fluid system? Although writers seem to agree that the self is a fairly stable organization at this point, it is still an extremely open system. The child seems to have evolved a basic orientation toward self and world, but this is by no means fixed and unalterable. The presence of this structure of self need not imply self is fixed, crystallized, and sealed in the book of doom.

The child's sense of self is still to be heavily influenced by further circumstances throughout life, particularly throughout childhood and adolescence. What is established is the basic framework from which the growing child will perceive and interpret his world. The self is now not merely a product of transactions but is an active participant in the transactional process, an active agent in the field.

The Meaning of "I" in Behavior
and Development

"Whatever the self is, it becomes a center, an anchorage point, a standard of comparison, an ultimate real. Inevitably, it takes its place as a supreme value. . . . In a fundamental sense, the self is right." (G. Murphy, 1966, p. 498) The child's sense of himself, his "I," the picture he holds of who he is, affect the way he organizes and assigns meanings to all his future experiences. His perceptions will be oriented toward enhancing and maintaining the self he has already developed. At birth he possessed potentialities to become many different kinds of persons; now he is more or less embarked upon a particular course. His "I" will now weigh and evaluate, choose and discard, interpret and integrate his experience to preserve, protect, and defend this ultimate value, this self that has emerged.

When we say that "the self is right," we do not mean this in any moral sense. Rather, the statement serves as an explanatory principle of behavior from a psychological perspective. Kohlberg (1966), for example, sees self-categorization of sex ("I'm a boy," "I'm a girl") as causal and pervasive in further personality development. In this sense, identification, especially sex-role identification, is a disposition to behave in certain ways.

The "I" thus assumes the key role in further development and behavior. Although the evaluations of others will continue to influence the child, these will now be perceived and screened by his own evaluational agency, his self-image.

How the child sees himself—in spite of its crudities, its lack of sophistication, its gaps and distortions—becomes by this third year of life a potent factor in influencing what he will become as a person.

REFERENCES AND ADDITIONAL READINGS

Ainsworth, M. D. S. Object relations, dependency and attachment: A theoretical review of the infant-mother relationship. *Child Development,* 1969, *40,* 969–1025.

Ainsworth, M., & Bell, S. Mother-infant interaction and the development of competence. In K. J. Connolly (Ed.), *Development of early competence.* London: Academic Press, 1972.

Ambrose, A. (Ed.) *Stimulation in early infancy.* New York: Academic Press, 1969.

Bandura, A., Ross, D., & Ross, S. Imitation of film-mediated aggressive models. *Journal of Abnormal and Social Psychology,* 1963, *66,* 3–11.

Beckwith, L. Relationships between attributes of mothers and their infants' IQ scores. *Child Development,* 1971, *42,* 1083–1097.

Bell, S. M., & Ainsworth, M. Infant crying and maternal responsiveness, *Child Development,* 1972, *43,* 1171–1190.

Bowly, B. *Attachment.* New York: Basic Books, 1969.

Bronfenbrenner, H. Freudian theories of identification and their derivatives. *Child Development,* 1960, *31,* 15–40.

Brown, R., Cazden, C., & Bellugi, U. The child's grammar from I to III. In J. P. Hill (Ed.), *Minnesota symposium of child psychology.* Minneapolis, Minn.: University of Minnesota Press, 1968.

Bzoch, K., & League, R. *The receptive-expressive emergent language scale (The REEL Scale).* Gainesville, Fla.: Tree of Life Press, 1970.

Chomsky, N. A. *Aspects of the theory of syntax.* Cambridge, Mass.: MIT Press, 1965.

Church, J. *Language and the discovery of reality: A developmental psychology of cognition.* New York: Random House, 1961.

Church, J. *Three babies: Biographies of cognitive development.* New York: Random House, 1966.

Corman, H., & Escalona, S. Stages of sensorimotor development: A replication study. *Merrill-Palmer Quarterly,* 1969, *15,* 351–361.

Decarie, T. *Intelligence and affectivity in early childhood.* New York: International Universities Press, 1965.

Elkonin, D. B. Development of speech. In A. V. Zaporozhets and D. B. Elkonin (Eds.), *The psychology of preschool children.* Cambridge, Mass.: MIT Press, 1971.

Erikson, E. H. *Childhood and society.* New York: Norton, 1951.

Ervin-Tripp, S. Language development. In M. L. Hoffman and L. W. Hoffman (Eds.), *Review of child development research.* Vol. 2. New York: Russell Sage Foundation, 1966. Pp. 55–106.

Escalona, S. K. Basic modes of social interaction: Their emergence and patterning during the first two years of life. *Merrill-Palmer Quarterly,* 1973, *19(3)*, 205–232.

Escalona, S., & Corman, H. Albert Einstein scales of sensori-motor development. (Ditto) Yeshiva University, 1968.

Fantz, R. L., & Nevis, S. Pattern preferences and perceptual-cognitive development in early infancy. *Merrill-Palmer Quarterly,* 1967, *13(1)*, 77–108.

Fein, G., & Clarke, S. A. *Day care in context.* New York: Wiley, 1973.

Flavell, J. *The developmental psychology of Jean Piaget.* Princeton, N.J.: Van Nostrand, 1963.

Friedlander, B. Receptive language development in infancy: Issues and problems. *Merrill-Palmer Quarterly,* 1970, *16,* 7–51.

Gewirtz, J. L. (Ed.) *Attachment and dependency.* New York: Wiley, 1972.

Goldstein, K. *Language and language disturbances.* New York: Grune & Stratton, 1948.

Gordon, I. J. *Early child stimulation through parent education.* Gainesville, Fla.: Institute for Development of Human Resources, University of Florida, February, 1967. Contract No. R-306, Children's Bureau, Department of Health, Education, and Welfare.

Gordon, I. J. *Baby learning through baby play.* New York: St. Martin's Press, 1970.

Gordon, I. J. What do we know about parents as teachers? *Theory Into Practice,* 1972, *11,* 146–149.

Gordon, I. J. The Florida Parent Education early intervention projects: A longitudinal look. A paper presented at the Merrill-Palmer Conference, Detroit, Michigan, February 8, 1973.

Hebb, D. The motivating effects of exteroceptive stimulation. *American Psychologist,* 1958, *13,* 109–113.

Hunt, J. McV. Toward a theory of guided learning in development. In R. Ojemann and K. Pritchett (Eds.), *Giving emphasis to guided learning.* Cleveland: Educational Research Council of Greater Cleveland, 1966. Pp. 98–145.

Huxley, R., & Ingram, E. (Eds.) *Language acquisition: Models and methods.* New York: Academic Press, 1971.

Kagan, J. Acquisition and significance of sex-typing and sex role identity. In M. Hoffman and L. Hoffman (Eds.), *Review of child development research.* Vol. 1. New York: Russell Sage Foundation, 1963. Pp. 137–167.

Kagan, J. *Change and continuity in infancy.* New York: Wiley, 1971.

Kagan, J. Do infants think? *Scientific American,* 1972, *226,* 74–82.

Kagan, J., & Moss. H. *Birth to maturity.* New York: Wiley, 1962.

Kohlberg, L. A cognitive-developmental analysis of children's sex-role concepts and behavior. In E. E. Maccoby (Ed.), *The development of sex differences.* Stanford, Calif.: Stanford University Press, 1966. Pp. 82–173.

League, R. Early language development in the normal child. In P. Satz and J. Ross (Eds.), *The disabled learner.* Rotterdam, The Netherlands: Rotterdam University Press, 1973. Pp. 45–78.

Lenneberg, E. H. *Biological formulations of language.* New York, Wiley, 1967.

Levenstein, P. Learning through (and from) mothers. *Childhood Education,* 1971, *47,* 130–134.

Lewis, M., & Ban, P. Stability of attachment behavior: A transformation analysis.

Paper presented at the meeting of the Society for Research in Child Development, Minneapolis, Minn., April 1971.

Maccoby, E., & Masters, J. C. Attachment and dependency. In P. H. Mussen (Ed.), *Carmichael's manual of child psychology.* (3rd ed.) Vol. 2. New York: Wiley, 1970. Pp. 73–158.

McCarthy, D. Language development in children. In L. Carmichael (Ed.), *Manual of child psychology.* (2nd ed.) New York: Wiley, 1954. Pp. 492–630.

McNeill, D. The development of language. In P. H. Mussen (Ed.), *Carmichael's manual of child psychology.* (3rd ed.) Vol. I. New York: Wiley, 1970. Pp. 1061–1162.

Mead, G. H. *Mind, self, and society.* Chicago: University of Chicago Press, 1940.

Mischel, W. Sex-typing and socialization. In P. H. Mussen (Ed.), *Carmichael's manual of child psychology.* (3rd ed.) Vol. II. New York: Wiley, 1970. Pp. 3–72.

Moreno, P. The assessment of attachment. *Selected Documents in Psychology,* 1973, *3,* 121.

Murphy, G. *Personality, a biosocial approach.* New York: Basic Books, 1966.

Myklebust, H. Language disorders in children. *Exceptional Children,* 1956, *22,* 163–166.

Nelson, K. Structure and strategy in learning to talk. *Society for Research in Child Development Monographs,* 1973, *38,* 1–135.

Papousek, H. Experimental studies of appetitional behavior in human newborn and infants. In H. Stevenson, E. Hess, & H. Reingold (Eds.), *Early behavior: Comparative and developmental approaches.* New York: Wiley, 1967. Pp. 249–278.

Piaget, J. *The origins of intelligence.* New York: Norton, 1963.

Piaget, J., & Inhelder, B. *The psychology of the child.* New York: Basic Books, 1969.

Razran, G. Observable UCS and inferable CS in current Soviet psychophysiology. *Psychological Review,* 1961, *68,* 81–147.

Resnick, M. Language ability and intellectual and behavioral functioning in economically disadvantaged children. Unpublished doctoral dissertation, University of Florida, 1972.

Rheingold, H. The social and socializing infant. In D. A. Goslin (Ed.), *Handbook of socialization theory and research.* Chicago: Rand McNally, 1969. Pp. 779–790.

Sayegh, Y., & Dennis, W. The effect of supplementary experiences upon the behavioral development of infants in institutions. *Child Development,* 1965, *36,* 81–90.

Schaefer, E., & Bayley, N. Maternal behavior, child behavior, and their intercorrelations from infancy through adolescence. *Monographs of the Society for Research in Child Development,* 1963, *28*(3), 127 pp.

Sears, R., Rau, L., & Alpert, R. *Identification and child-rearing.* Stanford, Calif.: Stanford University Press, 1965.

Shirley, M. The first two years, a study of twenty-five babies. Vol. I. *Intellectual Development.* Institute of Child Welfare Monograph Series, No. 8. Minneapolis: University of Minnesota Press, 1938.

Singer, J. L., & Singer, D. G. Personality. In P. H. Mussen and M. R. Rosenzweig (Eds.), *Annual review of psychology.* Vol. 23. Palo Alto, Calif.: Annual Reviews, Inc., 1972. Pp. 375–412.

Sullivan, H. S. *The interpersonal theory of psychiatry.* New York: Norton, 1953.

Uzgiris, I. C. Patterns of cognitive development in infancy. *Merrill-Palmer Quarterly,* 1973, *19(3),* 181–204.

Uzgiris, I. C., & Hunt, J. M. An instrument for assessing infant psychological development. (Mimeo) University of Illinois, 1966.

Watson, J. Smiling, cooing and "the game." *Merrill-Palmer Quarterly,* 1972, *18,* 323–340.

White, B. L. Fundamental early environmental influences on the development of competency. In M. Meyer (Ed.), *Third symposium on learning: Cognitive learning.* Bellingham, Wash.: Western Washington State College, 1972.

White, B. L., Castle, P., & Held, R. Observations on the development of visually directed reaching. *Child Development,* 1964, *35,* 349–364.

Yarrow, L., Rubenstein, J., & Pederson, F. Dimensions of early stimulation: Differential effects on infant development. Paper presented at the meeting of the Society for Research on Child Development, Minneapolis, Minn., April 1971.

Zaporozhets, A. V. The development of perception in the preschool child. In P. H. Mussen (Ed.), European research in cognitive development. *Monographs of the Society for Research in Child Development,* 1965, *30(2),* 82–101.

CHAPTER 5

FROM "I" TO THE "THREE Rs"

CHANGES IN BODILY FACTORS
Changes in Size and Rate of Growth

During the first few years of his life, the child grows in size slowly but steadily. Although published charts of height and weight may be slightly out of date because each generation shows gains in the rate of development, they offer indices from which we can learn about orderly development. Table 5.1 is based upon data originally assembled in the 1940s by Stuart and Meredith and adapted by Watson and Lowrey. It has been estimated that for the last 80 years gains in height have been at the rate of 0.5 to 1.0 centimeters (approximately 0.2 to 0.4 inches) per decade. Thus, to make Table 5.1 accurate for use in the 1970s, 0.6 to 0.8 inches should be added to each figure.

An important generalization can be induced from a study of the data in the table. First, the range of individual differences in body size increases with age, so that children in the tenth and ninetieth percentiles are further apart at age 6 than they were at age 2. Thus, each child becomes unique in his particular growth, although the overall group pattern is one of steady growth. The slow-growing (tenth percentile) boy of 6 resembles more the fast-growing (ninetieth percentile) boy of 4 in body size than he does his own age-mates. This fact about growth is often overlooked by parents, teachers, and other adults who tend to stress the age of the child and to neglect his actual developmental status, which is important to the child and influences his self-evaluation (see the section on self-evaluating in Chapter 6).

Another important generalization about growth during early childhood is that this is the time when the rate of growth in size levels off. Weight gains are stabilized at about 24 months and height increments are stabilized at about 3 years of age. Figures 5.1 and 5.2 graphically present these data. Simultaneous with the increase in linear size is the continued

TABLE 5.1 HEIGHT AND WEIGHT GAINS, AGES 2–6

	BOYS		GIRLS	
AGE*	10 PERCENTILE	90 PERCENTILE	10 PERCENTILE	90 PERCENTILE
	HEIGHT IN INCHES			
2	33.1	35.9	32.3	35.8
2½	34.8	37.9	34	37.9
3	36.3	39.6	35.6	39.8
3½	37.8	41.1	37.1	41.5
4	39.1	42.7	38.4	43.1
4½	40.3	44.2	39.7	44.7
5	40.8	45.2	40.5	45.4
5½	42.6	47.3	42.4	46.8
6	43.8	48.6	43.5	48.1
	WEIGHT IN POUNDS			
2	24.7	31.9	23.5	31.7
2½	26.6	34.5	25.5	34.6
3	28.7	36.8	27.6	37.4
3½	30.4	39.1	29.5	40.4
4	32.1	41.4	31.2	43.5
4½	33.8	43.9	32.9	46.7
5	35.5	46.7	34.8	49.2
5½	38.8	53.1	38	51.2
6	40.9	56.4	39.6	54.2

* See Table 10.1 for data on 6-year-olds that indicates a gain of about one inch at the ninetieth percentile in the years between the 1940s and the 1960s.
Source: Combined from Tables 4–4 and 4–5 in G. H. Lowrey, *Growth and Development of Children,* 6th ed., Year Book Publishers, 1973. Used by permission.

change in bodily proportions; thus, between ages 2 and 6 the ratio of head to trunk to legs alters. Figure 5.3 shows the changes from before birth to maturity.

Changes in Energy Needs

As the rate of increase in size levels off, there is also a reduction in the rate of gain in metabolism. During ages 3 and 4, there is a decrease in the rate of heat production as compared to the first two years. Generally, heat production increases throughout the growing years and then levels off, but at ages 3 and 4 it dips. Children, as a consequence, often cut down their food intake whereas parents often insist on increasing the amount of food that they expect the child to eat. Lack of understanding that this decrease

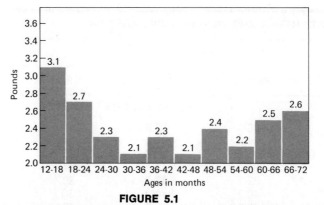

FIGURE 5.1

Expected increments in weight, 12 to 72 months. Created from data in *Growth and development of children,* 6th ed., G. H. Lowrey, Year Book Publishers, Chicago, 1973, p. 81. Used by permission.

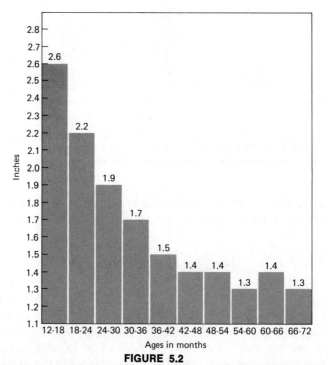

FIGURE 5.2

Expected increments in height, 12 to 72 months. Created from data in *Growth and development of children,* 6th ed., G. H. Lowrey, Year Book Publishers, Chicago, 1973, p. 81. Used by permission.

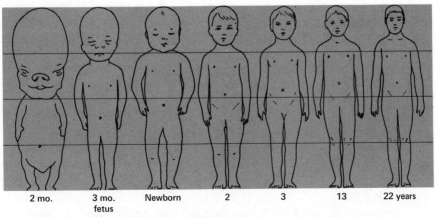

2 mo.   3 mo.   Newborn   2   3   13   22 years
        fetus

FIGURE 5.3

Changes in form and proportion of the human body during fetal and postnatal life. After Scammon, from L. B. Arey, *Developmental anatomy,* 6th ed., W. B. Saunders Company, Philadelphia, 1954.

in appetite is normal can lead to the creation of "food problems." Parents have grown accustomed to the child's previous increased demands for food, so during these two years, they become disturbed when the child begins to shove away his unfinished plate. If parents could learn to prepare wholesome food and take their cues concerning quantity from the child himself, some of the interminable dinner-table wrangles might be decreased or eliminated.

Increases in Motor Control

During these preschool years the child continues to develop rapidly his ability to manipulate the objects in his environment. The rate of increase in size slows down, but increase in complexity continues to be rapid.

The transactional nature of development becomes more obvious in the years between infancy and school. Opportunities for experience become increasingly important in determining the actual behavior and the actual uses to which the child will put his increasing coordination ability.

Generally, children go through a progression in which they first engage in activity simply, it seems on the surface, for the sheer joy of being active and finally arrive at a repetitive type of behavior in which they do and redo whatever they've just accomplished, such as going up and down stairs, climbing to the top of the jungle gym, or building a tower of blocks. This leads into the more sophisticated type of activity that emerges about the age of 4 or 5 in which the coordination task is only a tool in play or games of a social nature. At 3 the child climbs stairs to climb stairs; at 5 the child climbs stairs because he's a "good guy" and the "bad guy" is hiding up at the top. The same process of development holds for such other motor skills as block-building or drawing. Thus, children move from the stage of merely stacking blocks to the use of blocks in dramatic play and in attempts to build "real-looking" forts or garages or castles. Drawings change from the aimless scribbling of the toddler to the design stage and, finally, to the kindergartener's attempts to reproduce reality.

These developments represent not only the increasing control the child has over legs, arms, and small muscles but also the purposive aspects of behavior. He moves from use for the sake of use to use for social, communicative, symbolic, and interpretive purposes. Part of the new motor ability is used to handle feelings or fantasy; part is used to relate to other children; part is used as the child attempts to understand the culture that surrounds him.

In terms of pure "ability to do," we can observe in operation the growth principle of developmental direction. Control proceeds from large muscle to small muscle. For example, the order of leg development is walking, ascending and descending a few steps, jumping, hopping, and skipping. There is also an increase in strength. Studies of rhythmic activities also reveal that the ability to keep time with music develops with age.

The establishment of hand dominance is also usually completed during these years. The age-old dispute of heredity versus environment may be seen in the many articles devoted to the changing of left-handedness to right-handedness. Current thought would fit into our transactional approach, for our culture favors right-handedness and rewards right-handed behavior. Our tools, toys, and games are designed for the right-handed. Many children who might go either way, since to some degree "handedness" is learned behavior, become right-handed through the socialization process. It has been shown that most children can be oriented to using their right hand before age 6. We also know that no person is completely one-sided; he may carry on many activities with either hand.

Significance of These Changes

This increasing control over one's body is important in the evolution of selfhood. A major factor in the definition of the adequate self is the ability to assume tasks for oneself that formerly had to be done by others. As the child might express it: "Now I'm 6 I can tie my own shoes, dress myself, feed and wash myself, button some of my buttons (though maybe not those I cannot see), and go to the bathroom without help. Of course, I still need my mommy, but I don't need her to do all the things for me like she used to do."

Of course, mother may feel ambivalent toward this growing ability; she may be glad to see the child "growing up" but sorry to see him growing away from her. The increase in motor control thus operates, in relation to the self, as a force that enables the child to do more, and also, through the way people respond to his growth, influences his self-picture. He, too, makes his *own* response to his body, his *own* comparisons of his self with others. The child evaluates his own efforts at drawing, skipping, or whatever the task is. He evaluates himself against both his own aspirations and the achievement of others. A nursery school teacher once told the story of a 4-year-old, vigorously drawing, face close to the paper, tongue out, using a profusion of crayons. The teacher, steeped in the doctrine of encouragement, went up to him and said, ''Why Bobby, I think that's a fine drawing!'' To which Bobby replied, in the direct fashion of the 4-year-old, ''I think it stinks!'' In his eyes, he couldn't make the picture represent what he wanted it to, and the teacher's attempts at support were rejected.

The child's self-picture is influenced both by the way in which others respond to his growing abilities and by the way in which his already developed self-system responds. This differs in some degree from the previous stage in which the very development of self depended upon the development of motor control. Up to this time (the emergence of self-awareness), motor and mental development had been closely related. We saw in the last chapter that the development of motor control made it possible for the infant to develop more complex adaptive behaviors. Simultaneous with the emergence of self in the latter half of the second year of life, we find that ''the more adaptive intellectual functions are no longer closely limited by motor coordinations. The mental functions are free to differentiate and to expand pretty much on their own.'' (Bayley, 1955, p. 4)

There are, however, still links between cognitive and motor development. Fowler and Leithwood (1971) taught gymnastics to 4-year-olds and report that *cognitive regulation* was involved; that is, systematic verbal feedback by the instructors enhanced the children's performance. The children learned to control their bodies not simply by practice but by cognitive effort. Children have been taught violin by the Suzuki method, which requires careful listening to competent violinists, modeling the behavior of adults through use of small violins, and adjusting performance to a standard heard on a record. In this case, too, there is interaction of intellective and motor functioning. Cognition and motor activity used in concert enhance not only the child's competence in handling his body in intricate maneuvers but also his self-image.

THE EXPANSION OF ''MEANINGS''
Structuring the Physical World

Space.   Chapter 4 discussed the efforts of the infant in ordering his surroundings, in making a map, in creating a perceptual field. By the time he refers to himself as ''I,'' he has differentiated his own movements from the movements of objects in the field. He realizes that objects have permanence apart from their particular location in space at a particular time (the ball that was hidden behind the couch is the same ball that earlier was in the middle of the floor); he is able to perceive that the spatial field consists of more than those objects that have immediate utility to him; and, most significantly for his further development, the child can think of events and objects that are not present at the moment. He is capable of memory, of imagination, of pretending, of planning.

In structuring his world spatially, the child now includes symbolism as well as direct sensation. This symbolism, however, is limited to images of objects with which he has had direct concrete experiences. It is not symbolism in the sense of abstract thought. The child continues to structure his world around himself and is still highly egocentric. He can now think and talk of "ball," or "yard," or "house"; he can pretend to play ball; he can enjoy, by the age of 3, such a game as "hide the penny"— but all these lie within the immediate experience of the child. He cannot conceptualize about more distant objects. For example, Piaget and Inhelder (1956) reported that children of 4 or 5 had no notion of the fact that the mountain would look different from the opposite side.

Notions of the size of distant objects and their relationship to each other in space are likewise primitive. The child may know, if he has seen an airplane close by, that it is this same plane which appears so small high in the sky. However, size and space often get mixed up, and a small plane seen up close is perceived as actually being bigger than a huge jet bomber at high altitude. The size of the stars, the sun, and the moon are also beyond the comprehension of the preschool child. There is the delightful story of the young princess who wanted the moon and thought it was smaller than the trees because it could be hidden by the tree outside her window. Young children can realize that familiar objects can be stacked or fitted inside each other; they have some notions of space and size but they cannot handle distant objects (what Piaget calls "projective space").

The child gradually enlarges his understanding of how big is big and of the fact that the size of an object is constant despite its distance from the viewer, and he also struggles to establish an idea of how far is far. Is a mile in the car the same as a mile when he walks it? How far is a mile? Again, immediacy and concrete experience are the basis for the conceptualization. A walk around the block or a walk from home to some other landmark (such as the school, the store, or a friend's house) aids in establishing an understanding of distance. A mile becomes walking back and forth to a particular landmark. These early spatial anchorage points later enable the child to draw generalizations about new situations.

Pick (1972) has been exploring children's frames of reference in orienting themselves in space. One way he does this is by asking children to describe their homes: "What's on the other side of the bathroom mirror?" "How do you get from your room to the kitchen?" He has found that these are difficult questions for 4- and 5-year-olds but that 5-year-olds are superior to 4-year-olds in placing objects in a room and in knowing what's on the other side of the bedroom wall. Pick's concern is with the way the child learns and develops spatial frames of reference. Combining Piaget's theory of cognitive psychology and learning theory, he concludes that we can describe what a child knows but that we cannot yet fully explain how he learns it. He suggests that we let the child tell us what frame of reference he is using instead of imposing one.

In daily experience, adults often translate distance into the convenient direct terms through which they first established their concepts. Each of us probably still has an image of a mile as ''from my home to the grocery store and back'' or some similar image that we use as a measuring rod instead of conceiving of a mile as 5,280 feet.

By the time the child is ready for school, he has acquired concepts of space that grew out of his dealings with his surroundings. He has begun to conceptualize distance and can engage in using the objects in his field to solve problems. For example, he can do simple jigsaw puzzles that require understanding of shapes. Although he still may attempt to pound a piece into place, by and large he recognizes that the shape of the piece must correspond to the shape of the available space. Though he uses color and subject clues as aids in solving the puzzle, the child has a spatial orientation. Although he knows of the existence of objects outside his perceptual field, he is still mostly concerned with objects he can utilize, ones that are immediately related to him.

Time.   At the same time that the child is developing and enlarging his notions of the spatial environment, he is also developing the beginnings of understanding about his temporal environment. To the infant, life is lived completely in the present tense; truly, ''There is no time like the present.'' The young child recognizes more than the present, although there is still considerable confusion in his thinking about time. Perhaps one of the most difficult concepts for him to grasp is that time exists independently of him, his wishes, his needs. Although he recognizes that objects and people have an independent existence, he has also learned that he can affect their behavior. He can move a block, change (to some degree) his parents' behavior, or avoid an object that might hurt him. Time, however, is different; he can do nothing about it. If the child attempts to influence time, he finds out, alas, that it doesn't work. For example, the avid ''Captain Kangaroo'' fan, learning that his program is on television at 8 A.M., may ask his mother to set a timer to ring when it's time for the program. Getting impatient, he rings the timer by hand before the set time and then races to the TV set—but what's this? still no ''Captain Kangaroo.'' He can visualize objects as possessing permanency; this attempt by the child to manipulate time is an example of his still incomplete differentiation of self and world, his belief in his ability to influence the physical facts of the world by his own thoughts or efforts.

He is puzzled also by the relativity of time from his point of view. Why is it that when Daddy says he'll play with him "in a minute," the minute is so long, but when the child says he'll come "in a minute" from play, the time just disappears? Certainly concepts of day, week, month, and year hold no meaning at the beginning of this period of development. He first develops concepts of present time, then future time, and lastly past time. The child confuses time periods by assuming, for example, that it is a new day when he wakes up from his nap. It is only as he reaches 4 or 5 that he becomes really aware of clock time and calendar time although, of course, his concepts are still quite hazy.

Ames (1946) interviewed a small sample of children and found a consistent sequence of development; the child of 4 could separate morning and afternoon, and at 5 years of age he knew what day it was. Springer went one step further in studying 4- to 6-year-olds, asking them to tell various times on a clock face and to explain how they knew the answer. She also asked these children what time school started, what time lunch started, and what time school ended. She concluded, "First, the child is able to tell the time of activities which occur regularly in his daily schedule. . . . Second, the child is able to tell time by a clock: the hours, then the half and quarter hours." (Springer, 1952, p. 95)

Here again, in relation to time as to space, is the basic principle of developing understanding of the world in operation: The child moves from a concrete, action-oriented level toward a more abstract level. He first deals with time in terms of its utility, its relatedness to him, its function in enabling him to order his environment—that is, to routinize and predict the occurrence of events. Time, as well as space, serves the child as an anchorage point.

Age, time, and growth all become tangled together in the thoughts of the child. He conceives of people as continuing to grow bigger each year because he sees himself getting bigger. When he sees a tall grownup next to one of average size, he jumps to the conclusion that the taller grownup must be older. A taller tree, too, must be older. (Piaget, 1946) This relation between size (power) and age shows in his view of self. As the child approaches 4 or 5 or 6, a birthday possesses mystical power. The child sees a birthday as a landmark: "When I be 5, I go to kindergarten." His thinking about himself is oriented in relation to his size, his age, and the size of the people around him. "His size takes on meaning in terms of (1) the other aspects of his structural equipment; (2) in terms of the size of people with whom he is closely associated. . . ." (Macfarlane, 1939, p. 5)

Concepts of the self as big and, more particularly, as getting bigger are close to the core of the self of the child during these years. He is equally aware, however, of his own small size in comparison with that of adults and older siblings. Children of this age perceive their fathers as larger than their mothers, although they also perceive children of the opposite sex as being larger than themselves. (Katcher and Levin, 1955) The child may show this in a variety of ways as he seeks to change or comprehend this fact of life. A 4-year-old girl, for example, making a drawing, told the author, "I'm drawing me and my brother. He's really bigger, but I'm making *me* bigger." Children delight in standing on stools or chairs or other pieces of furniture, looking down on the heads of the adult below, and reporting gleefully, "Look, I'm bigger than you are!"

Quantity.   As in the child's concepts of space and time and, indeed, as in the development of all concepts including those of self, the child learns through the process of differentiating from his own direct experiences. In learning about quantity, this differentiating process goes through three stages before school and a fourth one beginning about the time he enters school. First, the child's behavior shows that he recognizes and *responds* to magnitude. The child can handle several objects and realizes that he has several objects. He then progresses to *naming.* It may sound to the proud parent as though the child were counting, and mother may brag how *her* 3-year-old can count to ten, but the child really has no concept of number. He may count objects, but he leaves out numbers; or he counts to ten when there are only five or six items to count; however, he keeps the rhythm of the counting irrespective of its accuracy. In the same way, children can memorize the alphabet without having the vaguest notion that it has anything to do with letters! The *ordering* function follows after naming. Here the child recognizes the existence of a system of numbers and can use the number system actually to count or to assemble a specified number of objects.

But the fact that the child can count does not mean he really understands numbers. An important Piagetian concept, conservation, has been much researched in recent years. *Conservation* means the understanding that certain properties, or aspects of an object, do not change when other visible features are changed. Thus, in a classical experiment, the child is given some plasticene and is asked to change its shape in some fashion. He is then asked whether or not there has been a change in the amount. According to Inhelder (1962), children below the age of 5 or 6 think that a change in shape means a change in the amount of material. The theoretical order of ability to conserve is amount of matter, weight, volume. Although the notion of conservation is accepted, there is still much disagreement about order, teachability, and the learning process behind the child's development.

There have been numerous experiments and attempts to train for conservation over the last dozen years. The results are mixed; some report success and some, failure. Those that succeed have usually used children who were close to the age of conservation. (Hartup and Yonas, 1971) Analyses of training methods indicate that the instructions to the participants are important. For example, Rothenberg (1969) reports that one must be sure that words such as "same" and "more" are understood (and disadvantaged children may not understand them fully) before assuming that it is conservation rather than vocabulary which is being assessed. The child's background of experience plays a major role: his opportunities to model and for manipulation (Goodnow, 1969), the emphasis that different subcultures place on certain skills such as space relations, and his opportunities for formal schooling are all significant.

Although the order of development of concepts about the physical world appears to be regular for groups of children—in each case proceeding from a self-centered base and developed through concrete experiences prior to the use of abstract reasoning—the child's concepts of the physical world are a function of the particular, unique transactions between his growing body and his environmental field. They are influenced by his needs and the way he has related himself to his environment in his earlier experiences. It must be reiterated that children of the same chronological age will vary widely in their concepts and that this wide variation is normal, natural, and expected. We can only, within gross limits, describe the general order by which certain concepts emerge, but even this order is subject to individual variation. The child differentiates these concepts through experience, particularly in the degree to which the concepts possess utility. He does not seek to comprehend space as space or time as time. Rather, he seeks to comprehend space so that he can use it, time so that he can control it. Concepts are meaningful; that is, they are guides and cues to action.

An understanding of how children conceive of their environment and of how their conceptions change as they develop makes it easier for us to conceive as they conceive, easier for us to understand the meaning of their behavior, and easier for us to supply opportunities for them to achieve their potentialities. This understanding may make the adult more tolerant of what otherwise might be viewed as "errors" on the child's part and enable him to relax and enjoy the child's behavior. The question of guidance has generated an important debate in the last half-dozen years because of numerous efforts to provide compensatory education for disadvantaged preschool children. Should such efforts be highly structured or more like the older traditional nursery school? The results are not all in, but at least in relation to conservation of number, Mermelstein and Meyer (1969) report that specific training efforts were not useful, and they suggest providing broader experiences in role playing and more contact with adults instead.

Language Development

We indicated in Chapter 4 that much remains to be learned about language acquisition. Yet it is clear that the preschool years are years of rapid growth in both the acquisition and use of language. We can look at the problem in three ways: descriptively, through the processes of language acquisition, and through the relationship of language to thought.

Table 5.2 shows the remarkable growth in language between age 2 and age 5. Vocabulary increases rapidly from 50 words to over 1000. Syntactically, the child's speech changes from ungrammatical utterances to those displaying a well-defined use of grammar. The level and the amount of communication increases rapidly during this time. (Lenneberg, 1969; McNeill, 1970; Brown, Cazden, and Bellugi, 1968) There are changes in the complexity of structure and in the use of questions and declarations as well as in vocabulary.

How does the child learn this? Although the issue is still unresolved (see Chapter 4), modeling, imitation, and adult reinforcement all provide cues to the child. For example, Moerk (1972) analyzed the language interaction between mothers and children in middle class families in which the children ranged in age from 20 to 60 months. He found that the mother provides opportunities for much modeling and also engages in correcting, expanding, and second-guessing what the child had in mind. As Moerk says, "Mothers in general seem to be very sensitive measuring instru-

TABLE 5.2 LANGUAGE MILESTONES

2	More than 50 words; two-word phrases most common; more interest in verbal communication; no more babbling.
2.5	Every day new words; utterances of three and more words; seems to understand almost everything said to him; still many grammatical deviations.
3	Vocabulary of some 1000 words; about 80 percent intelligibility; grammar of utterances close approximation to colloquial adult; syntactic mistakes fewer in variety, systematic, predictable.
4.5	Language well established; grammatical anomalies restricted either to unusual constructions or to the more literate aspects of discourse.

Source: E. Lenneberg, On explaining language, *Science,* 1969, *164,* 636. Copyright 1969 by the American Association for the Advancement of Science. Used by permission.

TABLE 5.3 THE MOTHER ASKS FOR REAFFIRMATION OF THE CORRECTNESS OF HER UNDERSTANDING

Jeffrey (2,4)	Wee, wee.
Mother	You want to read?
Jeffrey	Yeah.
Debbie	I made if fail.
Mother	You made it fall?
Jeffrey (2,4)	Ah wan taut. Ah wan taut.
Mother	You want toast?
Jeffrey	Ah wan taus.

Source: E. Moerk, Principles of interaction in language learning, *Merrill-Palmer Quarterly,* 1972, *18,* 246. Used by permission.

---

ments of the child's information processing capacities, as manifested by the fact that they can communicate with their children and that their children learn to speak in such a short time. Yet, nobody seems even to have asked what criteria these mothers use in measuring this information processing capacity and in deciding which type of feedback to provide." (Moerk, 1972, p. 244) An example of mother-child interaction is shown in Table 5.3. Moerk also found that nursery rhymes, even though they contain linguistic structures not commonly found in the child's language, are meaningful to the child, and he understands their structure. He concludes: "The phenomena of imitation through expansion, modeling, occasional questions, incomplete sentences, question-answer games, nursery rhymes, and structuring through picture books do not yet describe exhaustibly all the principles of interaction and teaching as applied by the mother." (Moerk, 1972)

We can see the critical importance of the adult as a provider of stimulation and opportunity for the child. No one technique or even a set of techniques should be expected to explain language acquisition. All of this variety can be categorized under interpersonal transaction. The unique combinations of procedures may vary widely, but a wide variety of approaches assists in development. As in the case of conservation, specific training is not the critical factor. Exposure, opportunity, and practice, particularly in the presence of a sympathetic adult partner, seem to be the common prerequisites. "Good language development is not contingent on specific training measures. A wide variety of rather haphazard factors seem to be sufficient." (Lenneberg, 1969, p. 637)

What is the relationship between language and thought? An acute observer of young children is rapidly aware that both grow apace. Our usual disposition when we see two things together is to investigate how one is affecting the other. We are always predisposed to hunt for causations. One view might be that thought depends upon language, but a number of research studies based on Piaget's viewpoints challenge that assumption. Furth (1966), in several studies of deaf children, found that they acquire Piagetian logical operations with only slight retardation as compared to normal children. Blind children, on the other hand, experience considerable difficulty. Sinclair-de-Zwart (1969) used conservation of liquids and two forms of verbal instruction to see whether learning the words and the linguistic forms would enhance conservation. She found it did not. Verbal training of subjects who were unable to conserve did not bring about conservation. She concluded that the development of linguistic skill runs parallel to the development of Piagetian cognitive development, but that one is not cause of the other. Piaget himself sees language as only part of the larger symbol system, and considers it neither a sufficient condition for the constitution of intellectual operation nor even a necessary one, in the early years at least. Both the growth in thought and the growth in language, according to Piaget, are part of a larger process, the growth of symbolic functioning in general. This is the ability of the child to transcend verbal language by engaging in symbolic play, by conjuring up mental images, by engaging in deferred imitation, and by manipulating objects.

On the other hand, Vygotsky (1962) and other Russian psychologists feel that words influence behavior. They hold that behavior is first influenced by words from the outside in the very young child and that as the child learns these, he uses them to control his own behavior. Language is seen as directing the child's attention both to his own behavior and to the effects of his behavior on the objects he is working with. The Soviet psychologists emphasize training what they call the *orienting response*— that is, the development of self-awareness and voluntary control of one's motor actions. The child is taught to imagine his actions and their effects through verbal instructions, demonstration, and imitation. (Zaporozhets, 1960) Sinclair-de-Zwart's (1969) research indicates that language does have the attending role but does not necessarily yield the cognitive payoff. Zaporozhets (1960) found that verbal instruction and imitation in motor tasks were more effective when children were taught to be aware of their motor activities, but this does not support the relationship between language and thought. A number of studies (Bruner, Oliver, and Greenfield et al., 1966) have indicated that children may behave in ways that show they understand a cognitive principle (such as grouping or conservation) when they cannot describe in words why they have done what they have done. These results suggest that in the preschool years, cognitive development is not equivalent to learning words but requires engagement in action that

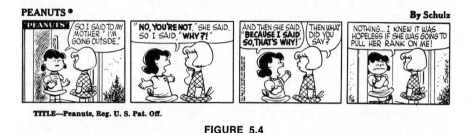

FIGURE 5.4

© 1956 United Feature Syndicate, Inc.

allows both for the development of words and for the child to see what effects his actions have on objects and on himself.

Reasoning

If reasoning is not equivalent to language, what are the ways that young children think, and what factors influence their reasoning? First, their thoughts are related to their experiences, to the personal meanings they have already derived, and to their continuing efforts to enlarge their understanding of what is taking place in and around themselves. This is the period Piaget has labeled the *preoperational stage.* It is the time when the child is still not able to conserve but is able to use symbols and to engage in what he calls *directional functions* with *unity of value.* (Piaget, 1970, p. 712) This means the child can deal with ordering and arranging and recognizes that objects have permanence (see Chapter 4). During this period, children's reasoning, as in the case of language, develops from their transactions with the environment. The process is an active one in which the child's concepts are not simply passively acquired but are created through his actions and through the feedback he receives.

Our view corresponds to Piaget's: "The main point of our theory is that knowledge results from *interactions* between the subject and the object, which are *richer* than what the objects can provide by themselves." (Piaget, 1970, pp. 713–714) In this sense, knowledge is both personal and public, but it can be understood psychologically only by inquiring into what the child conceives the facts to be. This is what influences his behavior toward objects. The young child, of course, from the external observer's point of view, makes errors in reasoning (as if adults did not!). For example, the rules of tag are bad because the child got tagged, but then they become good, and he enforces them when he tags another child. What is "fair" or "unfair" depends upon who is making the judgment rather than upon any abstract concept of fairness.

The urge to know, to understand, and to comprehend also influences children's thought. "Why" is the persistent and everlasting word of the preschool child. Unlike the little boy in *Alice in Wonderland* whose motives were assumed to be that "he only does it to annoy, because he knows it teases," the questioning of the young child is real and reflects his curiosity. He veritably lives in a wonderland and seeks answers. As Murphy says of curiosity: "Puppies, monkeys, men are forever poking their noses into what does not obviously concern them—that is, what does not concern any previously aroused drive, but very much concerns the completion of a perceptual or activity pattern." (G. Murphy, 1966, pp. 405–406) It is this curiosity that may lead children later to science but now leads them to think and to try to integrate experiences in order to answer the everlasting "why?"

From a linguistic orientation, Brown, Cazden, and Bellugi (1968) traced the development of Wh— questions by a child and demonstrated the increasing complexity of his syntax as well as his questions. Here we can see this development as parallel and related to reasoning.

Children perceive relationships between two events that occur close together in time, or share a common perceptual feature, or relate to a similar previous experience. For example, anyone who wears a khaki uniform is a soldier; you can tell a "bad man" on television or in the movies by his appearance, and so on. This is what Piaget calls *phenomenism.* The stereotyping of people and the beginning of class and caste role may have their origins in this type of thinking.

This *associative* process, this linking together of past and present, is a major way in which the child organizes his experiences and thinks about them. In the process, he invokes magic, he makes mistakes, he "mishears" words, and he tests his ideas by trial and error. This process, however, can be guided rather than left to chance or "nature." Ojemann and Pritchett (1963) demonstrated that kindergarten children could think about specific gravity in ways similar to adolescents if they had been led through a guided learning experience that was based upon their own desire to know and that used their present concrete level of thought. Such learning influences the child's development because it requires accommodation and does not allow for easy answers.

There has been a whole host of studies (some of which we referred to earlier in this chapter) on attempts to train or teach children to classify, order, arrange, and conserve. All such activities are signs that the child is moving out of the preoperational period (usually defined as ages 2 to 7) into the next stage. There have also been many attempts at teaching on concepts (such as number). In particular, there have been efforts to teach abstract-thinking skills (Blank, 1968) and classification skills to disadvantaged children who were conceived to lack them. A sample procedure from Olmsted, Parks, and Rickel (1970) gives the flavor of such efforts. This particular session concerns the attributes of a quarter, an American coin with a picture of George Washington on it. The results showed that the children were more able to group and used more criteria.

Teacher: *What do you see here, Janice?*
Child: *Money.*
Teacher: *Some money. Quentin, what do you want to tell about it?*
Child: *It's pink. . . .*
Child: *It's a nickel, no, a quarter.*
Teacher: *It's a quarter. Good for you!*
Child: *And it's gray.*
Teacher: *What, honey?*
Child: *It's gray and white.*
Teacher: *Oh, you're trying to tell about the color. Maybe if we figure out what it's made of, then you will know what color it is.*
Child: *Metal.*
Teacher: *It's metal. All right, and what color is metal?*
Children: *(All speaking at once) . . . White . . . Green . . . Red.*
Teacher: *Do you want me to tell you?*
Child: *Yes.*
Teacher: *It's silver. . . . It's silver colored. You could even say that it is metal-colored. . . . And what does it have on there, Janice?*
Child: *A man.*
Teacher: *All right, Quentin sees a man.*
Child: *With curly hair.*
Teacher: *With curly hair in the back.*
Child: *And it has a round shape.*
Teacher: *Good for you, you remembered it has a round shape! And what else do you want to tell about it?*

Source: P. P. Olmsted, C. V. Parks, and A. Rickel, The development of classification skills. *International Review of Education,* Special Number: Preschool Education, Aspects and Problems, 1970, 16(1), 71–72. Used by permission.

Glaser and Resnick's (1972) review concludes that there has been success in instruction on conservation if we consider that retention, transfer to a new task, and resistance to countersuggestion are criteria of success. However, there is no consensus on what instructional procedures are either necessary or sufficient, except that reversibility seems important. The ability to reverse—that is, to recognize that an act can be undone (clay pounded into a ball can be flattened, then repounded into a ball)—is one of Piaget's markers of operational thought. It does not seem inconsistent that children, especially if they are close to creating the concepts of reversibility and conservation from the welter of experiences they have had, can be assisted by a variety of instructional techniques to put it all together. The fact that they can be taught does not negate, to this author, Piaget's view that conservation rests on interaction; in fact, it tends to support it.

Classification, as indicated above, has also been studied. Here too, the results tend to support the notion that instruction can play a role, but the procedures used in studies are by no means uniform. From our point of view, reasoning processes and the products of such reasoning evident in the actions of a child are transactional, and the argument about learning is futile. We believe that children create their concepts from their contacts with the world; the provision of specific opportunities for such contacts, that is, instruction, is but another set of events upon which the child can draw. Didactic instruction seems to be neither a necessary nor sufficient cause for the enhancement of children's reasoning, but that does not mean it cannot play a role, particularly in those cases where we suspect that the child's other opportunities to learn are restricted.

Structuring the Interpersonal World

The child continues to develop his concepts of the interpersonal world as well as the physical world. Until the emergence of self-awareness, all his world was one. Now, however, he sees others as separate from him, and he needs to develop ideas about who these others are and how to behave in relation to them. Just as he differentiates aspects of his physical surroundings, he begins to make clearer distinctions in his interpersonal surroundings. He perceives that there are two worlds of people, an adult world and a child world. He belongs to both and still sees himself at the center of both. What images does he hold about the nature of both worlds?

The child is still working out his relationships with his parents. He goes through the very trying period of saying "no" to everything. His striving for selfhood throughout this period forces him to develop notions about his parents as well as himself in relation to his parents. Part of the development of "self" includes developing concepts of "others," and parents are "significant others." He must establish their identities while he works on establishing his own. He thus tests the limits of behavior and begins to form concepts of the role of "father" and "mother." We saw in Chapter 3 that the child learns his sex role first in the family. His concepts of parents are essential in this process.

In the studies by Mott, the 4- and 5-year-old white, middle class children, whose mothers were predominantly housewives, reported mostly that "mother is a working mother keeping the home running." (Mott, 1954, p. 100) A study of children of professional people (Finch, 1955) showed that these children conceived of both parents as playing roles connected with child-care activities, but saw the mother performing more of these activities as well as performing household duties. Fathers were seen in the role of economic provider. Both these studies, unfortunately, deal with small samples of middle class white children. The fact that the children see the father as playing an important role in relation to themselves points up the importance of seeing the family as a total social system in which all members make an impact upon the perception and behavior of the others. Clark (1967) indicates that the black lower class child does not see this view of the father role at all; father is a fleeting image. The male role is not that of provider of either economic or emotional support. Though the black boy in the ghetto must learn maleness through the same processes as his white middle class counterpart (through modeling, role playing, intermittent rewards and punishments), the result is different because the mother and grandmother wield the real power and maintain whatever family exists. Billingsley, however, points out that "There is no single uniform style of Negro family life, not even in the most depressed sections of urban ghettos." (Billingsley, 1968, p. 142)

That children this age perceive the differentiated role of male and female adult was demonstrated in a learning experiment in which kindergarten children were taught to solve problems. When the leader was a male, both sexes performed better than they did with a female leader, and the boys were more influenced than the girls by changes in the male leader's behavior. (Rosenblith, 1959) Koch, in her study of siblings, found that "girls were rated more affectionate, more obedient, and less resistant than were boys" by female teachers. (Koch, 1955, p. 37)

Children have clearly differentiated the male from the female adult. They respond with discrimination toward them, and their images of parents, although on a superficial "action" level, are essentially in keeping with their cultural experience. Further, the children themselves have identified with the appropriate sex role. They know that boys and girls act differently.

The child world, too, is taking on a differentiated character. It is not all one blur, one mass of kids to play with, where each child is equivalent to any other. The parallel play of the 3-year-old is superseded by the cooperative play of the kindergartner. This child is now aware of social pressures to conform, to be compliant, to give affection, to be discriminating. He even shows the beginnings of ethnic choice in playmates. (Lambert and Taguchi, 1956) Close friendships, not always of a temporary nature, develop during this time, and definite likes and dislikes appear. While there is no peer group in the formal sense of the word, there is certainly a world of peers in which the child is actively engaged in making his way.

A study of 124 nursery school children in Oklahoma, ranging in age from 2 to 5, found that boys display affection toward other boys rather than toward adults or girls. Using a time-sample observation procedure and categorizing behavior into physical and verbal aggression or affection, this study also disclosed that "at all age levels from 2 to 5 the children were more affectionate than aggressive in their response to others and more frequently employed affection than aggression in initiating contacts." (Walters, Pearce and Dahms, 1957, p. 25) Children's contacts with each other reveal that they are not "monsters" who need to be forced into social behavior; their love and affection are deep-rooted. They seek other children, want to be with other children, and look for friendship. The boys' behavior, as observed in both these studies, suggests that they use both affection and rough behavior as means for developing concepts of maleness.

Severy and Davis (1971) analyzed helping behavior in natural settings (a day-care center for retarded children, a University nursery school for young normals, and a school for older normals) and found that behavior could be classified as psychological helping and task helping. In the case of the former, they state that one has to perceive another's emotional states. They found that the young normal children made more helping attempts than the older and that retarded children made more attempts as they grew older. This study supports the above ones in showing helpful peer behavior in the preschool years. Of interest is the decrease of helpfulness in school-age children, which may be seen as the impact of the school in teaching children *not* to be helpful!

That such cooperation is learned and related to the culture is indicated in Kagan and Madsen's (1971) study in which Mexican, Mexican-American, and Anglo children were taught a game in which cooperation paid off. The study showed not only that the 4- to 5-year-olds were more cooperative than the older children (as in Severy's study) but also that there was a clear progression of cooperation from the Mexican being most to the Anglo the least in 7- to 9-year-olds.

We have indicated earlier that modeling is an important way in which children learn. This occurs also in the area of peer helping behavior. A study of kindergarten children, for example, Staub (1971), showed that they were more apt to help a child perceived to be in stress if the adult had modeled such behavior and if the adult had been warm and friendly toward them. Behavior toward peers, then, even in these early years, grows out of the pattern of treatment and perceived cultural values that surround the child. He has already moved to some awareness of the needs of others and his role in relation to them.

Another way to look at growth in the interpersonal realm is based upon Piaget's view of moral development. The standard procedure in studies based upon Piaget is to present children with stories that involve a moral question (guilt-innocence, motive, effect on others) and ask the children to complete them (see Chapter 11 for examples). Using such a technique, Irwin and Moore (1971) found that preschoolers had accepted the society's notions of social justice and had understandings of guilt and innocence as well as payment or apology. These were age-related, with the younger having poorer conceptions, but the movement from egocentrism toward recognition of others is clearly indicated.

By the beginning of school, the child knows that he is an individual and that all other people are not only separate from him but that they are individuals, too. He has also learned ways of coping with and dealing with other people that reflect his awareness of self and contribute to the future development of self.

SUMMARY

In this chapter we have seen how the interplay of maturation and experience has led to the expansion of the child's world. The preschool child has learned much about his immediate environment—about his parents, his neighborhood, and about such ever-present physical factors as space, time, and amount. He has learned to play alongside and with other children.

Although he knows much about his immediate environment, he is still living essentially in a world in which he sees himself as the central figure. He still has a long way to go on the path to maturity.

Chapter 6 will explore the processes used by the child in increasing his self-awareness as he moves along this path. Awareness of self and world go hand in hand, and the events discussed in the next chapter occur during the same time span as those presented above. The shift is one of focus, not time.

REFERENCES AND ADDITIONAL READINGS

Almy, M., Chittenden, E., & Miller, P. *Young children's thinking.* New York: Teachers College, 1966.

Ames, L. B. The development of the sense of time in the young child. *Journal of Genetic Psychology,* 1946, *68,* 97–125.

Bayley, N. Normal growth and development. In P. H. Hoch and J. Zubin (Eds.), *Psychopathology of Childhood.* New York: Grune & Stratton, 1955. Pp. 1–14. Reprinted by permission.

Beilin, H., & Kagan, J. Pluralization rules and the conceptualization of number. *Developmental Psychology,* 1969, *1,* 697–706.

Berlyne, D. Children's reasoning and thinking. In P. H. Mussen (Ed.), *Carmichael's manual of child psychology.* (3rd ed.) Vol. 1. New York: Wiley, 1970. Pp. 939–982.

Billingsley, A. *Black families in white America.* Englewood Cliffs, N.J.: Prentice-Hall, 1968.

Blank, M. A methodology for fostering abstract thinking in deprived children. A paper presented at the conference of the Ontario Institute for the Study of Education on Problems in the Teaching of Young Children, Toronto, Ontario, March 1968.

Brown, R., Cazden, C., & Bellugi, U. The child's grammar from I to III. In J. P. Hill (Ed.), *Minnesota symposium on child psychology.* Minneapolis, Minn.: University of Minnesota Press, 1968.

Bruner, J., Oliver, R., & Greenfield, P. et al. *Studies in cognitive growth.* New York: Wiley, 1966.

Caruso, J., & Resnick, L. Task structure and transfer in children's learning of double classification skills. *Child Development,* 1972, *43,* 1297–1308.

Clark, K. Explosion in the ghetto. *Psychology Today,* 1967, *1,* 30–38, 62–64.

D'Mello, S., & Willemsen, E. The development of the number concept: A scalogram analysis. *Child Development,* 1969, *40,* 681–688.

Finch, H. M. Young children's concepts of parent roles. *Journal of Home Economics,* 1955, *47,* 99–103.

Fowler, W., & Leithwood, K. Cognition and movement: Theoretical, pedagogical and measurement considerations. *Perceptual and Motor Skills,* 1971, *32,* 523–532.

Furth, H. *Thinking without language: The psychological implications of deafness.* New York: Free Press, 1966.

Glaser, R., & Resnick, L. Instructional psychology. In P. H. Mussen & M. R. Rosenzweig (Eds.), *Annual review of psychology.* Vol. 23. Palo Alto, Calif.: Annual Review, Inc., 1972. Pp. 207–276.

Goodnow, J. Problems in research on culture and thought. In D. Elkind & J. Flavell (Eds.), *Studies in cognitive development: Essays in honor of Jean Piaget.* New York: Oxford University Press, 1969. Pp. 439–462.

Gordon, I. J. (Ed.) *Readings in research in human development.* Glenview, Ill.: Scott, Foresman, 1965.

Gordon, I. J. (Ed.) *Readings in research in developmental psychology.* Glenview, Ill.: Scott, Foresman, 1971. (See articles by Sigel and Olmsted, Brison, Kohnstamm.)

Hartup, W., & Yonas, A. Developmental psychology. In P. H. Mussen & M. R. Rosenzweig (Eds.), *Annual review of psychology.* Palo Alto, Calif.: Annual Reviews, Inc., 1971. Pp. 337–392.

Inhelder, B. Some aspects of Piaget's genetic approach to cognition. In W. Kessen & C. Kuhlman (Eds.), Thought in the young child. *Monograph Society for Research in Child Development,* 1962, *27,* 19–33.

Inhelder, B., & Piaget, J. *The growth of logical thinking from childhood to adolescence.* New York: Basic Books, 1958.

Irwin, D., & Moore, S. The young child's understanding of social justice. *Developmental Psychology,* 1971, *5,* 406–410.

Kagan, S., & Madsen, M. Cooperation and competition of Mexican, Mexican-American and Anglo-American children of two ages under four instructional sets. *Developmental Psychology,* 1971, *5,* 32–39.

Katcher, A., & Levin, M. Children's conceptions of body size. *Child Development,* 1955, *26,* 103–110.

Kessen, W., & Kuhlman, C. (Eds.) Thought in the young child. *Monograph Society for Research in Child Development,* 1962, *27.*

Koch, H. The relation of certain family constellation characteristics and the attitudes of children toward adults. *Child Development,* 1955, *26,* 13–40.

Kohlberg, L. Early education: A cognitive-developmental view. *Child Development,* 1968, *39,* 1031–1061.

Kohlberg, L. Stage and sequence: The cognitive-developmental approach to socialization. In D. A. Goslin (Ed.), *Handbook of socialization theory and research.* Chicago: Rand McNally, 1969.

Lambert, W. E., & Taguchi, Y. Ethnic cleavage among young children. *Journal of Abnormal and Social Psychology,* 1956, *53,* 380–382.

Lenneberg, E. On explaining language. *Science,* 1969, *164,* 635–643.

Lloyd, B. Studies of conservation with Yoruba children of differing ages and experience. *Child Development,* 1971, *42,* 415–428.

Lowrey, G. H. *Growth and development of children.* (6th ed.) Chicago: Year Book Publishers, 1973.

Macfarlane, J. W. The guidance study. *Sociometry,* 1939, *2,* 1–23.

McNeill, D. The development of language. In P. Mussen (Ed.), *Carmichael's manual of child psychology.* (3rd ed.) Vol. 1. New York: Wiley, 1970. Pp. 1061–1162.

Mehler, J. Studies in language and thought development. In R. Huxley & E. Ingram (Eds.), *Language acquisition: Models and methods.* London & New York: Academic Press, 1971. Pp. 201–224.

Mermelstein, E., & Meyer, E. Conservation training techniques and their effects on different populations. *Child Development,* 1969, *40,* 471–490.

Moerk, E. Principles of interaction in language learning. *Merrill-Palmer Quarterly,* 1972, *18,* 229–258.

Mott, S. M. Concept of mother: A study of four- and five-year-old children. *Child Development,* 1954, *25,* 99–106.

Murphy, G. *Personality, a biosocial approach.* New York: Basic Books, 1966.

Mussen, P. H. (Ed.) *Carmichael's manual of child psychology.* (3rd ed.) Vol. 1. New York: Wiley, 1970.

Ojemann, R., & Pritchett, K. Piaget and the role of guided experiences in human development. *Perceptual and Motor Skills,* 1963, *17,* 927–940. Reprinted in I. J. Gordon (Ed.), *Human development: Readings in research.* Glenview, Ill.: Scott, Foresman, 1965.

Olmsted, P., Parks, C., & Rickel, A. The development of classification skills in the preschool child. *International Review of Education,* 1970, *16,* 67–80.

Piaget, J. *Le developpement de la notion de temps chez l'infant.* Paris: Presses Universitaires de France, 1946.

Piaget, J. *The origins of intelligence in children.* New York: International Universities Press, 1952.

Piaget, J. *The construction of reality in the child.* Translated by M. Cook. New York: Basic Books, 1954.

Piaget, J. Piaget's theory. In P. H. Mussen (Ed.), *Carmichael's manual of child psychology.* (3rd ed.) Vol. 1. New York: Wiley, 1970. Pp. 703–732.

Piaget, J. & Inhelder, B. *The child's conception of space.* London: Routledge & Kegan Paul, 1956.

Pick, H. Mapping children—mapping space. Paper presented at the meeting of the American Psychological Association, Honolulu, Hawaii, September 1972.

Radke-Yarrow, M., Scott, P., & Waxler, C. Learning concern for others. *Developmental Psychology,* 1973, *8,* 240–260.

Rosenblith, J. F. Learning by imitation in kindergarten children. *Child Development,* 1959, *30,* 69–80.

Rothenberg, V. Conservation of number among four and five year old children: Some methodological considerations. *Child Development,* 1969, *40,* 383–406.

Severy, L., & Davis, K. Helping behavior among normal and retarded children. *Child Development,* 1971, *42,* 1017–1032.

Sigel, J. The attainment of concepts. In M. L. Hoffman & L. W. Hoffman (Eds.), *Review of child development research.* Vol. 1. New York: Russell Sage Foundation, 1964. Pp. 209–248.

Sigel, L. The sequence of development of certain number concepts in preschool children. *Developmental Psychology,* 1971, *5,* 357–361.

Sinclair-de-Zwart, H. Developmental psycholinguistics. In D. Elkind & J. H. Flavell (Eds.), *Studies in cognitive development, essays in honor of Jean Piaget.* New York: Oxford University Press, 1969. Pp. 315–336.

Springer, D. Development in young children of an understanding of time and the clock. *Journal of Genetic Psychology,* 1952, *80,* 83–96.

Staub, E. A child in distress: The influence of nurturance and modeling on children's attempts to help. *Developmental Psychology,* 1971, *5,* 124–132.

Vygotsky, L. *Thought and language.* Cambridge, Mass.: MIT Press, 1962.

Walters, J., Pearce, D., & Dahms, L. Affectional and aggressive behavior of preschool children. *Child Development,* 1957, *28,* 15–26.

Wright, C., & Kagan, J. (Eds.) Basic cognitive processes in children. *Monograph Society for Research in Child Development,* 1963, *28.*

Zaporozhets, A. V. *Razvitie prozvol' nykh dvizhenii* (*The development of voluntary movements*). Moscow: Academic Pedagogical Sciences, 1960. (To be published in English.)

CHAPTER 6
THE DEVELOPING SELF

"I never did, I never did, I never did like
'Now take care, dear!'
I never did, I never did, I never did want
'Hold-my-hand';
I never did, I never did, I never did think much of
'Not up there, dear!'
It's no good saying it. They don't understand."

IDENTIFYING

A major task of early childhood consists of identification with one's own sex—learning the appropriate male or female adult role. We know that the child enters school with fairly clear ideas about who "momma" and "daddy" are; we know that the child differentiates between boy and girl roles. How does he accomplish this? He does so primarily through the process of identifying with the parent of the same sex. Identification before "I" and at the beginnings of the self were with the mother. The boy in early childhood needs to redirect his identification pattern to the father. He perceives the way his father walks and talks, the clothes he wears, the way he relates to the mother, the things he talks about, and the activities he engages in around the house. The boy, using his father as a model, borrows his father's clothes, picks up his language, and "works" around the house. The father, usually pleased by the obvious efforts of the son to emulate him, aids in the process by playing with him, by letting him assist in chores, by buying him junior-size versions of the father's tools, golf clubs, or razor. Often the child doesn't care for the make-believe; he wants to use Daddy's equipment. The toy isn't rewarding to him; he cannot fantasize adequately with it. Wearing Daddy's own shirt, dragging to the floor, is far better than wearing a shirt "like Daddy's," although that is better than nothing.

In our culture, most boys are far removed from seeing fathers at work and have only vague notions of what father does away from home. In our discontinuous society, this phase of the sex role must be learned at a later date. In either a rural or more primitive society, the work life can be seen by the child, and his play includes imitating the work of the father. In such a continuous culture, play blends into work. Boys in our urban, industrial society identify with a partial image of "man."

There seem to be three levels of identification, according to Lynn (1959). These are (1) sex-role preference, the wish to be a particular sex (Brown, 1958, and Chapter 13), (2) sex-role adoption, the acting out in behavior of an aspect of the role of a particular sex, and (3) sex-role identification, the "internalization of the role considered appropriate to a given sex and to the unconscious reactions characteristic of that role." (Lynn, 1962, p. 555) Lynn (1959) postulated that the pattern of development proceeds through these stages. An adaptation of his idea is represented in the following diagram for the development of boys:

identification with mother → male preference → male adoption → male identification.

The girl growing up in a home, if the mother is present, is perhaps in a better position to identify with her own sex than a boy is. For her the culture is more continuous. She can participate in the work life as well as in the home and recreational life of the mother. Much of learning is accomplished through observation and does not necessarily require that the child behave and be reinforced for his behavior. Children see and hear what goes on between the adults around them; they pick up the tones of voice, the actions, and the actual language. Again, adopting Lynn's 1959 framework, identification for girls follows the path indicated below:

identification with mother → male adoption → identification with aspects of the mother's role.

During early childhood, both boys and girls are in the second stage. Identifying includes more than copying the activities, gestures, and speech of the parent. Attitudes and values are also learned through this process. The boy learns not only how to act like a man but also how to think and feel like a man. The girl learns not only to behave as her mother behaves but also to adopt attitudes toward both her own and the opposite sex. Children learn through identifying with the parents and through accepting themselves as "male" or "female."

The issue of parent-parent relationships or the absence of a parent seems to be vital. Hetherington and Frankie (1967), for example, found that when the father was the dominant person, both boys and girls tended to imitate him (which may account for Lynn's "male adoption" for girls) but that when the mother was dominant, girls identified more with her, and boys were less strongly identified with the father. They also indicate that maternal warmth seems important for the girl and paternal power for the boy. Since our society is in rapid flux, we cannot be sure how these patterns will change or even how they apply in the many homes with single parents. What we can say is that "The socialization process by means of which sexual identification is accomplished seems to be a highly complex one in which learning (reward and punishment), role-playing, child rearing practices, modeling and general social expectations all play roles." (Gordon, 1969)

In identifying with parents, children take over and incorporate into their selves a wide range of attitudes and values beyond those concerned with the sex role. Both masculinity and femininity, according to Sears, Rau, and Alpert (1964), are functions more of attitudes about control of sex and aggression than of imitation of parental behavior, freedom being related to masculinity. Protective behavior by mothers feminizes both boys and girls. (Kagan and Moss, 1962) Concepts are learned through identification and, because of the emotional setting in which they are learned, may be difficult to change. Close identification with family values may lead to a narrow view of other people's ideas, values, and ways of life. Studies of prejudice, for example (Trager and Radke-Yarrow, 1952), demonstrate that the seeds are sown during these preschool years. Knowledge of race develops before the child's third birthday.

Although there has been much rhetoric and too little research and although attitude measurement of preschoolers who cannot respond to conventional questionnaires is a problem, there is some work (Sowder, 1972) which suggests that children can identify their own ethnic membership and that, in the selection of dolls for playmates, they reveal ethnic and social class biases, including attitudes toward their own group. Porter (1971) found that such attitudes toward self are influenced by contact, by skin color within the black group, and by the child's sex. Her overall conclusion on the basis of her study of Boston, however, is that "It is clear that many black children have low esteem for themselves on a racial basis; white children are positively attracted to the favored status." (Porter, 1971, p. 138)

Identification is a major process by which roles and attitudes are learned. The early childhood period, it seems clear, is the period of the greatest intensity of identification, of the greatest need to identify. (Kagan, 1958) Since these roles and attitudes are learned early in life in a close interpersonal setting, they become a basic part of the core of the child's self and are fairly stable elements in the way he will feel and behave throughout life.

Role Playing

Concurrently and as a part of identifying, the young child engages in role playing. He acts out the behavior he perceives to belong to certain roles. These may be culturally stereotyped, such as the boy playing milkman, fireman, policeman, cowboy, or "Daddy" and the girl playing house and talking to her dolls as she perceives her mother talking to her. Listening to young children playing a role lends credence to the idea that they are consciously working on being their perception of the other person. Watch them work on being their perception of the other person. Watch how the boy plays Daddy. He kisses Mother goodbye (or uses whatever goodbye ritual, if any, is observed in his home), grabs his briefcase, or lunchbox, or whatever it is that Daddy takes with him, and says, "I'm off to work." He leaves the room. Dead silence follows (because of his lack of concepts of work), and he returns shortly to play the role of Daddy at home. What is he doing? He is trying out, through behavior, how it feels to be Daddy. Children devote many hours of what adults call playtime to this activity; it is essential to their development. With the emergence of new modes of parent relationships, both boys and girls may play a variety of roles. Often Mommy leaves for work as well as Daddy, and often Daddy as well as Mommy cooks and cleans.

G. H. Mead saw this role playing as being intimately connected with the development of language and social meanings. He said, in effect, that by assuming a role, the child takes within himself stimuli for action and response that formerly were possessed by the real person. For example, when the real mother talks to her daughter, she is providing the girl with stimuli for action. When the daughter, playing the role of mother, talks to her dolls, she is learning to respond to her self. "In the play period the child utilizes his own responses to these stimuli which he makes use of in building a self." (Mead, 1934, p. 150) The girl learns what her mother means when she talks to her. By role playing, she increases her understanding of both her mother and herself.

E. Maccoby (1959) analyzed role playing from the viewpoint of instrumental learning and arrived at a position similar to Mead's. Through role playing, the child engages in covert role practice by which he learns how to respond as his parent responded. Maccoby discusses two additional ideas, however, that should not be overlooked when attempting to comprehend the process of role playing in the young child: (1) As we noted earlier, one can never really "take over" the role of another. (2) The child may misunderstand the parent's behavior. He may select the wrong cues, but he has no way of knowing this.

Further, the child may learn behavior in a setting other than the home

—the street, the nursery school—that is more satisfying to him than that which he learns at home, and thus he may act in conflicting ways. The adult may also set up a conflict by overly rewarding one type of behavior while displaying different behavior himself. For instance, mother may tell the child to tell the truth at all times and yet may engage in obvious social lies in front of the child. Also, there may be differences between the verbal content and the nonverbal message. To which should the child attend?

Deciding through role playing is one technique he may use. Role playing is a cognitive as well as an affective process. The child sorts out and arranges what he sees and makes his own sense of it all. In role playing, self-development is the integrated activity of both cognition and affect. As Piaget so aptly stated, "The formation of personality is dominated by the search for a coherence and an organization of values that will prevent internal conflicts. . . ." (Piaget and Inhelder, 1969, p. 158) He reconciles the different messages by testing them out in his own play—a fairly safe way to solve his dilemma. Role taking and identification also prepare the way for truly socialized play and for organized games. We will see in Chapter 9 how concepts of "other" and "self" learned through identification and role playing contribute to the child's ability to play games, to communicate effectively with peers, and to further his self-development.

SELF-EVALUATING

Differentiating "self" from "other," distributing "other" into discrete categories, and learning the roles associated with "significant others," as we have indicated, is affective as well as cognitive. It is the sense of well-being or discomfort accompanying or following shortly after action that conveys to the child what degree of satisfaction or dissatisfaction is associated with this concept of self. For example, on a hot summer day a group of children may be playing on the lawn, dashing back and forth through the sprinkler. They enjoy not only the interaction with peers but also the sheer fun of getting wet and cooling off, working their legs by running, and perhaps most important, playing with the mud and puddles they can create by stopping the sprinkler and letting the water go all in one place. Tactile stimulation, good companions, and an acceptant parent who observes the play from a distance all combine to give the child a sense of well-being. As a part of each experience, the child evaluates its impact upon himself. He evaluates personally, so that he creates over time a picture of his own self-worth.

How realistic are these self-evaluations at this stage of the game? Perhaps not very, by adult standards. Nevertheless, the child has definite images of what he can and cannot do, what his skills and abilities are. A group of youngsters may be climbing a tree, but one child, who looks completely capable to the observer hangs back. Upon questioning, he says in effect that he doesn't like to try it; he'd rather watch. Another child, watching his older brother do something, jumps into the act with "me, too." He almost can't conceive that his older brother might be able to do something he can't do. Of course, when parents make evaluations of performances, as they so often do, the child incorporates their estimate into his. But independently of parents, he makes, by the age of 4 or so, his own estimate of his capabilities.

Although it is easy to subscribe to this idea, it has been very hard to develop effective procedures for assessing the self-concepts of young children. (Coller, 1971) What can we ask them? How can we infer meaning from their behavior? Several different approaches have been used, but all have problems. One approach is to observe behavior and then to infer what perception of self and situation might have influenced the behavior. Let's take an example: Billy, a three-year-old, is playing by himself in a day-care center. Joe comes over and grabs Billy's toy. Think of all the things Billy can do—he can grab back, hit, bite, cry, go to an adult, get another toy, etc. Which behavior indicates a positive view of self? A second approach is to use paper-pencil means. Some of these require the child to mark a happy or sad face (Yeatts and Bentley, 1970), place an X on a line of circles (Long, Henderson, and Ziller, 1967), or in other ways indicate his feelings. But does the child really understand such abstract instructions? Does choosing the top circle in a row of circles mean anything? A third approach has been to use doll play. The study by Porter (1971) cited earlier used doll selection.

One of the critical problems in the study of early child development is the lack of adequate assessment tools. But even with crude measurement, relationships have been found to exist between self-concepts inferred from behavior and first-grade reading success (Lamy, 1962) and between self-reports and such success. (Wattenberg and Clifford, 1962) We need far more work in refining and relating affective measures, such as self-esteem, to other measures before we can really define the importance of self-evaluating in the total picture of development.

STRIVING TOWARD INDEPENDENCE

The poem at the beginning of this chapter states in capsule form how the child at the end of this developmental period might feel about all the pushes and pulls, do's and don'ts, and safety precautions with which we surround him. While he is still strongly emotionally dependent upon his parents, he feels ready to try his wings, to conquer new territory, to reach out on his own. This striving for independence has been manifest throughout this period. Although the early years, ages 2 and 3, are perhaps the most critical times in the child's movement away from overdependence, the nature of the transactional field, and particularly the parents' attitudes throughout the preschool years, will strongly influence the success or failure of the child's efforts to achieve independence.

By about the age of 6, the development of motor control and the development of language have given him the basic skills to use. He can dress himself, make his wants known verbally, control his eliminative processes, etc. But what good are these capabilities unless he can exercise them? What good is a good climbing-tree if Momma says, "Not up there, dear"? The child demonstrates his need for independence by his efforts to find out about himself through what has been labeled negativism. His first response is often "No!" even before he may be clear about what is being asked of him. He is attempting to test the limits, to establish his identity through this (to parents at least) distressing technique.

Baumrind (1967) studied, by means of observations on home visits and during structured mother-child play and by parent interviews, the background of a group of middle class white children who had been classified by nursery-school teachers and psychologists as self-reliant, self-controlled, explorative, and content in contrast to children not so grouped. She found that the former came from homes where parents "were markedly consistent, loving, conscientious, and secure in handling their children." (Baumrind, 1967, p. 80) The children knew what was expected of them, yet parents respected their independence and, indeed, trained them for it. They gave the child a set of expectations—and the reasons for them —and held the child to them in a loving way.

Striving for independence, then, requires parental support, which is not best made manifest through neglect and laissez-faire adult behavior. We do not mean that the independent preschooler is not attached to the family by strong, positive ties; there are ways in which the child seeks independence while still being emotionally close to his family. He plays farther from home, no longer confined or confining himself to hearing distance of the house. He reports back to the family that other parents do things differently, other children can stay up later, other friends have new toys. The basic melody of the adolescent refrain, "All the others are doing it," is played during the end of early childhood.

HANDLING FEELINGS

We have seen that the evaluation process is a feeling as well as a thinking process (if such a dichotomy can be made). The bridge is the concept of *cognitive style,* that is, the way the child approaches a task. As in the use of self-concept, cognitive style has been studied by several means, mostly by asking children to find a shape embedded in a larger pattern (Witkin et al., 1962) or to select objects that go together (Kagan, Moss & Sigel, 1963), and by observing play behavior (Kagan & Kagan, 1970). In her review of these studies and of the antecedents of child performance in parent-child interactions, Olmsted (1972) indicates not only that children can be seen as impulsive or reflective, as analytical or global in their thinking, and as dependent or independent of the surrounding perceptual field but also that these patterns were related to parent-child interactions early in life. The picture is not completely clear, but Witkin's measure of field dependence seems to have been especially reliable over time and across cultures. (Singer & Singer, 1972)

In his transactions, the child runs into situations that frustrate and upset him as well as situations that please and delight him. He has to learn to express these unpleasant feelings in ways that are acceptable to his parents and peers. The infant has no such difficulty. Everyone accepts crying as a legitimate response, even though they may deal with the crier differently. The young child must learn what patterns, in terms of age and sex, the culture deems appropriate.

Early responses to frustrating situations are reflected by temper tantrums, direct physical aggression, crying, and similar reactions. These are "all-out" responses, usually thought by the adult to be completely out of proportion to the situation. The young child's tolerance of frustration and delay is much less than the adult's. When he wants something, he wants it *now*. When he's engaged in an activity, he wants to complete it. Postponing current pleasure for future satisfaction is too difficult. Most young children's negative feelings, then, are evoked by an interference with his activity.

Similarly, children's fears are related to their growing awareness of self and their awareness of others as separate and distinct from them. Their fears change from concern about sudden noises to fear of the dark, of being alone, of "bad men." (Jersild and Holmes, 1935) We know little of the consistency of such feelings as fear. Bronson (1970), in a longitudinal study of 60 children from the time they were 6 months old until they were 8 years old, found that boys were consistent but that girls were not. There was a relationship for the boys between fear of new situations at 6 months and fear at 8. Why this should be is not at all clear. We need further longitudinal studies of many aspects of feelings before we will be able to chart the consistency and changes and to comprehend the how and why.

Each child evolves to some degree his own methods for dealing with tension, frustration, fear, and other unpleasant feelings. He protects his self in a variety of ways. Perhaps the best term to describe these ways is *defense mechanisms*. One major way the child (and the adult) protects himself is through perceptual means. He either denies or distorts the perception or assigns such a personal meaning to the event that his interpretation allows him to preserve the status quo. We're all familiar with the sour-grapes type of response. This is perceptual distortion. The child is not so skillful. He distorts and denies more vigorously. When Daddy says,

"It's bedtime," the child says, "No, it's not!" as if saying it loud enough will change the fact.

Protecting the self and communicating feelings go together. The acute observer can recognize the behavioral clues that indicate that the child is under stress. His behavior is a language that reveals his self to us. Since young children live more "on the surface" than adults, we can more easily interpret their behavior. Of course, knowledge of the situation is essential; otherwise misinterpretation is easy. But, we can watch for denial and distortion, strong negativism, temper tantrums, withdrawal and avoidance activities, or outright physical aggression. They are signs by which the child tells us that the pressure of environment is causing tension within his self. Remember our earlier caution: inference about meanings is a tricky business.

EXPRESSING THE SELF THROUGH
CREATIVE ACTIVITY

The child expresses his self not only through behavior and language but also through creative activity. During the period of early childhood, he begins to handle and manipulate clay, mud, sand, blocks, and boxes. He pounds and piles, feels and smears, shapes and destroys. He derives pleasure from the forms he creates, the texture of materials he uses, the activity itself. The action is as important to him as the product. He also begins to use paints and crayons and produces "works of art" on two-dimensional surfaces. His concern is not with the reproduction of reality as the adult perceives it but with the sheer pleasure of making things.

The child's imaginative play is stimulated by the presence of play materials and natural materials that can be used for play. The games and activities have high emotionality. As Repina reports, "The preschooler reproduces the objects and events that arouse his imagination or emotionally involve him . . . a characteristic feature of a child's imagination is its vividness, its intense emotionality." (Repina, 1971, p. 262)

Although play undoubtedly involves a maturational factor (that is, the child now has greater motor control and coordination), it does not emerge spontaneously from the child. The transactional nature of the situation must be kept in mind. The role of parents in providing opportunities, materials, and themselves as stimuli for the development of dramatic play has been demonstrated. (Smilansky, 1960) Intervention research, such as that by Gordon (1973), has also shown that parents who would not ordinarily provide these materials or experiences will learn to do so and that this has a positive effect on both cognitive and affective child development.

Figures 6.1, 6.2, and 6.3 show examples of methods by which par-

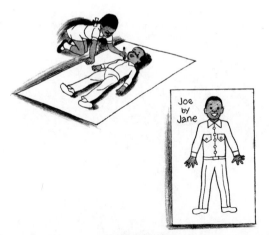

FIGURE 6.1

From I. J. Gordon, B. Guinagh, and R. E. Jester, *Child learning through child play,* St. Martin's Press, Inc., New York, 1972, p. 94. Used by permission.

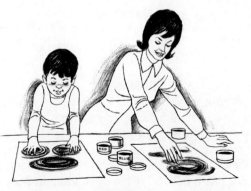

FIGURE 6.2

From I. J. Gordon, B. Guinagh, and R. E. Jester, *Child learning through child play,* St. Martin's Press, Inc., New York, 1972, p. 88. Used by permission.

ents were encouraged to enhance children's play in ways that related to self-identity.

Creative activity requires more than the provision of experience. It requires, at this age, a nonjudgmental attitude. As G. Murphy says so well, "It may be necessary to encourage a long period of groping and gloating, messing and manipulating. . . . he [the child] must richly experience, richly interweave, richly integrate." (Murphy, 1958, 168) Creative activities help the child relate the cognitive and affective as parts of self; they are necessary to adequate self-development. Although it is a cliché, success does breed success.

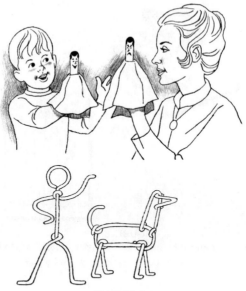

FIGURE 6.3

From I. J. Gordon, G. Guinagh, and R. E. Jester, *Child learning through child play,* St. Martin's Press, Inc., New York, 1972, p. 82. Used by permission.

SUMMARY

The preschool years are highly important in the formation and development of self. The child has differentiated self from other and spends these years building and elaborating his self-structure, learning who he is, who others are, and how to behave. He learns, primarily through his experiences with his family, what to expect of the world and what the world expects of him. His basic notions of his own adequacy are established. He learns ways of coping with his environment and protecting and expressing the self. He has not surrendered his egocentricity, but he has learned that other people have separate personalities.

Throughout the chapter, we have indicated threads of research that highlight the vital importance of parent-child transactions as influencers of self-development. Although there is much still to learn, we are developing sound concepts of what is involved in providing children with sound psychological beginnings. In addition to American research (Hess et al., 1971; Schaefer, 1972; Gordon, 1970, 1972), there is research on the relationships between family variables and scholastic performance in English schools that shows the following conditions to be positively related to school performance: homes in which independent thinking and freedom of discussion occur, in which there are values conducive to intellectual effort, in which children's curiosity and academic aspirations are supported, and in which there is harmony between home and school values. (Miller, 1971)

In a study made in Utrecht, Holland, Rupp indicated the "cultural-pedagogical aspects of upbringing" and found that when high achievers were compared with low achievers within the lowest socioeconomic class, the high achievers came from homes in which parents held this cultural-pedagogical point of view. They saw themselves as educators. They practiced this by "reading to the child, playing table games and word games with him, providing educational toys and books, reading and possessing books themselves, telling their children informative things of their own accord, teaching their children preschool skills, going to places of interest." (Rupp, 1969, p. 176) It is evident from these results and from the material presented in earlier chapters that self-development is influenced by what parents do as information givers, modelers, stage setters, and direct teachers.

During these preschool years, self-awareness has grown from the dim, vague image labeled "I." The child's self-picture now includes many differentiations: self as son or daughter, self as playmate, self as imaginary hero, and many other selves. These are not crystallized but are still fluid. They serve as the framework upon which further concepts will be built. Because of what has already been established, the child is prepared for these new adventures. He is ready now to leave his first safe base and emerge into the larger world, the world outside the family.

REFERENCES AND ADDITIONAL READINGS

Baumrind, D. Child care practices anteceding three patterns of preschool behavior. *Genetic Psychology Monographs,* 1967, *75,* 43–88.

Bronson, G. Fear of visual novelty: Developmental patterns in males and females. *Developmental Psychology,* 1970, *2,* 33–40.

Brown, D. Sex-role development in a changing culture. *Psychological Bulletin,* 1958, *55,* 232–242.

Coller, A. *The assessment of "self-concept" in early childhood education.* Urbana, Ill.: ERIC Clearinghouse on Early Childhood Education, 1971.

Gordon, I. J. Social and emotional development. In R. Ebel (Ed.), *Encyclopedia of education research.* (4th ed.) New York: Macmillan, 1969.

Gordon, I. J. *Parent involvement in compensatory education.* Urbana, Ill.: University of Illinois Press, 1970.

Gordon, I. J. What do we know about parents as teachers? *Theory Into Practice,* 1972, *11,* 146–149.

Gordon, I. J. The Florida Parent Education early intervention projects: A longitudinal look. A paper presented at the Merrill-Palmer Conference, Detroit, February 1973.

Gordon, I. J., Guinagh, B., & Jester, R. E. *Child learning through child play.* New York: St. Martin's Press, 1972.

Hess, R. E. et al. Community involvement in day care. In *Day care: Resources of decisions.* Washington, D.C.: U.S. Office of Economic Opportunity, 1971.

Hetherington, E. M., & Frankie, G. Effect of parental dominance, warmth, and conflict on imitation in children. *Journal of Personal and Social Psychology,* 1967, *6,* 119–125.

Jersild, A. T., & Holmes, F. Children's fears. *Child Development Monographs,* 1935, No. 20.

Kagan, J. The concept of identification. *Psychological Review,* 1958, *65,* 296–305.

Kagan, J. Acquisition and significance of sex-typing and sex-role identity. In M. I. Hoffman & L. W. Hoffman (Eds.), *Review of child development research.* Vol. 1. New York: Russell Sage Foundation, 1964. Pp. 137–168.

Kagan, J., & Kagan, N. Individuality and cognitive performance. In P. H. Mussen (Ed.), *Carmichael's manual of child psychology.* Vol. 1. New York: Wiley, 1970. Pp. 1273–1378.

Kagan, J., & Moss, H. *Birth to maturity.* New York: Wiley, 1962.

Kagan, J., Moss, H., & Sigel, I. Psychological significance of styles of conceptualization. In J. C. Wright & J. Kagan (Eds.), Basic cognitive process in children. *Monograph Society for Research in Child Development,* 1963, *28,* 73–112.

Lamy, M. Relationship of self-perception of early primary children to achievement in reading. Unpublished Ed.D. dissertation, University of Florida, 1962. Reprinted in I. J. Gordon (Ed.), *Human development: Readings in research.* Glenview, Ill.: Scott, Foresman, 1965.

Levin, H., & Warwell, E. The research uses of doll play. In R. Herron & B. Sutton-Smith (Eds.), *Child's play.* New York: Wiley, 1971.

Long, B., Henderson, E., & Ziller, R. Self-social correlates of originality in children. *Journal of Genetic Psychology,* 1967, *111,* 47–57.

Lynn, D. B. A note on sex differences in the development of masculine and feminine identification. *Psychological Review,* 1959, *66,* 126–135.

Lynn, D. B. Sex-role and parental identification. *Child Development,* 1962, *33,* 555–564. Reprinted in I. J. Gordon (Ed.), *Human development: Readings in research.* Glenview, Ill.: Scott, Foresman, 1965.

Maccoby, E. Role-taking in childhood and its consequences for social learning. *Child Development,* 1959, *30,* 239–252.

Mead, G. H. *Mind, self and society.* Chicago: University of Chicago Press, 1934.

Miller, G. W. *Educational opportunity and the home.* London: Longmans, 1971.

Murphy, G. *Human potentialities.* New York: Basic Books, 1958.

Murphy, L. et al. *The widening world of childhood.* New York: Basic Books, 1962.

Mussen, P., & Rutherford, E. Parent-child relations and parental personality in relation to young children's sex-role preferences. *Child Development,* 1963, *34,* 589–607.

Olmsted, P. Cognitive style in children: A review of the research. (Mimeo) Gainesville, Fla.: Institute for Development of Human Resources, College of Education, University of Florida, 1972.

Piaget, J., & Inhelder, B. *The psychology of the child.* New York: Basic Books, 1969.

Porter, J. *Black child, white child.* Cambridge, Mass.: Harvard University Press, 1971.

Repina, T. Development of imagination. In A. Zaporozhets & D. Elkonin (Eds.), *The psychology of preschool children.* Cambridge, Mass.: MIT Press, 1971.

Rupp, J. C. C. *Opvoeding tot school-weerbaarherd (Helping the child to cope with school).* Groninger, The Netherlands: Wolters-Noordhoff, 1969.

Schaefer, E. Parents as educators: Evidence from cross-sectional, longitudinal and intervention research. *Young Children,* 1972, *4,* 227–239.

Sears, R., Rau, L., & Alpert, R. *Identification and child rearing.* Stanford, Calif.: Stanford University Press, 1964.

Singer, J. L. *The child's world of make-believe: Experimental studies of imaginative play.* New York: Academic Press, 1973.

Singer, J., & Singer, D. Personality. In P. Mussen & M. Rosenzweig (Eds.), *Annual review of psychology.* Vol. 23. Palo Alto, Calif.: Annual Reviews, Inc., 1972.

Smilansky, S. *The effect of sociodramatic play on disadvantaged children.* New York: Wiley, 1968.

Sowder, B. Socialization determinants in the development and modification of intergroup and intragroup attitudes and behaviors. In B. Sowder & J. Lazar (Eds.), *Research problems and issues in the area of socialization.* Washington, D.C.: George Washington University, September 1972.

Sutton-Smith, B., & Herron, R. *Child's play.* New York: Wiley, 1971.

Trager, H., & Radke-Yarrow, M. R. *They learn what they live.* New York: Harper & Row, 1952.

Wattenberg, W., & Clifford, C. *Relationship of self-concept to beginning achievement in reading.* Final Report, 1962, Wayne State University, CRP #377, United States Office of Education.

Witkin, H. A. Origins of cognitive style. In C. Scheerer (Ed.), *Cognition: Theory, research, promise.* New York: Harper & Row, 1964. Pp. 172–205.

Witkin, H. A. et al. *Psychological differentiation.* New York: Wiley, 1962.

Yeatts, P. P., & Bentley, E. L., Jr. *I feel, me feel; self-concept appraisal.* Athens, Ga., 1970.

THREE

EMERGENCE
FROM HOME

CHAPTER 7

THE CULTURAL SETTING

*American children are growing up within the most
rapidly changing culture of which we have any
record in the world, within a culture where for
several generations each generation's experience has
differed sharply from the last, and in which the
experience of the youngest child in a large family
will be extraordinarily different from that of the first
born. . . . So long standing and so rapid have been
these processes of change that expectation of
change and anxiety about change have been built
into our character as a people.**

THE IMPACT OF THE CULTURE
Cultural Factors at Work

One cannot understand the behavior of the child without understanding
the situation (in this case, culture) in which it occurs. This is why we are
looking at the external situations—family, culture, school, peer group. One
way of studying this external situation, or cultural milieu, was devised by
cultural anthropologists who lived with a society and studied its ways in
detail. Psychologists have adapted these procedures to the study of
smaller aspects of life, such as child-rearing practices. For example,
Caudill and Weinstein (1969) compared the amount of verbal interaction
and physical contact between mother and infant in Japanese and American homes. Their technique was observation in the home. They found
that by as young as 3 to 4 months of age, the children were adapting to
the cultural pattern of more emphasis on verbal interaction in the American sample and physical in the Japanese. Another technique has been to

* Margaret Mead, "The Impact of Culture on Personality Development in the United
States Today," *Understanding the Child*, 1951, *20*, 17.

observe behavior in structured mother-child situations. Greenglass (1971), for example, had Canadian-born and Italian-born mothers engage in a discussion with their preadolescent and adolescent children and reported that Italian mothers used fewer reasons and more imperative statements toward their preadolescents than the Canadian mothers did. Although both groups tended to increase the use of justifications to the adolescents, the Canadian mothers' justifications were more normative (rule-like); the Italian mothers' were more concrete and specific. Hess and Shipman (1965), Streissguth and Bee (1972), and Olmsted and Jester (1972), among others, have analyzed maternal teaching behaviors with the critical social variable being social class rather than ethnicity.

Steward and Steward (1973) found that ethnicity was more important than class in differentiating the maternal teaching behavior of Anglo-, Mexican-, and Chinese-American mothers interacting with their 3-year-old sons in a standardized teaching setting. The Mexican-American mothers used more original instructions and a slower pace; the Chinese provided the most specific instructional feedback and enthusiasm. The middle class Anglos provided much preparation and informative feedback. The only social class difference was found with the Anglos in the type of feedback. Others, notably Rainwater (1970), Coles (1971), and Polansky, Borgman, and DeSaix (1972), have used mixtures of observations, interviews, and questionnaires to increase our understanding of the life of the poor dwelling in Appalachia and in a city project. Such investigations indicate that family size, living conditions, crowding, and other life-space variables affect maternal behavior, child-rearing practices, and child development. Psychologists too, have used a broad approach. Perhaps the best single example of this approach is in the work of Barker and Wright (1954). They used the term *psychological ecology* to describe the field research into the psychological living conditions and behavior of the children in a particular small town they called "Midwest." The method is not only described in the reference cited above but also in their *One Boy's Day* (1951), which illustrates how behavior is recorded with attention to all the factors in the psychological setting.

To understand the role of the cultural setting as a factor influencing development, we may borrow from Barker his realization of the importance of the behavior setting. He reports:

In our efforts to sample this universe [of individual behavior] adequately, we found that our behavior sample was improved if, in addition to using the usual stratification guides—ages, sex, social class, race, education, and occupation—we sampled behavior in such divergent places as the drug store, the Sunday School classes, the 4H Club meeting, and the football games. Early, we made the not very startling discovery that if we collected behavior in a variety of

*behavior areas, the variability of our behavior sample was greatly
increased, . . . and saw for the first time . . . that behavior comes
not only in particle form, but in extra-individual wave patterns that
are as visible and invariant as the pools and rapids in Slough Creek
west of town. The Presbyterian worship services, the high school
basketball games, and the post office, for example, persist year after
year with their unique configurations of behavior, despite constant
changes in the persons involved. These persisting, extra-individual
behavior phenomena we have called the* standing behavior patterns
of Midwest. [Barker and Wright, 1954, p. 7]

In this chapter, we will be concerned with some of the "standing behavior patterns" as revealed in the mass media and in class behavior. In
Chapter 8, we will look at the school, and in Chapter 9, at the peer world.
Each of these investigations will, of necessity, highlight only certain aspects of the total situation in which the child finds himself. The child is
constantly exposed to the general culture in which his family lives. As he
plays with other children, visits other homes, goes to school, his horizons
widen, his exposure increases, and his views and attitudes become influenced by all he experiences. How he will feel about others, how well he
will do in school, what he will learn, how he will evaluate himself—all this
is influenced by the culture. He will, of course, interpret his experiences
in a personal manner, but the very experiences themselves are cultural.

We often hear of the American Way of Life. Although it may be an
idealized image that ignores the diversity of subcultures existing within
our general society, there is some truth to the notion of an American Way
of Life. The old melting pot notion has given way to one of cultural plural-
ism, reflected daily in the conflicts and cooperative endeavors that cross
race, age, sex, regional, and class lines. America is still defining its way
of life, and the process is sometimes bloody. The notion of diversity is
basic and is reflected in the research by Morris in which various "ways"
were ranked by college students in many parts of the world. American students from various sections of the country gave top rank to the following
"way":

*We should at various times and in various ways accept something
from all other paths of life, but give no one our exclusive allegiance.
At one moment one of them is the more appropriate; at another
moment another is the most appropriate. Life should contain
enjoyment and action and contemplation in about equal amounts.
When either is carried to extremes we lose something important for
our life. So we must cultivate flexibility, admit diversity in ourselves,
accept the tension which this diversity produces, find a place for
detachment in the midst of enjoyment and activity. The goal of life
is found in the dynamic integration of enjoyment, action, and
contemplation, and so in the dynamic interaction of the various paths*

of life. One should use all of them in building a life, and no one alone.
[Morris, 1956, pp. 15–17]

Culture and counterculture groups, potheads and squares, black power advocates and anti-blacks, Indians and Chicanos, Birchites and their opposites, hawks and doves, long and short hairs (and who knows what additional antithetical groups by the time this book is read)—all compete for attention, support, and control, and all reflect the flexibility, diversity, and tension described by Morris. How is the diversity of American life communicated to the child? How is he presented with his own subculture's norms in the midst of the "standard" culture? Major purveyors of the latter are the mass media: TV, radio, books, papers, and magazines.

Mass Media

Social psychologists skilled in the study of propaganda techniques have long been aware of the messages to children contained in comic strips, children's books, and TV programs. Analyses of comic strips made in the 1950s and 1960s to determine what image of America they present to the child indicated that "100 percent Americans," as distinct from those identifiable as members of ethnic groups, played the dominant roles in adventure series. By 1973, the picture was somewhat better but still essentially the same. Just as there had been token integration in the schools, there had been token integration in the media. The use of black actors in TV commercials increased considerably, and series such as *Julia* and *Sanford and Son* were introduced. Children's commercial television, the infamous Saturday schedule, still pays little attention to minorities (7 percent black and 2 percent others were characters), and "all figures of authority or sources of information were white . . . non-American and non-white cultures were referred to negatively almost every time they were mentioned." (ACT, 1973)

The family situation depicted in comic strips and TV shows has also been scrutinized. Father has been depicted as a comic character—weak and easily outmaneuvered by his clever wife. In other cases, a wife is seen as a "dingbat." Teachers, too, are either stereotyped old maids or ineffectual men. Commercials and many of the regular programs convey women in distorted and/or stereotyped fashion and limit their roles as well as their intellect. Gerbner (1966) analyzed stories that included teachers and found that the image of the teacher was higher in Eastern Europe and the Soviet Union than it was in Western Europe and the United States. Further, he found that teachers in the United States were dramatized as less professional and more frustrated by their society than their counterparts in Europe.

The antihero or nonhero is present not only in the literature of the times but also in the films, TV shows, and other media likely to be seen and heard by the young. Attitudes toward right and wrong and justice and evil are also demonstrated in the mass media. On television, for example, "the hero, personalizing virtue, and armed with the impregnable armor of 'right' as well as the six-shooter, confronts evil, personalized by the villain; there is a violent physical struggle; and right ultimately triumphs. . . . In such programs the incidence of violence and threats of violence is great indeed." (*Television for Children,* pp. 11–12) But does this affect the children? The Surgeon General's Report (1972), based upon commissioned studies and reviews, equivocates, stating that the effect of violence "is small compared with many other possible causes, such as parental attitudes or knowledge of and experience with the real violence of our society." (SPHS, 1972, p. 7) Liebert and Baron (1972), Eron et al. (1972), and Stein (1972), among others, present much stronger cases for the negative impact of much of TV on children. Stein, for example, concludes that "most current media content reinforces immature aspects of children's thought and behavior, such as aggressive stereotyping. . . ." (Stein, 1972, p. 199)

The mass media directed at children present a narrow image of American life, a hedonistic, pleasure-principle view. This view does not depict our cultural diversity, and to a great extent it ignores the ideas that all people are worthy, that the use of law is preferable to force, and that values are complex. The media present an ethnocentric, stereotyped view that fails to represent our cultural ways; family and teacher roles are highly artificial, and justice is often extralegal.

But, as the Surgeon General's Report indicated, the role of interpersonal relations and the interpretation of the image of the world by the people they know and trust are more significant in determining children's attitudes than are the media. The chances are good that the printed word or the television screen can reinforce what is already believed or create images where none are present but may not change substantially attitudes and values learned through identification. As in so many areas, research does not necessarily clear up the issue but demonstrates instead the complexity of human behavior and development. We still have much to learn about what the media do to us.

Social Class Membership

The following excerpts from fieldworkers' reports of efforts to work with rural and small-town, lower class women give the flavor of life that cannot be conveyed through statistics. These workers were asked to describe the difficulties they encountered in implementing a parent education program aimed at infant and early child development. (Gordon, 1967)

In Mrs. Jones' home, her friends come over. They like parties. They just don't care what type language they use, and many times I go in

*the home and the baby's on the floor, crawling. They don't change
the baby or anything. There's about 13 people living in the home. The
oldest of the children is 9 with a lot of very young ones. Usually
there's a husband and another woman's husband and a girl friend
and her boy friend. They all come over. They all butt in and ask smart
aleck questions. For example, they say, "Well gee, who would ever
thought of the stupid idea of going and using cans to show an infant
that young anything? What does the baby know?" They thought it
was somewhat stupid for me and the mother to sit there and explain
and show the baby different objects.*

.   .   .

*Mr. Brown is a mechanic and Mrs. Brown is a plain spoken person.
The house is too small for the needs of this family because they have
four daughters. It consists of the parents, four daughters, a girl friend
about 17 years old, the husband's father who lives with them—he
drinks quite heavy—and also Mrs. Brown's father who lives with
them. The friend will not stay with her divorced parents so they are
content to allow her to live with them. The home consists of a living
room with a sofa, a dining room, a kitchen, a small back porch with a
washing machine, two bedrooms and a screened front porch . . .
[the house has] city utilities. The children sleep in the friend's room
which contains two double beds. The master bedroom has one
double bed and a crib. The front screened porch has a single cot in
it. In all, there are only two available sleeping quarters because of
the two bedrooms. The grandfather is 49, but he can't hold a job
because he is an alcoholic.*

.   .   .

*This is a mother where the husband spends his time mostly at the bar
and his money on alcoholic beverages. But she is a fine mother. She
is a mother of eight kids; she's a very busy mother. The husband
makes enough money to support his kids, to put his wife in a good
home, to give his children the kind of clothes they will need for
summertime and wintertime and school and going to church. They
could have these different clothes to wear if the husband would put
his money to a good use. And when I say, "to a good use," I know
that he doesn't, because he drinks this wine. Well the money that I
know he spends on beer, liquor, and wine, if he took to spending it
for his children, the mother could do a lot with it. She told me that she
does a lot of sewing by hand and she sews well. Whenever she sews
and people come to pay her, she has to hide the money because if
he knew that she had any kind of money, he'd go there and bug her
and bug her until he got it. And if she doesn't give it to him, it'll be a
whole mess. She wanted to get the baby a pair of shoes, so she
asked me if I'd go downtown and get them for her. She gave me
some money and told me that when I bring the shoes and change
back, if her husband's there, to please leave the shoes in my car and*

*keep the change for her until I saw her another day or came back
later when I thought he was gone. This type of thing is wrong and
she knows that it's wrong, but there's nothing she can do about it.
She just sits and sews and sees that the children have something to
eat. She knows that they could do better if her husband would come
home and act like a husband should. She tells me he gets this check
from the army because he's retired plus he's working. From the way
she sits down and talks to me, I think she's unhappy with the way
her life is. She doesn't let it show with the children; she said when
she puts the children to bed, this is her time for thinking and wishing
that she could do something better. During the day she doesn't even
have time to sit down and think, or sit down and drink a cup of coffee.
She's always busy. If she's not doing housework, she's sewing, trying
to make another dollar. So she is unhappy, but she doesn't let it show
around the children.*

In contrast, the following example taken from the same general social
group indicates the danger of oversimplification by labeling a family by
social class.

*I started with Mrs. Adams by interviewing her at the hospital. She
indicated to me that she would be leaving rightaway and go to
another part of the state within about three months. Afterward I told
her I would like to meet her at her home. After she left the hospital
and went home I made an appointment to visit. After we talked and I
explained more about the project, she became very interested and
thought it was the right program for her baby. She decided to try and
make other changes to stay here for this project. She said she would
contact me later and let me know if she could work out something so
her baby could still be in this project. I waited for a month and
checked back with her. This time I had great news. She had insisted
in moving here. She and her husband both moved here. I'm not sure
at all if it was the program, but I do think that it played a part. This I
enjoyed most of all, because I felt that I had really encouraged this
mother about the project. After being in the project, this mother was
so interested that after we started she looked forward every week for
my coming in. I do feel very earnestly that this mother is working with
her baby. From time to time we would go to the theories about child
development and these exercises. This mother would always ask
questions about the theories. She let me know she was interested in
what she should do about the theories for her baby. When we did the
testing on her baby, she was delighted to know that the baby would
do as much for the tester as she would do for herself and me. I
enjoyed very much working with Mrs. Adams, and I think she
enjoyed, too, the improvement of the baby. Mrs. Adams is now
working, but she is still interested in how and in what ways she can
get me to cooperate with her, so that she may be home on her days
off for me to continue work with her baby. We tried working with the*

TABLE 7.1 ETHNIC GROUPS IN THE UNITED STATES, 1971 SURVEY

GROUP	SIZE
English, Scotch, Welsh	29,500,000
German	25,500,000
Black	22,600,000*
Irish	16,400,000
Spanish (including Mexican, Puerto Rican, Cuban, Spanish, Latin American)	9,200,000
Italian	8,800,000**
French	5,400,000
Polish	5,100,000
Russian	2,200,000
American Indian	793,000*
Japanese	591,000*
Chinese	435,000*
Filipino	343,000*

* From 1970 census data. Scandinavian not represented in survey, which covered only the listed eight ethnic groups.
** Had highest median family head income at $11,646, national average, $10,359.
Source: Census Bureau data released through Associated Press and appearing in the *St. Petersburg Times,* May 13, 1973.

grandmother, but the baby doesn't respond as well for the grandmother as it does for the mother. So I have arranged to go on her off days even though it might interfere with my schedule. I do hold back this time for them because she is very interesting and I enjoy it very much.

There is a vast body of literature descriptive of social class. The controversy at this time is the old chicken-egg one: Do personal characteristics "cause" poverty or does the state of poverty lead to the symptoms of behavior called lower class? Is lower class behavior denigrated because the research has been done by middle class researchers? Is it a function of societal oppression? Whatever it is, there are group differences in ways of life, and these differences in adult behavior influence the following generation.

Ethnic Membership

Further complicating the picture of a single American society is the rich variety of ethnic groups that exist (see Table 7.1). Each ethnic group preserves certain aspects of its own particular heritage and follows, perhaps unwittingly, the Old Testament injunction, "And thou shalt teach them diligently unto thy children." In a study of Jewish and southern Italian families in New Haven that investigated the dynamics of achievement in America,

Strodtbeck and his colleagues found differences between Jewish and Italian families in terms of expectations. Jewish parents set higher educational and occupational expectations for their sons and had no notions of submitting to fate. The Italian parents set lower educational and occupational expectations, felt that children should remain close to home rather than seeking their fortunes as individuals, and were more willing to believe that one could not influence his own destiny. (Strodtbeck, 1958) But note in Table 7.1 that by 1971 the Italian family head was making a higher income than any other nationality group, including the WASPS (White, Anglo-Saxon Protestants) covered in the survey!

Coleman (1966) in an extensive study of many schoolchildren throughout the United States reported that black lower class youngsters tended to feel externally controlled, victims of luck, chance, or fate; that is, they did not, at the time Coleman conducted his study, have much belief in their own ability to control what would happen to them either in interpersonal relationships or in education. Whether this finding based upon data collected in 1964 is still valid in 1974 is not clear, for certainly there have been tremendous changes in these ten years. The data of black families' expectations for their children seem to indicate that they value education and wish their children to do well in school but that lower class families, both white and black, lack the knowledge of school itself to provide children with specific expectations for school performance.

Studies of day-care centers in New York City revealed that German-American mothers and grandmothers focused on problems of discipline, whereas Italian-American mothers worried less about discipline and more about nudity, sin, and sex. Public showers for preschool boys and girls were accepted by Czech and German mothers, who perceived them as related to cleanliness, whereas Irish mothers rejected the showers. (Opler, 1955) Such ethnic attitudes are not confined to the eastern seaboard or to the big cities of the North. They exist in varying degrees throughout the country. The Puerto Rican in New York, with his problems of adjusting to both an industrial and an urban culture (Lewis, 1965), has his counterpart in the Cuban in Tampa and Miami and the Mexican in the Southwest.

The way of life of an ethnic group is compounded of a mixture of old and new, class and economic variables, and the dynamics of acculturation. The Polish-American in Detroit leads a different life from the Pole in Warsaw; the Jew in New York leads a different life from the Jew in Savannah; the Irishman in Boston is not the mirror image of the Irishman in San Bernardino.

Studies of the American blacks reveal similar social class and regional variables. Northern blacks react to frustration differently from southern blacks; middle class blacks' values and ways of life are quite distinct from lower class ones and are essentially similar to white middle class values. Davis and Havighurst's study of child rearing in Chicago in the

1940s led them to conclude, "The striking thing about this study is that Negro and white middle-class families are so much alike, and that white and Negro lower-class families are so much alike." (Davis and Havighurst, 1946, p. 708)

We cannot talk of a group without placing it in its situation, in much the same way that we cannot understand the behavior of the child without knowing the setting for his behavior. The urban ghetto increases the sense of frustration of those who have to cope with overcrowded, dilapidated dwellings, limited city services, high rents, and the total pressures of what is experienced as a dead-end path. As Hall (1966) indicates, the urban setting, because of the density of population, compounds the problems of the lower class family.

Rainwater, for example, describes parent-child relationships in the St. Louis high-rise project that has since been demolished. A few excerpts suffice:

> Whatever the events that produce the child, he is usually treated with warmth and loving attention, despite his instrumental care being perhaps insufficient or erratic by pediatric standards. . . . Among lower-class Negro women, taking care of babies is regarded as a routine activity which is not at all problematic. There is no great concern with the child's development, little anxiety about the appearance of crawling, talking, walking, and other signs of growth and maturation. These things come as they come, with little more than passing comment on the part of the mothers and others who care for the child. . . . [p. 218] Children enter into household affairs at a very early age. Homes in Pruitt-Igoe are "adult centered," . . . the important matters are those of adult concern, and there is little effort to base household activities on the children and their needs. At the same time there is relatively little effort made to insulate children from adult activities and events. They are generally allowed to observe whatever is going on within the home, and their presence is simply ignored when important adult activities are taking place.
> . . . Adult interest in and interaction with children declines rather sharply as they move toward the school years. Children of four, five, and over seem to be regarded as much less interesting than babies and toddlers, and adults and older siblings are more likely to ignore them, to push them into the background of the family activities. . . . [p. 219]
> Mothers in Pruitt-Igoe introduce children into the instrumental organization of the family at early ages, to help with the heavy demands of homemaking. Girls in particular may take on significant responsibilities—caring for babies, cleaning the house, cooking. As such patterns of responsibility become established, they help to solidify the relationship between girls and their mothers. Boys live in a more anxious and ambiguous situation. There is less for them to

do; they may undertake chores such as going to the store or occasionally cleaning up, but in general they are not expected to take so much responsibility as girls. It is not considered fitting that they do woman's work, and their mothers generally regard males as basically irresponsible. . . . [p. 221] Here is the beginning of a long sequence of development that leaves adult women feeling more in control of their intimate social world than men, that leaves men feeling more vulnerable in that intimate world. [p. 222] [Rainwater, 1970]

An understanding of the individual child requires an understanding of the many subcultures to which he belongs and, more particularly, a knowledge of the specific combination of subcultures. The organization, the arrangement of these, is a clue to understanding behavior. For example, a single child may be middle class, white, Presbyterian, born in New England but schooled in California, second-generation Scotch, and so forth. Each of these factors contributes something to his development—the particular "whole" unique to him.

THE EFFECTS ON CHILDREN

Just what effects do cultural influences have upon the child? Of course, we can make the sweeping generalization that culture and personality are part and parcel of each other, but that does not help us very much. We need to get beyond this anthropological truth to seek out the more specific effects. If we could but look at ourselves, particularly when we travel abroad, we would see the mark of our national character—what cultural anthropologists call our basic personality structure—upon us. It permeates our complete being. If we turn our focus upon the growing child of school age, we see it manifested not only in the total behavior of the child but also in many particular ways: in scholastic performance, self-concepts, attitudes toward others. The child is not purely a cultural being, but he cannot be viewed in isolation from his culture.

Test and Scholastic Performance

Many studies have been made concerning the effects of social class and ethnic membership on performance on intelligence and achievement tests and on the ability to learn academic materials in school. Two major problems that confront us in understanding the relationship between cultural factors and test performance are (1) the degree of bias built into the tests or the school situations themselves and (2) the control of all the other variables that influence test performance. Can we really say that cultural differences cause test differences?

This issue is not only of scientific concern; it also has great political and social significance. The battle among scientists and politicians concerning the wisdom of the "war on poverty" of the late 1960s and the disputes over its results reflect varying views about the relationships between cultural factors and intellectual, academic, and cognitive development. Hess (1969) centered the controversy around two conflicting hypotheses, the deficit hypothesis and the difference hypothesis. In the former, performance by children in school is seen as a function of the inadequacy of the cultural environment, especially the home, in providing the basic underpinnings for school success. In the latter, the culture is seen as providing what the child needs for survival in his culture and as providing him with adequate tools for cognitive and intellectual development, but these tools are seen as different from those possessed by the major culture. This incompatibility thus creates a problem. Whichever view one takes, the effects seem clear; lower class children do worse on standardized tests and perform worse in school than do middle class children. From the point of view of the child, this places him at a disadvantage in the school situations in which he finds himself. While experts offer remedies such as doing away with schools, changing schools, changing the parents, or pumping learning into the child, the individual child faces a difficult time.

A study of black children in southeastern United States (Kennedy, Van de Riet, and White, 1961) reveals that black elementary school children scored significantly lower on intelligence tests than whites. A New York City study (Lesser, Fifer, and Clark, 1965) indicates that there are social class and ethnic group differences in level of ability and ethnic group differences in patterns of performance. On four scales of the Hunter College Aptitude Tests (verbal, reasoning, number, and space conceptualization) given 6- and 7-year-old children, middle class children were significantly superior on all scales and subtests. Middle class children were more like other middle class children of different ethnic groups than they were like lower class children from their own ethnic backgrounds.

Cole and Bruner (1972) elaborate on the deficit versus difference concept and describe differences between competence (the ability a child may possess) and performance (the behavior he produces in a given situation). They state that "those groups ordinarily diagnosed as culturally deprived have the same underlying competence as those in the mainstream of the dominant culture, *the difference is in performance being accounted for by the situations and context in which the competence is expressed.*" (Cole and Bruner, 1972, p. 168) They cite, for example, the comparison of the performance of African children versus Yale sophomores (Gay and Cole, 1967) in which the rice farmers were far more accurate than Yale students in estimating the amount of rice in a container. Evans (1970) reviewed the psychological research on the development of African children and pointed out that whether one used Piaget types of measures or standard intelligence tests, one found that the basic competence was there but was manifested in different ways, depending upon the values and economic system and the cultural experiences in the tribe or region. Several of these studies found that schooling was an important variable in the utilization of abstract thought. Her data offer support for the difference hypothesis and certainly support for the rejection of any genetic hypothesis to account for differences. The problem faced by culturally different children, whether a function of ethnicity or social class, or a combination of the two, is that whereas they may possess basic competence and may have performance skills for being effective within their culture group, they must survive in the larger complex industrial society. It is here that difference may function as deficit.

Language appears to be a key variable. "The most crucial difference between middle-class and lower-class individuals is not the quality of language, but in its *use.*" (John and Goldstein, 1964, p. 269) The middle class child develops more flexible usage. There is considerable investigation of language development at the present time. Such research seems to indicate that standard English as taught in schools is not necessarily the language of the home or the street.

The work of Labov has been perhaps the most significant in restructuring our understanding of the language performance of black ghetto children. (Labov, 1970–1972) His view is that "the concept of verbal deprivation has no basis in social reality; in fact Black children in the urban ghettos receive a great deal of verbal stimulation, hear more well formed sentences than middle class children, and participate fully in a highly verbal culture; they have the same basic vocabulary, possess the same capacity for conceptual learning, and use the same logic as anyone else who learns to speak and understand English." (Labov, 1972, pp. 59–60) However, he indicates that the grammar of the black English vernacular differs from that of standard English. It is in the performance of the child when he must operate with standard English that he is judged inferior. He concludes, "There is no reason to believe that any non-standard vernacular is in itself an obstacle to learning. The chief problem is ignorance of language on the part of all concerned." (Labov, 1972, p. 67) While all this is true, the use of BEV (black English vernacular) in situations that require the use of standard English creates problems for the child in school and for the adult when he seeks certain job opportunities in the larger culture. The problem we face is complex: How do we encourage cultural diversity, benefit from the richness of plurality, and still provide children with the skills necessary for communicating effectively across groups? The culture leaves its impact, and while one may take a position scientifically, political and value ramifications translate difference into deficit.

Sex differences also reflect cultural expectations. Anastasi and Cordova used the nonverbal Cattell culture-free test on bilingual Puerto Rican children in New York. They found that not only did these children score lower than the norms but also that sex and order of language instruction affected results. The girls did better when they received instructions first in Spanish and then in English on the retest; the boys reversed this order. They report, "Each culture stimulates the development of certain abilities and interests and inhibits others. The resulting psychological differences will be inevitably reflected in test performance, as in any other behavior of individuals reared in diverse cultural settings." (Anastasi and Cordova, 1953, p. 6)

The Lesser study indicated that the Chinese children ranked first on reasoning and space, second on numerical ability, and third on verbal ability. The Jewish children ranked first on verbal and numerical abilities, second on reasoning and space. Black children ranked second on verbal ability, third on reasoning, and fourth on numerical and space. The Puerto Rican children ranked third on numerical ability and space, fourth on verbal ability and reasoning. Jewish girls were superior to Jewish boys for both verbal and space scales. Otherwise, boys were higher than girls in the other ethnic groups on these scales. Lesser et al. (1965) interpret these findings to support the notion that different cultures reinforce different abilities.

Although in the above study the race of the examiner was controlled, often black children suffer on tests because of problems of racial awareness. Even preschool children seem to be affected by their awareness of being black and faced with a white tester. Language scores at age 2 were "apparently due to lack of verbal responsiveness, rather than poor comprehension of language." Further, "this apparent early awareness of racial differences and loss of rapport has serious implications . . . particularly in the use of verbal items on intelligence testing." (Pasamanick and Knobloch, 1955, p. 402)

School achievement, as we would expect, is also affected by the cultural background of the home. Regardless of social class membership and, to a certain extent, regardless of ethnicity, a number of parental factors have been found to be related to school success in Western societies. Reviews by Gordon (1970) and Hess et al. (1971) indicate that academic guidance, cognitive operational level and style in the family, educational aspirations, verbal facility, and in the emotional area, parents' own sense of self, belief in their control of their destinies, willingness to devote time to their children, and consistency of management and discipline all relate to child performance. The presence of books in the home is also a strong indicator.

Miller's review of English research (1971), Keeve's (1970) Australian study, and Rupp's (1969) Dutch study all present similar findings. Although there is variability within groups, the above factors seem to be related to social class membership; that is, middle class homes are more likely to provide academic guidance in an intellectual framework, to be homes in which freedom of discussion occurs and in which there is harmony between home and school values. However, as Gordon indicates, "There is tremendous variability within social class groups. If we are interested in identifying particular desirable parental attributes, then social class is not a usable label." (Gordon, 1972, p. 148)

The cultural standing and level of aspiration of the parents play fundamental roles in affecting both the academic performance of their children in school and the development of the child's intellectual powers. It is no great wonder, then, that we see performance differences in children and recognize that these differences are not wholly biological in origin but owe their presence to cultural opportunities for developing perceptions and self.

Attitudes toward Self and Others

Cultural forces affect not only intellectual performance but also the total behavior of the child. What does it mean to the child to be lower class, or black, Chicano, Polish, Jewish, or even a Southern white? Each group that is either a minority or perceives itself to be one mobilizes its energies and defenses in keeping with its concept of itself as a group. Just as the individual denies or distorts perceptions to preserve his self, so does the group. The child learns early that he is living in a somewhat alien world, a world hostile to his group, a world from which he must shield himself. "They" are different from "us," he is told by the actions of his parents, his older siblings, and the other adult members of his group. We noted above that even 2-year-olds were aware of color difference. Northern children rarely fight the Civil War in play activities and are not even highly aware that they are "Yankee"; Southern white children, on the other hand, are highly aware of their "Rebel" status. The early 1973 disturbances in Florida schools over the singing of *Dixie,* the display of the Confederate flag, and the use of the name Rebel reveal that these are still powerful emotional symbols.

The first effect of ethnic or class group membership is a heightened awareness of oneself as different and a corresponding perceptual defense for interpreting the vicissitudes of fortune. The child learns to expect unequal treatment and develops concepts of himself that often tend to reinforce the stereotype. Since one's self-image is learned through evaluational interaction with adults, the child learns from his experiences with nonmembers of his group to evaluate himself in a certain way. He tends to take over the majority's attitude and thus keeps the cycle going. Of course, he learns self-image from the other members of his own group. Considerable effort is presently being expended, for example, to help young black children to enhance their self-image through the notion that "black is beautiful." This, however, reflects the defenses that a minority group establishes because of the overwhelming effect of the majority's view on the self-concept of the minority group child. A comparison of Northern and Southern white and black preschoolers indicates that not only are they aware of differences but also that all groups tended to prefer the white. (Morland, 1966) This view is carried into the school, where black children are more sensitive to the language and behavior of the teacher as indicating racial attitudes. Harlem children, for example, were aware of both the overt means by which teachers threatened their self-esteem (calling them stupid or commenting on their capabilities, race, and the like) and the more covert means of avoidance and distance-maintaining techniques. (Fuchs, 1966) Similarly, studies of Jewish children show early awareness of their Jewishness and increased sensitivity to environmental presses. (Clark, 1954)

Performance may be influenced because the perceptual field is reduced when threatened and also because the particular culture may or may not value certain types of activities or may teach certain ways of dealing with situations. For example, the Navajo, when faced with a novel situation, tends to sit tight and do nothing, to be what Americans might term "rigid" in shifting his level of aspiration. (Bruner and Rotter, 1953) Middle class Americans approach testing situations with a firm belief in competition, individuality, and the value of achievement. Achievement in school reflects this basic approach to life.

There are other ways of evaluating oneself in addition to assessment of skin color or ability. The literature generally indicates that lower class youths measured on whether they feel they control their own fate score lower than middle class youths. A person's sense of control over his own destiny has been shown by Coleman (1966) to be related to academic achievement. At the risk of overanalogizing, it sometimes seems as if lower class black youths see themselves as being on a conveyer belt. "They" do things to you and on you, they put you through a system, and you are shaped and molded. This analogy, of course, can be challenged by the new militancy of ghetto youth. However, even their demand is for instant change from the outside without necessarily a corresponding change in skill, performance, or behavior from the inside. As E. Gordon states, "It is in the area of attitude towards self and others that the crucial determinants of achievement and upward mobility may lie, and it is in these areas that our data are least clear. . . ." (E. Gordon, 1970, p. 303)

The individual's self-concept, his self-evaluation, is strongly influenced by the cultural factors in his life situation. An understanding of what it means to be a member of a particular culture can only be inferred by the nonmember, but an attempt to understand is necessary for any full comprehension of behavior.

Just as self-concepts are based upon cultural experiences, so are concepts of others. Each culture is somewhat ethnocentric; that is, it teaches and believes that it has found the "good life," the "right" way to live, and that persons from other societies are either misguided or inferior. If they could only see "our" way, and if they had the intelligence, they would become like "us." The United States' efforts in Germany and Japan after World War II reflected this belief, as did the earlier colonial attitudes of the major European powers. Since the American culture is not a completely unified one, the various subcultures also reflect this ethnocentrism. Indeed, one of the major concerns of teachers is the presence in their classrooms of large numbers of lower class children who do not wish to become middle class like their teachers! Even the learning of standard English is perhaps influenced by a conflict in values. (Labov, 1964) The child might be saying, "I'll talk my way, and you talk yours."

One of the attitudes that develops is the predisposition on the part of the child to see people from other groups as being all alike, whereas he recognizes the range of differences within his own group. This can be seen not only across national lines but also between generations. Adults tend to perceive all adolescents as alike; pupils tend to perceive all teachers as alike. Although individual members may be exempted with the usual, "You're not like the others," the stereotype tends to be maintained.

Cultural perceptual distortion exists in all of us; it can be understood through our understanding of the process of differentiation and the role of experience. Children growing up in any society are limited to experiences within it and cannot clearly perceive other ways of life. When they do have opportunities to meet and be with people of other cultures, these contacts may either be on a nonegalitarian or artificial basis or may be interpreted so as to reinforce their current attitude. (Campbell, 1967)

SUMMARY

The self of the child is, to a great extent, a product of the experiences that his culture provides for him. It gives him ways to organize his perceptions through its language structure and communications, it brings him into contact or prevents him from having relationships with certain people, it teaches him the values he should hold as "good" and the attitudes he should hold toward self and others.

The culture is taught primarily through the people who surround the child, and he learns through the processes of identification with these people and through differentiation. As he emerges from the home, he carries with him his family culture, a distillation of the various subcultures to which he belongs. His experiences in school and in the world at large continue to both enhance and modify his concept of self and his *Weltanschauung,* his view of the world.

REFERENCES AND ADDITIONAL READINGS

Action for children's television. *ACT Newsletter*, 1972–1973, *3*, 1–6.

Anastasi, A., & Cordova, F. Some effects of bilingualism upon the intelligence test performance of Puerto Rican children in New York City. *Journal of Educational Psychology*, 1953, *44*, 1–19.

Anastasi, A., & D'Angelo, R. A. A comparison of Negro and white preschool children in language development and Goodenough Draw-a-Man IQ. *Journal of Genetic Psychology*, 1952, *81*, 147–165.

Arnheim, R. The world of the daytime serial. In W. Schramm (Ed.), *Mass communications*. Urbana, Ill.: University of Illinois Press, 1949.

Bandura, A., & Walters, R. *Social learning and personality development*. New York: Holt, Rinehart & Winston, 1963.

Barker, R., & Wright, H. *One boy's day*. New York: Harper & Row, 1951.

Barker, R., & Wright, H. *Midwest and its children*. New York: Harper & Row, 1954.

Bernstein, B. Social structure, language, and learning. *Educational Research*, 1961, *3*, 163–176.

Bruner, E., & Rotter, J. A level-of-aspiration-study among the Ramah Navaho. *Journal of Personality*, 1953, *21*, 375–385.

Bruner, J. The cognitive consequences of early sensory deprivation. In J. Frost & G. Hawkes (Eds.), *The disadvantaged child: Issues and innovations*. Boston: Houghton Mifflin, 1966. Pp. 137–144.

Campbell, D. Stereotypes and the perception of group differences. *American Psychologist*, 1967, *22*, 817–829.

Caudill, W., & Weinstein, H. Maternal care and infant behavior in Japan and America. *Psychiatry*, 1969, *32*, 12–43.

Cazden, C. B. Substructural differences in child language: An interdisciplinary view. *Merrill-Palmer Quarterly*, 1966, *12*, 185–220.

Chilman, C. A. Child-rearing and family relationship patterns of the very poor. *Welfare in Review*, January 1965, *3*, 9–19.

Clark, K. Jews in contemporary America, problems of identification. *Jewish Social Service Quarterly*, 1954, *31*, 12–22.

Cole, M., & Bruner, J. Preliminaries to a theory of cultural differences. In I. J. Gordon (Ed.), *Early childhood education*. NSSE, 71st Yearbook, Part II. Chicago: University of Chicago Press, 1972. Pp. 161–180.

Coleman, J. *Equality of educational opportunity*. HEW, USDE, Washington, D.C.: GPO, 1966.

Coleman, W., & Ward, A. A comparison of Davis-Eells and Kuhlmann-Finch scores of children from high and low socio-economic status. *Journal of Educational Psychology*, 1955, *46*, 465–469.

Coles, R. Migrants, sharecroppers, and mountaineers. In *Children of crisis*. Vol. 2. Boston: Little, Brown, 1971.

Colfax, J. D., & Sternberg, S. F. The perpetuation of racial stereotypes: Blacks in mass circulation magazine advertisements. *The Public Opinion Quarterly*, 1972, *36(1)*, 8–18.

Davis, A., & Havighurst, R. Social class and color differences in child-rearing. *American Sociological Review*, 1946, *11*, 698–710.

Deutsch, M. Facilitating development in the preschool child: Social and psychological perspectives. *Merrill-Palmer Quarterly*, 1964, *10*, 249–264.

Deutsch, M., & Brown, B. Social influences in Negro-white intelligence differences. *Journal of Social Issues,* 1964, *20,* 24–35.

Duncan, O., Featherman, D., & Duncan, B. *Socioeconomic background and achievement.* New York & London: Seminar Press, 1972.

Eron, L. et al. Does television violence cause aggression? *American Psychologist,* 1972, *27,* 253–263.

Evans, J. *Children in Africa, a review of psychological research.* New York: Teachers College, Columbia University, 1970.

Fuchs, E. *Pickets at the gates.* New York: Free Press, 1966.

Gay, J., & Cole, M. *The new mathematics and an old culture.* New York: Holt, Rinehart & Winston, 1967.

Gerbner, G. Images across cultures: Teachers in mass media fiction and drama. *School Review,* 1966, *74,* 212–230.

Gill, L. J., & Spilka, B. Some nonintellectual correlates of academic achievement among Mexican-American secondary school students. *Journal of Educational Psychology,* 1962, *53,* 144–149.

Gordon, E. Problems in the determination of educability in populations with differential characteristics. In *Needs of elementary and secondary education in the seventies.* Washington, D.C.: House Committee on Education and Labor, March 1970. Pp. 298–313.

Gordon, I. J. Early child stimulation through parent education. (Mimeo) Gainesville, Fla.: University of Florida, 1967. P. 25.

Gordon, I. J. *Parent involvement in compensatory education.* Urbana, Ill.: University of Illinois Press, 1970.

Gordon, I. J. *On early learning: The modifiability of human potential.* Washington, D.C.: ASCD, NEA, 1971.

Gordon, I. J. What do we know about parents as teacher? *Theory Into Practice,* 1972, *11,* 146–149.

Greenglass, E. A cross-cultural comparison of maternal communication. *Child Development,* 1971, *42,* 685–692.

Hall, E. T. *The hidden dimension.* New York: Doubleday, 1966.

Havighurst, R. J. Social class perspectives on the life cycle. *Human Development,* 1971, *14,* 110–124.

Hertzig, M., Birch, H., Thoman, A., & Mendez, O. Class and ethnic differences in the responsiveness of preschool children to cognitive demands. *Monograph Society for Research in Child Development,* 1968, *33* (Whole No. 117).

Hess, R. Parental behavior and children's school achievement: Implications for Head Start. In E. Grotbert (Ed.), *Critical issues in research related to disadvantaged children.* Princeton, N.J.: Educational Testing Service, 1969. P. 76.

Hess, R. E. et al. Community involvement in day care. In *Day care: Resources of decisions.* Washington, D.C.: U.S. Office of Economic Opportunity, 1971.

Hess, R., & Shipman, V. Early experience and the socialization of cognitive modes in children. *Child Development,* 1965, *36,* 869–886.

Himmelweit, H. et al. *Television and the child.* New York: Oxford, 1958.

John, V., & Goldstein, L. The social context of language learning. *Merrill-Palmer Quarterly,* 1964, *10,* 265–276.

Keeves, J. P. The home environment and educational achievement. Unpublished manuscript, Australian National University, October 1970.

Kellaghan, T. Preschool intervention for the educationally disadvantaged. *The Irish Journal of Psychology,* 1972, *i,* 160–176.

Kellaghan, T., & uHallachain, S. A preschool intervention project for disadvantaged children. *Oideas,* 1973, *10,* 38–47.

Kennedy, W., Van de Riet, V., & White, J., Jr. The standardization of the 1960 revision of the Stanford-Binet scale of Negro elementary school children in the southeastern United States. *Cooperative Research Program Bulletin,* Project #954. Washington, D.C.: Department of Health, Education, and Welfare, Office of Education, 1961.

Kvaraceus, W. C. (Ed.) *Negro self-concept.* New York: McGraw-Hill, 1965.

Labov, W. Stages in the acquisition of standard English. In L. Shuy (Ed.), *Social dialects and language learning.* Champaign, Ill.: National Council of Teachers of English, 1964. Pp. 77–103.

Labov, W. The logical non-standard English. In F. Williams (Ed.), *Language and poverty.* Chicago: Markham Press, 1970. Pp. 153–189.

Labov, W. Academic ignorance and black intelligence. *Atlantic Monthly,* 1972, *229,* 59–67. Copyright © 1972, by The Atlantic Monthly Company, Boston, Mass. Reprinted with permission.

Lavin, D. *The prediction of academic performance.* New York: Russell Sage Foundation, 1965.

Lesser, G. Problems in the analysis of patterns of abilities: A reply. *Child Development,* 1973, *44,* 19–20.

Lesser, G., Fifer, G., & Clark, D. Mental abilities of children from different social-class and cultural groups. *Monograph Society for Research in Child Development,* 1965, *30.*

Lewis, O. *La vida.* New York: Random House, 1965.

Liebert, R., & Baron, R. Some immediate effects of televised violence on children's behavior. *Developmental Psychology,* 1972, *6,* 469–475.

Lloyd, B. Studies of conservation with Yoruba children of differing ages and experience. *Child Development,* 1971, *42,* 415–428.

Makarenko, A. S. *The collective family: A handbook for Russian parents.* New York: Doubleday, 1967.

Mead, M. The impact of culture on personality development in the United States today. *Understanding the Child,* 1951, *20,* 17–18.

Miller, G. W. *Educational opportunity and the home.* London: Longmans, 1971.

Morland, J. K. A comparison of race awareness in northern and southern children. *American Journal of Orthopsychiatry,* 1966, *36,* 22–31.

Morris, C. W. *Varieties of human value.* Chicago: University of Chicago Press, 1956.

Neubauer, P. (Ed.) *Children in collectives: Child rearing aims and practices in the kibbutz.* Springfield, Ill.: Charles C Thomas, 1965.

Olmsted, P., & Jester, R. E. Mother-child interaction in a teaching situation. *Theory Into Practice,* 1972, *11,* 163–170.

Opler, M. K. The influence of ethnic and class subcultures on child care. *Social Problems,* 1955, *3,* 12–21.

Pasamanick, B., & Knobloch, H. Early language behavior in Negro children and the testing of intelligence. *Journal of Abnormal and Social Psychology,* 1955, *50,* 401–402.

Pinneau, S. R., & Jones, H. E. Development of mental abilities. *Review of Educational Research,* 1958, *28,* 392–400.

Polansky, N., Borgman, R., & DeSaix, C. *Roots of futility.* San Francisco: Jossy-Bass, 1972.

Rainwater, L. *Behind ghetto walls.* Chicago: Aldine, 1970.

Rupp, J. C. C. *Opvoeding tot school-weervaarherd (Helping the child to cope with school)*. Groninger, The Netherlands: Wolters-Noordhoff, 1969.

Schwebel, A. Effects of impulsivity on performance on verbal tasks in middle- and lower-class children. *American Journal of Orthopsychiatry,* 1966, *36,* 13–21.

Sheldon, W., & Carrillo, L. Relation of parents, home, and certain developmental characteristics to children's reading ability, I. *Elementary School Journal,* 1952, *52,* 262–270.

Sheldon, W., & Cutts, W. Relation of parents, home and certain developmental characteristics to children's reading ability, II. *Elementary School Journal,* 1953, *53,* 317–521.

Shuey, A. Stereotyping of Negroes and whites: An analysis of magazine pictures. *Public Opinion Quarterly,* 1953, *17,* 281–287.

Spiegelman, M., Terwilliger, C., & Fearing, F. The content of comic strips: Goals and means to goals of comic strip characters. *Journal of Social Psychology,* 1953, *37,* 189–203.

Stein, A. H. Mass media and young children's development. In I. J. Gordon (Ed.), *Early childhood education.* NSSE, 71st Yearbook, Part II. Chicago: University of Chicago Press, 1972. Pp. 181–199.

Steward, M., & Steward, D. The observation of Anglo-, Mexican-, and Chinese-American mothers teaching their young sons. *Child Development,* 1973, *44,* 329–337.

Streissguth, A., & Bee, H. Mother-child interactions and cognitive development in children. *Young Children,* 1972, *27,* 154–173.

Strodtbeck, F. L. Family interaction, values and achievement. In D. C. McClelland (Ed.), *Talent and society.* Princeton, N.J.: Van Nostrand, 1958. Pp. 135–195.

Television for children. Boston: Foundation for Character Education, undated (circa 1959).

Ten Houten, W. The black family: Myth and reality. *Psychiatry,* 1970, *33,* 145–173.

United States Public Health Service. *Television and growing up: The impact of televised violence.* Report to the Surgeon General, Washington, D.C., 1972.

Williams, F. (Ed.) *Language and poverty.* Chicago: Markham, 1970.

CHAPTER 8

"SCHOOL DAYS, SCHOOL DAYS"

THE SCHOOL AS A
SOCIAL INSTITUTION

The school is second only to the family in its impact upon the self of the child. Up until the time of the child's entry into school, the family has constituted a buffer that is constantly at hand to interpret experience. When playing, watching TV, or being read to, the child has virtually immediate access to a parent or parent-surrogate for explanation, support, and information. Going to school changes all this. He moves into a new society, with its own way of life—the school culture. He must come to grips with it all alone, without the aid of parents. Truly, he is on his own for the first time. Of course, in the modern school there are such institutions as the PTA and parent-teacher conferences, but the ability of the parent to intercede directly in the experiences of the child is limited. To some parents and to some children, this is a distressing thing; to others, it is a cheerfully accepted sign of growing up.

We know that schools teach not only the "fundamentals" but also values and behavior patterns, concepts of the world and self, and the whole gamut of information, both formal and informal, that is deemed necessary to the child in the process of becoming an adult in contemporary society. In this chapter we shall only attempt an overview of the school; subsequent chapters will provide further details.

What Schools Are versus What Schools
Ought To Be

As with any social institution in a changing, pluralistic culture, there is considerable disagreement as to what schooling should be. The mass media often contain both attacks and praise (although far more of the former). Labels are pinned on points of view, such as "traditional" and "progressive," and parents ask, "Why isn't arithmetic taught the way I learned it?"

or "Why do they have family life courses in high school?" Trends of concern for the gifted dominate educational literature, followed by waves of concern for the retarded. No one seems to be satisfied with the school as it is; everyone wants to remake it in terms of his own ideas.

The important fact to the child is that attitudes toward school held by his parents are communicated to him. He knows school only as it is today for him. He cannot comprehend, if he goes to a school with movable furniture, that his father's school had nailed-down desks lined up in rows. He cannot comprehend that his parents' reactions toward school may stem from their uncertainties or from their own unfortunate experiences with school as it was. Controversies over phonics, ungraded schools, and grouping may rage around him; he only knows what he experiences and what his parents communicate to him.

Educational literature, full of suggestions for what schools *should be,* offers little help in knowing what schools *are.* In order to understand school as it is experienced by the child, we need to look at what practices currently exist—what schools *are.*

Schools as Reflecting
the Community's Values

By and large, what is taught in a school and how it is taught is governed not only by the educational theoreticians and the classroom teachers but also by the local community and the state. School administrators are not independent agents but are influenced by the power structure of the community. Often they have no tenure as administrators and must conform to what boards of education, composed of laymen, demand. Various groups within the community attempt to influence a board. No school is free of this, so no school is purely progressive or traditional; it reflects the total of all the varying ideas and pressures placed upon it and is usually an unintegrated compromise. Actually, for the child, it is a rare school that possesses (and follows) an integrated philosophy of education. Each teacher in turn helps to shape the image of school by his own interpretation of life and his concept of the role that schooling plays in living.

Changes in curriculum require the mutual consent of school and community personnel. The school acts to teach and reinforce those values and skills perceived by the community as desirable, or at least those so perceived by the power elements of the community. Studies of the power structure of the community and the school (Hines and Curran, 1955; Kimbrough, 1963) reveal that each community, to a certain extent, has its own particular alignment but that, generally, newspapers and organizations bring pressure to bear and that the lower class and ethnic minorities have less than proportional influence. School board members are usually well-educated business or professional people with children in school. The control of education thus rests in the hands of middle class, conservative people. Schools reflect their views. Not only historical national forces but also current forces play roles. Mobility patterns are such that parents at PTA meetings in one state refer to what schools were doing in the state they just left.

Textbook publishers, too, help to shape what happens in the classroom through their books, their extra guides and other publications, and through the resource people they furnish to school districts for in-service teacher training. In addition, the merger of "hardware" (IBM, RCA) and "software" book companies (SRA, Random House) to form large-scale educational corporations is another force shaping the school.

The federal government, through its establishment of research and training programs, its regional laboratories, and its direct aid to school systems under the Elementary and Secondary Education Act of 1965 also influences the curriculum, materials, and organization patterns of schools. One example of how the picture is changing a little is to be found in a special research and development program, originally funded under the Economic Opportunity Act (also the source of Head Start), called the Follow Through Program. In this program a unique pattern of teaming outstanding early-childhood projects with school systems was employed to implement planned variations of programs throughout the country. These programs have diverse philosophies and delivery systems, but those involved as program sponsors agree that the concept of an external, accountable agency working with school and parents is a successful device for change. In the Florida Parent Education Program (Gordon, 1972), for example, home visits by paraprofessionals are functional for both poor and middle income parents. Parents are able to work effectively in a variety of fashions as decision makers regarding staff and curriculum and as volunteer teachers in classrooms in ways that shape the school to better meet the needs of those formerly excluded from power.

The reintroduction of parents into schools transcends Follow Through and the earlier parent-involvement activities of Head Start. States such as California and Florida are moving toward mandated parent involvement by going so far as to have a parent advisory committee for each school. In addition, the court-ordered desegregation of schools has had a major impact. Emotions ran high in the 1972 primaries over bussing, and there has been a degree of "white flight" from desegregated schools. The issue of how best to provide good and desegregated education is far from resolved. (Weinberg, 1970)

Generally, what the child will experience in school is a conglomerate of the American culture, with certain middle class, conservative values and behavior patterns receiving more emphasis. No school teaches a culture alien to the "American way." The child of middle class parents will generally find the school reinforcing the values being taught in the home while it also presents him with the 3 Rs.

We mentioned above that the individual teacher in the classroom takes the generalized institution of "school" and modifies it in his own terms. Today, this may lead to conflict between teacher and administrator as teachers push for true professionalization and a voice in the decision-making process through their organizations.

Studies of the social origins of teachers show that they come from a wide variety of backgrounds despite the stereotype of white collar, middle class background. Although the stereotype has some validity for elementary teachers, it is not true for high school teachers in urban areas, whose family backgrounds may be lower class.

Cohen's (1967) review of social status led her to conclude that teachers are drawn from all elements of the society, with lower blue collar groups underrepresented and professional and managerial groups contributing more than their share. For those from low-status backgrounds, teaching is a path for upward social mobility. (Davis, 1965)

What does this mean in classroom practice? Even though we cannot and should not stereotype class membership, teachers are usually either middle class or upwardly mobile. "In any event, however, no matter what their initial social status, almost all teachers give allegiance to the basic middle-class values in the areas of personal ambition and morality. . . . Children from families lowest in the socioeconomic scale tend to find school a place of alien standards." (Wattenberg et al., 1957, p. 69)

Teachers tend to encourage and favor those children whom they "understand"—those children whose homes are like theirs, whose dress and speech are like theirs, whose "manners" are "good," whose parents value what the teachers value. These biases show in their behavior. Among other examples, third-grade teachers seemed to behave differently toward middle class and lower class children, having a more favorable "mental health" relationship with the former. (Hoehn, 1954)

In addition to social class, sex role has an influence. The elementary school, with some few exceptions in urban areas, is largely a feminine institution. Teachers tend to favor "good" behavior and to make similar demands upon boys and girls. Girls are more able to meet these demands, and all indices of difficulty in school show a significantly greater number of boys than girls. Primary teachers in a suburban area, for example, favored achieving girls over achieving boys, and preferred dependent girls the most. (Levitin and Chananie, 1972) It is generally known that teachers have more negative interactions with boys than with girls. Even sex differences in language development may rest partly on this base. (Waetjen and Grambs, 1963)

A word of caution must be inserted here. The assumption that the social class of the teacher relates to particular behaviors has not been tested. A teacher's behavior is influenced by situational classroom factors, by his own perceptions of self and others, and by the external demands of the system (see Chapter 11 for some specific examples of this). Nevertheless, he cannot overlook the impact of his own particular subculture.

SCHOOLS HAVE A CULTURE

Perhaps the best way to understand the role of the school is through the adoption of the concept that the school is a culture, a way of life, and that it can be studied as such. The school has values and ways of communicating these; it has a series of expectations and a series of routines of communicating these; it has an interpersonal climate in which socialization occurs; it operates in a physical setting that also conveys its value system.

Each school may be viewed as a subsociety possessing its own way of life. Students entering this school must learn its culture, which may or may not be in harmony with the culture learned at home. Through the socialization process taking place in the school culture, each child broadens his self-picture and either modifies or strengthens it. He learns, in addition, the culturally approved patterns of thought and either accepts, modifies, or rejects these, based upon the self with which he came to school. As in any culture, there are mores and folkways, both written and unwritten, that govern the behavior of most of the members and systems of rules to discipline those who do not conform. The child leaving home and entering the school thus has a whole range of new cultural experiences to integrate into his growing self.

Grouping and Grading, School Organization

In the street on the way to school or in the school bus or in the neighborhood, the child mixes with children of various ages. He is conscious of his own age, but it isn't until he steps inside the door of the school building that age becomes a crucial fact. If he is born a day too late, he waits a whole year to enter. Being in the first grade, or second grade, or whatever grade becomes a dominant factor. What grade he is in governs his access to certain age-mates or peers; it influences his status within the school; it even affects what time he may eat lunch! The concept of grade level, although a number of school districts are attempting to use ungraded classes, is a major factor in influencing expectations and identifications. Even the teacher identifies himself by the grade he teaches.

Grade levels based on chronological age create a false impression of homogeneity. Both parents and teachers tend to think of the "typical" or "average" second-grader and lose sight of the wide range of individual differences among the children. Testing programs and other administrative devices all share in attempting to create homogeneity where little exists. In spite of much research on promotion and grade-level standards, schools are still basically grade-level oriented, and as much as one-third of a class of first-graders may be repeaters.

The data indicate that nonpromotion is not an effective technique for the setting of standards (Prescott, 1957) and that achievement or ability grouping per se does not lead to differential achievement. (Abramson, 1959; Goldberg & Passow, 1966)

Within a class, teachers group for reading, with three groups being the typical pattern. One wonders here, too, what impact being in the slow reading group has upon the self-concept of the child. Many teachers use systems of individualized reading or flexible grouping, and these would seem to be more desirable.

It is not only in the elementary school that grouping and grading present the child with a set of hurdles that influence his self-picture. The secondary school, in its attempts to meet individual needs through separate "tracks" for academic, general, commercial, and vocational students, its accelerated classes and its general math courses, demonstrates a hierarchy of values to the adolescent. He may perceive that the academic student is worth more than the vocational student in the eyes of the community. The student who is shunted into general math or general science or denied admission to accelerated programs may see high school as a threatening, defeating experience. Conversely, the gifted youngster may wonder whether anyone is interested in him as a person rather than as a natural resource. He may be counseled into advanced algebra in the eighth grade when he has little desire for a scientific career.

New organizational forms, such as team teaching, the middle school, and independent study programs, are all presented as efforts to reach individuals; yet there is no solid body of research at present to support these changes. Automated classrooms, with portions of the work on a computer-assisted basis, present the child with new images of the world in which he lives.

The very organization of the school—its promotion policies, the methods used by teachers to organize their classes, class size, hardware—provides guideposts for the child's behavior. All of these show the pupil what and who is important in this new culture. He soon learns the ropes. He sees cues to his behavior in the behavior of his teachers. The teacher and the school become new anchorage points in his perceptual field. The school grounds can be placed upon the child's psychological map as well as on a physical map. The way of life of the school and its culture become incorporated into his way of life.

This school culture may be examined by studying its status arrangements, its physical environment, its daily pattern of activity, and its stated goals. Each of these impart information to the child about how he should behave, what he should learn, what his self should become.

Status Relationships

Three kinds of status relationships exist in a school culture—those between administrator and faculty, those within the faculty, and those within the student body. Our concern is not the status relationship per se but its effect upon children's development.

The way in which the principal plays his assigned status role has direct bearing on the behavior of the students. Two studies may serve to illustrate this point.

The first study was in an elementary school described by its faculty and by research observers as rigid and authoritarian. The teachers, observers recorded, "in a way, seemed to be afraid of her [the principal], reporting like children on what they had done and how they managed." (Taba, 1955, p. 63) The children's value patterns were found to present a picture of social distance, immature interpersonal perceptions, and overemphasis on competitive comparison.

Second, as a part of the Kellogg studies in educational administration, it was found that pupils' attitudes were influenced by the principal's behavior. In an investigation of principal, teacher, and pupil behavior in Tampa, Florida, it was found that if the principal were autocratic, pupils expressed unfavorable attitudes toward self, school, and other students. The more democratic the principal, the more favorable the attitude of pupils. (Maynard, 1955)

Status relationships among faculty members are influenced by length of service, degrees held, social origins, and the subject taught. Many school systems now employ aides, who are paraprofessionals and often drawn from the community. This introduces a whole new status group that is usually ranked below teachers. This status arrangement in a faculty affects its morale and productivity, which, in turn, affect the learning climate for youngsters.

School policies often reflect the status situation. For example, children may be excused from certain classes for trips or other extracurricular activities but are not allowed to cut some other classes. The students soon learn what subjects are considered really important by the school. In one high school, for example, chemistry laboratory space was reduced so there could be more room for driver-education classes; in another, the core period (combined English and social studies double period) was the one always affected by extra band practice, rehearsals for the junior play, and the like. What possible concepts could students develop other than that chemistry and core were less significant than driver education and band?

Children are exposed to these status relationships because the teachers often make them explicit. In an intermediate-grade classroom, the following incident occurred:

Mrs. Jones announced, "Today for physical education we will have a rhythm lesson." Mark's hand went up. "Yes, Mark?" "Coach Harris told us boys we could play football today." Mrs. Jones replied, "Coach Harris made a mistake. Each Friday at 10 o'clock will be your rhythm lesson."

On the other hand, teachers have pushed the notion of equality of pay and status in their dealings with the public. They view themselves as almost interchangeable parts and do not know how to plan, delegate responsibility, and differentiate function. Even in team teaching, it was found that 90 percent of the work was planned by individual teachers. (Norwalk, 1963) As Joyce indicates, teachers resist a formal hierarchical structure within the teacher group. (Joyce, 1967) However, they do have a highly developed, informal structure, and the child gets the message.

The most significant status relationships, however, are not the ones among adults but the ones among the pupils themselves—the peer status hierarchy. This is so vital that Chapter 9 is focused on the peer culture itself, and the chapters on adolescence will include material on peer relationships during that period.

Physical Plant

In building new schools, there is a definite relationship between the philosophy of education held and the type of building erected.

The physical plant reveals the culture of the school as much as skyscrapers reveal the culture of a city. The relationship is perhaps even more direct with schools, because the building occurs by design. The people pass bond issues to build school buildings, but not to build commercial structures. Decisions are made to build gymnasiums before libraries, auditoriums before kindergarten rooms, teaching auditoriums rather than individual classrooms, removable rather than fixed walls, administrative wings at a sacrifice to other uses of space. All these choices reflect what the powers controlling school budgets believe to be important. They present in brick and steel the adults' notions of what schools ought to be. The changes in thought about the nature of the learning process and the increased knowledge about child and adolescent development have wrought changes in school buildings.

The analytical observer can deduce from his observations of the building itself something about the adult world's beliefs about how children learn and what children should learn. Of course, old buildings still much in use may not reflect the changes in attitudes toward children and learning. Many a teacher has been frustrated in his attempts to provide a good, flexible learning situation in a room in which all the chairs are nailed to the floor.

The Hidden Agenda—Routines
and Procedures

Although all the above factors influence the child, the actual day-to-day operations of his classroom—the interpersonal relations, the rules and regulations, the experiences that are provided—are the most crucial factors, but they are often taken for granted by both teacher and pupil. The many routines that permeate the daily activities are almost a part of the scenery.

Beginning with the first day in nursery school or kindergarten and extending through graduate school is the unending concept of clock time: The student is expected to learn that there is a time to play, a time to rest, a clean-up time, a time to listen, etc. The older child or adolescent in the departmentalized situation is expected to learn in 40- or 50-minute intervals, shift his focus, and learn something different in the next period. The lesson of the clock is perhaps essential in a modern, industrial world. Unfortunately, it may mean that young children are prevented from staying with a highly interesting task and forced to shift their focus to other activities.

If we realize that motivation is self-oriented, then we might well question the highly time-oriented, compartmentalized approach to education that is so widespread. Children soon learn, it is true, to adjust to time pressures, but this does not mean that such pressures are desirable. "If there is any single issue on which the school system has been most at odds with its slums it is on the matter of time. If you can look forward to spending your whole life unemployed and draped on a street corner, what's the rush? Schools don't see it that way. They are obsessed with time." (Miller, 1966) Notions of attention span being related to age might also be questioned when we can observe children thoroughly engrossed for long periods of time in activities that are meaningful to them. Many good elementary classrooms provide for variable scheduling of activities within the classroom to allow children to express and meet their individual needs. The concept of the open school, which is based somewhat superficially on the British Infant School, is an example of efforts to break the lockstep. Concepts of modules are appearing in high schools. These allow for flexible scheduling and reflect a more sophisticated approach to learning.

A standard activity in virtually all schools is the opening exercise. The following is an excerpt from an observation in a primary grade—the first class meeting in January 1959. (One can see the same activity in January 1975!) The observer, seated in an observation booth, writes:

The class was sitting crosslegged on the floor and Mrs. Hall was collecting money for something. Mrs. Hall said, "Mark owes 3 × 30 cents and he has a dollar, how much does he get back in change?" Jeff raised his hand and yelled, "Ten cents." Mrs. Hall said, "That's very good, Jeff." Another boy said, "Joe said ten cents too!" Mrs. Hall said, "Oh, I didn't hear him." The class said, "Yes, I heard him," and "Joe said it too." Joe said, "Yes, I knew that answer." The class then took turns going to the front of the room and telling the class what Santa gave them for Christmas and their experiences over the holidays. (I didn't see any sign of ending the math lesson and beginning the story telling.) Sally explained a certain game she had received for Christmas. Joe sat crosslegged in the front row and said, "Does the game have beads on which to count?" Sally said, "Yes, it does." Joe said, "Oh, well, I've seen one like that before."

Mrs. Hall said, "Class, let's help Karen so she can . . . [take the] roll." The girls all stood up and counted off, then they sat down and the boys did the same thing. Joe said, "Warren isn't here today." Mrs. Hall said, "Thank you, Joe; now, Karen, take the list to the office." The class then continued the story telling. Mrs. Hall said, "Ann will be the last one to share her experience over Christmas with the class." Joe sighed and said, "Oh, gosh." Mrs. Hall said, "We have to start something else, Joe." Joe sighed again and put his fingers in his mouth. Mrs. Hall said, "Everyone stand," after Ann had finished her story. The class stood and started singing, "The Grand Old Flag," "My Country 'Tis of Thee," and "America." Mrs. Hall said, "Stand straight." Joe straightened up and put his hands behind him. The class then said the "Our Father" and the "Pledge of Allegiance" while Hal held the flag at the front of the room. The class sat down on the floor after pledging the flag.

An analysis of this observation reveals a number of values and concepts being presented—the child's image of Christmas, patriotism, time, numbers, support for each other, obedience to adult authority, the sharing of experiences. Of course, some of these are not explicit, but they are still present. Frequently a teacher will put a more explicit statement of values on the chalkboard or bulletin board, often one that contains the standards (or at least the teacher's standards) of conduct for the room. One such list, labeled "Good Citizens in the Fourth Grade," contained these items: "A good citizen listens, is responsible, pays attention, sticks to his job, is thoughtful of others, is honest, is helpful, shares with others."

Outside the classroom the extracurricular life of the school also demonstrates values to the child. Club membership, cliques, student activities, elections of officers all serve either to spread the school's culture or to isolate certain segments of the school population. This seems to be true in elementary schools as well as in high schools.

Based upon an analysis of class and ethnic status and the culture of several schools, Taba concludes, "Usually there is a correlation between the parental economic status and school participation; students whose families have community status have status in school. Their chances of developing their self-expectations, both in school and at home, are great, while others are deprived of such chances in both." (Taba, 1955, p. 67)

Academic Expectations

Nowhere in the above discussion have we dealt with the question of what, specifically and consciously, the school sets out to teach the child. Schools traditionally teach subject matter and intellectual skills. These are certainly perceived by both teacher and pupil as the main job of the school. In the modern world, each child needs to know as much as he can about other peoples, about science and technology, about effective communication with others, about his cultural heritage, his system of government, and the like. Both the pupil and his teachers expect him to learn these things at school.

Although the pupil may not use the teacher's words to describe his view of school, he does know that there are, and should be, certain academic expectations. The child entering first grade expects to learn how to read and write and may expect to learn these the first day. The youngster entering junior high expects to move into a departmentalized subject-matter system in which English is taught separately from math and even the social studies may be divided into history, geography, civics, economics, etc.

But subject matter is a poor definition of academic expectation. The curriculum reforms of the 1960s were based on psychological notions of discovery, activity, and "learning to learn," on social notions of what was valuable and desirable for all to know, on political notions of the cold war, on changing ideas about the organization of the subject matter itself. Academic expectations, therefore, include ways of thinking and learning as well as the content learned.

Just what, specifically, are schools expecting their pupils to learn? Again, no generalizations can be made that apply to all schools. With the American concept of decentralized, local school control, two schools in the same city may have somewhat different curriculums. With this reservation in mind, we can gain some insights into what schools are teaching.

Behavioral and Attitudinal Expectations

We have already mentioned some of the behavioral expectations taught through routines and regulations, but again, any list of expectations would be applicable only to a given school. One source of information is the textbooks, which provide some idea of what is being stressed. (We cannot know, of course, whether these materials are being used in any given situation; only a local study could establish that.) Textbooks can be analyzed to reveal their biases. Kane's (1970) review of social studies texts revealed their sins of omission and commission in the treatment of Jews, blacks, Chicanos, Indians, Orientals, and all who are not white Anglo-Saxon Protestant. The state of Florida in 1973 dropped two of its major texts on Florida history because of their distorted presentations about blacks.

Although materials can reveal value expectation, the teacher is the key. Pupil behavior is influenced in many ways by the behavior and perceptions of the teacher. Often the teacher is unaware that he is influencing his pupils by his tone of voice, his choice of children for activities, his selection of materials to display, and the like. Hall's *The Silent Language* (1961) illustrates how classroom culture is conveyed. Kounin and his colleagues (1966, 1967) have shown how the teacher's classroom management procedures influence pupil conduct. Soar (1967) has indicated that teacher behavior can be observed in at least two dimensions, hostile-nonhostile and direct-indirect control, and that these relate to pupil change in vocabulary, reading, and creativity. The indirect, nonhostile classroom produced the most growth in vocabulary, but for reading, optimum growth occurred under either the indirect, hostile or the direct, nonhostile teacher. Although these are academic outcomes, they are presented as examples of the subtle influence of teacher behavior. The Soars' (1972) analysis of teacher-pupil behavior in Follow Through classrooms indicates further that patterns of teacher behavior influence skill learning and concept learning in complex ways. Rosenshine and Furst's (1973) review further amplifies the methodological issues involved in observing classrooms as well as the current findings.

The host of researchers working on the school and its effects on the achievement, attitudes, self-concept, and behavior of its pupils all reflect the growing awareness that the school as an institution communicates far more than a neutral knowledge of reading, writing, and arithmetic. There have been some efforts to attend the nonacademic side of school by building units that stress attitudes and values. Glaser (1969) has proposed ways in which teachers can move from stressing memory to emphasizing commitment, values, and responsibility.

The Ojemann work in Iowa is an excellent example of teaching consciously for the creation of attitudes. The purpose of this program is to help children to develop a causal orientation toward behavior, an orientation that "recognizes that human behavior is produced by many factors and that one can distinguish between an approach to a given behavior incident which recognizes and takes into account the variety of factors that may have produced it as compared with an approach that considers mainly the overt form of the behavior." (Ojemann et al., 1955, p. 95)

There have also been suggestions about completely revamping the educational system (Fantini and Young, 1970) or even eliminating it. (Illich, 1971) Nevertheless, schools seem to be pretty much the way they were and will probably remain essentially the same for some time to come.

SUMMARY

The school culture demonstrates constantly to the child how it expects him to behave and what values the adults who mold the culture believe to be important. This is done through the organization and daily way of life of the school. The school itself reflects the attitudes and values of the community, state, and nation or, at the least, the attitudes of the middle class segment of the general population. The school, far from being radical and extreme, is essentially a conservator of the cultural values and serves as society's agent in passing these values to the child.

If the self develops through transactions with the environment, it would certainly follow that most children learn to behave and to view themselves in the way in which their teachers expect. Although each child perceives the school in his own way, the school situation that is provided for him plays a tremendous and often overlooked role in influencing the self-concept of the child.

REFERENCES AND ADDITIONAL READINGS

Abramson, D. The effectiveness of grouping for students of high ability. *Educational Research Bulletin,* 1959, *38,* 169–182.

Cazden, C., John, V., & Humes, D. (Eds.) *Functions of language in the classroom.* New York: Teachers College, 1972.

Cohen, E. Status of teachers. *Review of Educational Research,* 1967, *37,* 280–295.

Dahlke, H. O. *Values in culture and classroom.* New York: Harper & Row, 1958.

Davis, J. *Undergraduate career decisions.* Chicago: Aldine, 1965.

Fantini, M., & Young, M. *Designing education for tomorrow's children.* New York: Holt, Rinehart, & Winston, 1970.

Fleming, E., & Anntonen, R. Teacher expectancy as related to the academic and personnel growth of primary-age children. *Monographs of the Society for Research in Child Development,* 1971, *36* (Serial No. 145), 1–31.

Glaser, W. *Schools without failure.* New York: Harper & Row, 1969.

Goldberg, M., & Passow, H. *The effects of ability grouping.* New York: Teachers College, 1966.

Gordon, I. J. An instructional theory approach to the analysis of selected early childhood programs. In I. J. Gordon (Ed.), *Early childhood education.* NSSE, 71st Yearbook, Part II. Chicago: University of Chicago Press, 1972. Pp. 203–228.

Gordon, I. J. *The Florida parent education follow-through program.* Gainesville, Fla.: Institute for Development of Human Resources, 1972.

Hall, E. T. *The silent language.* New York: Fawcett, 1961.

Havighurst, R., & Neugarten, D. *Society and education.* Boston: Allyn & Bacon, 1957.

Hernandez, N. V. Variables affecting achievement of middle school Mexican-American students. *Review of Educational Research,* 1973, *43,* 1–40.

Hines, V. A., & Curran, R. L. The school and community forces. *Review of Educational Research,* 1955, *25,* 48–60.

Hoehn, A. A study of social status differentiation in the classroom behavior of nineteen third grade teachers. *Journal of Social Psychology,* 1954, *39,* 269–292.

Holt, J. *The underachieving school.* New York: Pitman, 1969.

Illich, I. *Deschooling society.* New York: Harper & Row, 1971.

Joyce, B. Staff utilization. *Review of Educational Research,* 1967, *37,* 323–336.

Kane, M. *Minorities in textbooks.* Chicago: Quadrangle Books, 1970.

Kimbrough, R. B. *Political power and educational decision-making.* Chicago: Rand McNally, 1963.

Kounin, J. An analysis of teachers' managerial techniques. *Psychology in the School,* 1967, *4,* 221–227.

Kounin, J. *Discipline and group management in classrooms.* New York: Holt, Rinehart & Winston, 1970.

Kounin, J., Friesen, W., & Norton, A. Managing emotionally disturbed children in regular classrooms. *Journal of Educational Psychology,* 1966, *57,* 1–13.

Kounin, J. S., & Gump, P. V. The comparative influence of punitive and nonpunitive teachers upon children's concepts of school misconduct. *Journal of Educational Psychology,* 1961, *52,* 44–49. Reprinted in I. J. Gordon (Ed.), *Human development: Readings in research.* Glenview, Ill.: Scott, Foresman, 1965.

Levitin, T., & Chananie, J. Responses of female primary school teachers to sex-typed behaviors in male and female children. *Child Development,* 1972, *43,* 1309–1316.

Maynard, H. A study of pupil human relations within a school as influenced by the principal's pattern of behavior. Unpublished doctoral dissertation, University of Florida, 1955.

McCarthy, D. Some possible explanations of sex differences in language development and disorders. *The Journal of Psychology,* 1953, *35,* 155–160.

Miller, R. Is it always the child? *Saturday Review,* 1966, *49,* 76–77, 93–94.

Norwalk Board of Education. *The Norwalk plan of team teaching.* Fifth report, 1962–1963. Norwalk, Conn.: The Board, 1963.

Ojemann, R. H. et al. The effects of a "causal" teacher-training program and certain curricular changes on grade school children. *Journal of Experimental Education,* 1955, *24,* 95–114.

Ortego, P. D. Montezuma's children. *The Center Magazine,* 1970, *3*(6), 23–31.

Prescott, D. *The child in the educative process.* New York: McGraw-Hill, 1957.

Rodehaver, M. W., Axtell, W. B., & Cross, R. E. *The sociology of the school.* New York: Crowell, 1957.

Rosenshine, B., & Furst, N. The study of teaching in natural settings using direct observation. In R. Travers (Ed.), *Second handbook of research on teaching.* (2nd ed.) Chicago: Rand McNally, 1973. Pp. 122–183.

Smith, G., & Kniker, D. (Eds.) *Myth and reality.* Boston: Allyn & Bacon, 1972.

Soar, R. S. Observed teacher-classroom behavior and changes in pupil achievement, creativity, and anxiety. (Mimeo) Gainesville, Fla.: Institute for Development of Human Resources, 1967. P. 22.

Soar, R. S., & Soar, R. M. An empirical analysis of selected Follow Through programs: An example of a process approach to evaluation. In I. J. Gordon

(Ed.), *Early childhood education.* NSSE, 71st Yearbook, Part II. Chicago: University of Chicago Press, 1972. Pp. 229–260.

Stiles, L. J. (Ed.) *The teacher's role in American society.* New York: Harper & Row, 1957.

Taba, H. *School culture.* Washington, D.C.: American Council on Education, 1955.

Torrance, E. P., & Myers, R. E. Teaching gifted elementary pupils research concepts and skills. *Gifted Child Quarterly,* 1963, 1–3. Reprinted in I. J. Gordon (Ed.), *Human development: Readings in research.* Glenview, Ill.: Scott, Foresman, 1965.

Travers, R. M. W. (Ed.) *Second handbook of research on teaching.* Chicago: Rand McNally, 1973. (See chapters by Bidwell, Dreeben, and Lortie.)

Waetjen, W., & Grambs, J. Sex differences: A case of educational evasion? *Teachers College Record,* 1963, *65,* 261–271.

Wattenberg, W. et al. Social origins of teachers and American education. In L. J. Stiles (Ed.), *The teacher's role in American society.* John Dewey Society, Fourteenth Yearbook. New York: Harper & Row, 1957. Pp. 61–70.

Weinberg, M. *Desegregation research: An appraisal.* (2nd ed.) Bloomington, Ind.: Phi Delta Kappa, 1970.

CHAPTER 9

THE WORLD OF PEERS

THE PEER SOCIETY

In our efforts to comprehend the various environmental forces that exert their influence upon the developing self of the child, we have investigated the adult world—the family, the mass media, and the school. The child, however, lives in two worlds: an adult world and a child world. In Chapter 5, we saw that he begins to live in a world of peers before he goes to school; but it isn't until he is in school that this world assumes a commanding position in his life. In terms of his perceptions, peers move from being at fairly low levels of awareness and importance to a very high level of awareness and importance. His peers exert tremendous influence upon his behavior, his attitudes, and his view of self. If all the world's the stage that Shakespeare claimed, children and adolescents are playing primarily to an audience of their peers. Their peers sit in the front rows and the box seats; parents and teachers are now relegated to the back rows and the balcony.

Particularly in an urban, industrial society, the world of peers assumes an important cultural role. In order to understand the behavior of the child and adolescent, we need to gain some general knowledge of the society in which he lives—the peer society.

This chapter will discuss the concept of the peer society in general. It will also present information mostly about preadolescent peer groups. Later chapters will include sections on the adolescent peer society as it relates to the total self-development of early and late adolescence. The preadolescent's perceptions of his peers will be included in the next chapter. This will permit us to get an overview of the peer world and then see this peer world at work in the life of the individual.

Every society possesses language, shared values, standards of behavior, rituals, tasks that need to be performed for survival, an organizational framework, a sense of "we-ness." Every society possesses a culture —a way of life. The peer society is a subsociety in the general American scene. In turn, it is divided into subsocieties that are essentially develop-mental-age-graded. A peer subsociety might be defined as containing all the children of a particular developmental age who have communication with each other, although not necessarily in a face-to-face relationship. Within this peer society is the more intimate and more vital subgroup—the peer group. Any peer society contains a number of peer groups. These are the face-to-face, more organized and integrated, selective groups in which the peer culture is carried and taught.

Reasons for Formation

Why do these groups form? What pushes children to join? What do they get from them?

One reason can be seen in the very name sociologists have given these groups. They are the *peer* groups, a society of people on a par with each other. Needs for acceptance, for belonging, for experiencing are all provided after a fashion by the adults, but it is only in the peer society that the child can meet these needs as an equal. "In the shadow of superordinate adults he cannot gain recognition, play differentiated roles, practice social skills or interact with others except as a dependent and subordinate figure." (Ausubel, 1958, p. 458)

A second reason for the creation of these groups lies in the dis-continuity that exists in an industrial culture. Children are expected to be children, they are presented with really few models for adult economic behavior, and they have virtually no productive role to play in the econ-omy. Parents expect them to become emancipated, to belong to organiza-tions outside the home, and to grow up (which means to grow away). At the same time, the children are provided with no participation or status in the adult world. They turn to the society of their peers to gain this sense of productivity and achievement.

The child is also still establishing his own personal identity. He needs experiences with equals, he needs try-out time with new roles, he needs the warmth, support, and acceptance of a nonfamily group as he strives for self-expression and self-understanding.

The need for identity leads to the strange paradox that the child, in seeking independence from the adult world, becomes dependent upon his peers. The peer society becomes the security base from which the child's private war for independence can be fought. Even though the group may demand, in early adolescence particularly, the utmost con-formity to its standards, the child is willing to pay this price for what he gains—a sense of being on his own.

The push of the adult world toward joining certainly exists in the American culture. In other cultures as well, peer groups are affected in their development by the adult pressures for group living and group ac-tivity. In the Israeli *kibbutz* (cooperative farm), where children are reared in a "children's house" although they also have a family, peer group life begins earlier than in the general Israeli culture, and "early . . . [the group] becomes the most important praising figure." (Rapaport, 1957, p. 593) The effects are seen in studies of cooperative behavior such as that made by Shapira and Madsen (1972), which indicated that kibbutz-reared children (ages 6 to 10) were more cooperative, even in a situation designed for competition, than were city-raised Israelis.

In France, where the family is the arbiter of social behavior and the school does not stress group living, peer groups such as we know them do not exist. The preschool child is tied to the extended family. The peer life in school is *sub rosa,* unknown to both teacher and parent. Its main function seems to be to provide "a clearing house for individual interests. . . . The French peer group is, much more than the American peer group, a source of relaxation and defense of the member's identity." (Pitts, 1960, p. 277) Bronfenbrenner (1967, 1970) shows how the peer group is manipulated by the Soviet authorities to influence character development. It acts as a part of the social system, not an escape from it.

In a rapidly changing world, the experiences of the child are greatly different from the experiences his parents had as children. Communication between the generations becomes more difficult, because communication depends upon common perceptual experience. The child needs to share his experiences, to reflect upon them, to relive them. He can do this today only with his peers. The lament of the adolescent, although ancient, was never more true or tragic than today; his parents really don't understand.

Another factor in the formation of peer groups is the development of the child. He has reached the point in neuromuscular development where highly active group games requiring skill are not only possible but are highly satisfying experiences. He has reached the time in his development of self where he has some comprehension of "other." He could not engage in group play before he realized the interaction between his own behavior and that of others, before he had some concept of rules, before he could visualize how others might behave. By the time he enters the second or third grade, he has reached this point in his self-development. He will continue, through his peer group activity, to grow in these concepts; thus, membership not only requires the rudimentary development of concepts of other but also provides the opportunity for their further development.

CHARACTERISTICS OF A PEER GROUP

A peer group is characterized by being an intimate, selective group in which admission is by mutual choice, and status within the group is a func-

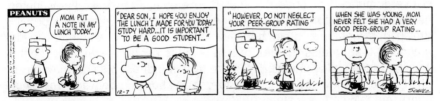

FIGURE 9.1

© 1966 United Features Syndicate, Inc.

tion of the group's values and the individuals' roles. There is a rapid organization of the social structure of the classroom, which, once formed, possesses considerable stability from grade to grade. However, an individual's position in the group can change with time. (Glidewell, 1966)

Organization

Factors affecting individual acceptance tell us about the particular value systems these groups hold. Although all children of a given age are members of the peer society, they do not all belong to groups or to the group of their choice. What does a child need to gain belonging in the group of his choice? What contributes to status?

Intelligence is a requirement in the way we might expect. Sells and Roff (1967) found that there was a low but reliable relationship between IQ and popularity within social class groups. They studied a large number of children in Minnesota and Texas, from grades 4 to 7. They also found, however, that rejection was related to IQ in almost the same degree. In technical terms, the amount of predictability from IQ to peer opportunity was about 5 to 10 percent; that is, that percentage of whatever influenced popularity was contributed by IQ. The same findings held for school achievement, and popularity and rejection. Brightness may make a child more visible in a classroom, and it may be this that produces both acceptance and rejection. There is some evidence (Torrance, 1963; Long et al., 1967) that highly creative children are seen as oddballs and are less accepted.

Family background influences peer status, although again not always in an expected way. Research seems to indicate that the popularity of children from broken homes is not adversely affected by this, that ordinal position means little, and that only children do not lose out in the struggle for status. As an echo of Chapter 3, the family, rather than any objective, external variable, seems to be the contributing factor status and membership. Feinberg found that parental interest and participation in athletic and social activities was related to high peer status. (Feinberg, 1953) The dominance-submission pattern in the home, as it affects the self-development of the child, also influences peer acceptance. If at home the child is overdominated or underdominated, overevaluated or underevaluated, he develops self-concepts that are reflected either in aggressive or withdrawn behavior or in other behavior (such as crying, whining, and demanding) that creates trouble for him with his peers. We would expect to find the family influence exerted more in this indirect fashion through the child rather than in any direct one-to-one relationship between any single family variable and peer status.

The *social class* position of the family plays a role in the peer culture. It influences the circle of friends with whom the child will associate. Although age, school values, and the nature of the larger community are mitigating factors, children of the same social class generally choose each other on sociometric tests, and children from the middle class are perceived as possessing more favorable personality traits than lower class children. Since the peer culture mirrors the adult culture, we would expect that the degree of importance children attach to social class position, race, or ethnic background varies with the degree of importance their parents attach to these variables. However, well-designed research is still slim.

Ethnicity is a key factor in acceptance. Hartup (1970) summarizes the research by indicating that results depend upon whether the groups are segregated or integrated, upon the racial composition of neighborhoods, and upon the degree of the subjects' ethnic identification. In one study that examined both ethnic and social class cleavage among young children, Stodolsky and Jensen (1969) report:

> *While there are both racial and social-class correlates of liking and disliking other children in the program, we do not typically see nor do our results suggest that children of either racial or social-class groups isolate themselves into cohesive, exclusive groups even though occasional instances of this sort of behavior do occur. A large proportion of the social interaction in the Ancona classrooms, and of the friendship choices of the children in the program, occurs across racial and social-class lines. [Stodolsky and Jensen, 1969, p. 44].*

Since ethnic awareness increases with age, we would expect that the picture might change. Studies reviewed by Sowder (1972) indicate that this is what tends to happen but that the results, as Hartup (1970) also indicated, are inconclusive. We need more work, better techniques, and a mixture of anthropological and sociopsychological insights if we are to understand the complexity of class and ethnic factors in peer relationships.

Appearance has prestige value, particularly for girls, and it has more in the secondary school than in the elementary school. In Tryon's study of adolescents, to be "good looking" was important for prestige in both 12-

and 15-year-old girls, unrelated for 12-year-old boys, but very important for 15-year-old boys. (Tryon, 1943, p. 565) A study of preadolescents found that the factor of height was not related to social status. (Heber, 1956) Youth seems to mean by appearance the whole person and not a single factor.

Skill, one of the reasons for the formation of these groups, plays a major role in determining acceptance. Of course, the criteria for which skills are acceptable are functions of the age, sex, and social background of the group, but the child who fails the skill test will not be admitted. Again we have the circle: It takes skill to belong, and belonging provides the experience for the further development of skill. Athletic prowess for boys is the *sine qua non* at all age levels for favorable rating by peers. Social skills, including dancing and the art of conversation, are important for adolescent girls, whereas preadolescent girls resemble the boys in their interest in athletic ability. Social power is more closely related to emotional acceptance than to competence. Bonney and Powell found that to first-graders, being cooperative and following teacher's direction are the skills that bring acceptance. (Bonney and Powell, 1953, p. 492) We shall see the role of skill more clearly in subsequent chapters when we focus again upon the self of the child.

Age also seems to be a factor in acceptance in classroom peer groups. The overage child in the intermediate grades is not accepted by his classmates (Morrison and Perry, 1956), although the factor of age in the junior high grades does not seem significant. We should remember that no single factor is the only causative agent. The viewpoint of teachers, the self-concept and behavior of the overage child, and parental attitudes are all involved. In the secondary school, a time when the relationship between chronological age and physical maturity is low, age is not an important factor. Physical maturity is important because of the change in heterosexual relations.

Even though we are discussing each of these variables somewhat in isolation from one another, they do not function this way. They are all mediated by the self-organization of the child and the particular organization of his peer and adult worlds. Intelligence, family, ethnic, and social class background, the development of skill, appearance, and the degree of achievement required to keep up with one's classmates are all functions of the particular, unique self of the child. This is why all correlations, although positive and valid, are never near the 1.00 mark. How the child feels about his intelligence, his family, and so forth, determines the amount of drive he has for peer group membership, the choice of group he will make, and the behavior he will perceive as appropriate in attempting to gain acceptance. His peers will not evaluate him so much on separate external criteria as they will on his *total* behavior. If his values approximate theirs, if they see that his interests resemble theirs, if he can contribute to the development of the group, they will accept him. Even though some of his behavior patterns are different, his peers will perceive him to be like them. They will distort their image of him to make him resemble them more than he does.

What behavior do peers consider important? Friendliness, expressiveness, ability to show emotion, "outgoingness," cooperation, daring and enthusiasm, emotional stability, and dependability are given by various researchers as important traits. On the other hand, in middle class groups, hostility is related to rejection.

Research on delinquency and delinquent gangs shows that these groups have expectations for personal values that tend to be similar to those of other peer groups. "Members of lower-class street-corner groups are often the most fit and the most able youngsters in their community, for this is a tough league in which to make the grade. One must possess both stamina and perseverance, as well as the capacity to interact and to subordinate self to the overall needs of the group." (Kvaraceus, 1959, p. 16) They differ from the middle class boy only in valuing belligerence and dominance. (Glidewell, 1966)

Sex Cleavage. Peer group organization is generally characterized by sex cleavage. Beginning in preadolescence, the groups are split on sex lines. Sociometric studies show that boys and girls rarely pick each other for activities. Observations of classroom behavior reveal that children, when given the choice, segregate themselves on sex lines. When children's responses are elicited by means of the incomplete-sentences approach, in which they finish a stem such as "most boys ———," they are always more favorable to their own sex. (Harris and Tseng, 1957) Teachers' attempts in the fourth grade, for example, to have children dance with each other are met with horseplay and subversion by the boys along with the mild compliance that must be shown in school. An unpublished study by Gordon and Spears of more than 150 children's self-reports from grades 3 through 12 in one school shows that wanting to be liked by the opposite sex is rated lower than wanting to be liked by the same sex in preadolescence. Adolescent boys say they want girls to like them more than boys, and the girls favor both sexes equally. Same-sex choice reaches its high point in grades 5 and 6 and declines somewhat after that.

We know far more about the peer life of boys than of girls. "Our knowledge of peer influences and group behavior among girls is appallingly weak." (Hartup, 1970, p. 437) With the emergence of women's liberation, we may begin to get some needed solid research.

If we see the peer group as a place where children can safely work on appropriate sex-role behavior, in which they can talk over experiences safely with their peers, then we can understand this cleavage. When we study adolescence in more detail, we can see how youth belongs to several groups, some heterosexual and some continuing to reflect the preadolescent cleavage.

Membership Roles.   Any organization must have certain members perform certain duties if it wishes to survive. Formal organizations have presidents, secretaries, and the like; informal organizations such as peer groups have similar roles. A *role* is an organized pattern of behavior in an interpersonal setting. (For an interesting discussion of role in relation to behavior setting, see R. Barker and H. Wright, *Midwest and Its Children,* pp. 50 ff.) When one plays a role, it enables others, to some degree, to predict behavior and to pattern their own behavior. As we observe children in groups, we can see these behavior patterns in operation. They are essential for group process. In a ball game, a position on the team may be considered a role: pitcher, outfielder, shortstop, center, end, halfback. Other roles are cheerleader, coach, and umpire or referee.

The more pervasive roles in terms of self-structure are played through time and in a variety of situations. In any group, there is always an operator, an idea man, an argument settler, a diplomat, an arranger, a spark plug who actually gets the group moving, a daredevil, and so on. There are always those who supply information or materials, who set the style, who act out in behavior the way others feel but don't quite dare to do. The group is organized so that different roles are accorded varying degrees of status. In the delinquent gang of boys, the fearless defier of adult authority may have high status; in the middle class suburban group, the style setter, the fashion leader, may be the high status role in the adolescent girl group. Individual behavior in a peer group setting is functional for both.

Certain roles need to be performed for group survival; membership in the group provides experiences for learning these roles; role performance brings status; and status provides new opportunities for individual and group enhancement. The individual learns in the group setting, but his behavior also molds the group culture.

An external observer can comprehend much about the self-structure of the group members by analyzing the roles being played and by evaluating the status attached to each role. He will see that some youngsters are able to perform a wide range of roles, whereas others have a limited repertoire. Status position in the group shifts as one adapts himself to the group demands, as he conforms to group pressures. Roles that may have had high status lose value as the group matures; new roles become important.

It should not be construed that adaptability of an "other-directed" nature, in which the youngster loses his uniqueness and conforms for the sake of belonging, is desirable. Highly acceptable youngsters with an ideal self are children with strength, values, and self-regard. It is the insecure youngster with feelings of inadequacy who is willing to sacrifice himself to gain identity. To be sure, all group members gain some sense of identity through affiliation, but not in the same way or to the same degree as the youngster to whom the group is the center of his existence.

In summary, the roles played in the group are an outgrowth of individual and group needs. They reflect the unique organization of roles that members perceive themselves as capable of fulfilling and the group as a whole perceives as desirable for group existence.

Codes and Customs

The culture of the peer group is carried on and conveyed through its language, rituals, activities, and tools. Just as the archeologist can learn about ancient civilization from examination of its objects of art, its writings, its utensils for both production and leisure, and just as the cultural anthropologist can do the same in his study of primitive cultures, so the sociologist and social psychologist can study the culture of the peer group by examining its means for accomplishing its cultural objectives.

The *language* of the peer society changes to some degree with each generation. Because a primary purpose for formation of peer groups is establishment of an identity apart from the adult world, youngsters need to create a language their parents can't quite understand. A second purpose of peer language is to create a bond, a "we-feeling," through being able to communicate thoughts and feelings to each other in a special way. We've had "slang," "jive" talk, "bop" talk, "rock 'n roll" talk, talk that's "way out there, man," and "hippie" talk. We've had the stylized language, such as pig Latin in its various forms, that each generation learns from the one preceding it as it begins its life as a group. The language of any society enables its members to think in certain ways; there is a relationship between language structure and thought. It also allows for certain feelings to be expressed that are shared by members. What can be more eloquent than his own language to describe the ultimate in ecstasy to the teenager? Mystics, theologians, and some psychologists talk of "cosmic experience." Does this convey the same intensity as the peer jargon? Peer language has a richness, a flavor all its own, and its power is indicated by the many attempts of adults to copy it and comprehend it.

Activities

"Standing on the Corner, Watching All the Girls Go By," a song title circa 1955, describes one of the rituals of adolescent boy groups, particularly of the upper-lower and lower-middle classes. To show that life does, after all, have *some* stability, a 1967 favorite was "Music to Watch Girls By." Rituals might be said to be the stylized, repetitive group activities that serve to cement relationships among members, increase the feelings of identity and belonging, and provide experience in new ways of behaving distinct from adult-supervised patterns. Groups develop stylized greetings and leave-takings, usually not too different from the fraternity handclasp or the drinker's toast. The group meeting place, whether it be street corner, pool hall, pizza parlor, teenage night club with psychedelic music, or somebody's back porch, is a part of the ritual group life. Street-corner gangs have their "pad" or home ground, their bit of territory on which outsiders can set foot only through permission or warfare; more socially acceptable groups have similar home bases. The word goes out along the peer grapevine, and the clan gathers at its meeting place to transact its affairs. Huge clusters of many groups may meet, almost in convention.

Another type of ritual is the initiation ceremony. Crane identified five types in preadolescent gangs in Australia, all of which can be seen in the United States as well. They are:

1. *Phallic—genital rather than sexual.*
2. *Ordeal—endurance of pain, fear, indignity.*
3. *Demonstration of skill.*
4. *Signing a document and taking an oath.*
5. *Social aggression.* [*Crane, 1952, p. 115*]

Why such ceremonies? They serve to impress the newcomer with the power of the group, to demonstrate group values, and to increase feelings of identity. They teach the new member the group's rules, history, and symbol system.

Group rituals shade off into activities that are often repetitive but are not stylized or loaded with the emotional overtones of rituals. Crane's study, using the reminiscences of students at teachers colleges in Australia, divided the activities of boy gangs (age 9 to 13) and girl gangs (age 11 to 13) into the following categories:

a. Predatory activities. *Amongst boys, forty-four percent of all gang occupations were of this type, e.g., arranging fights, raiding orchards or melon-patches, throwing stones, birds' nesting and bush-roaming, pulling down fences, lighting bush fires. The girls' predatory activities were mainly confined to teasing others not in the gang, and trying to upset other gangs.*
b. Social activities. *These may be divided into the socially disapproved and the socially approved.*
   (1) Disapproved. *Here boys' gangs exclusively were represented in such a behavior as smoking, telling sex yarns ("smut sessions") and swearing.*
   (2) Approved. *Only one boys' gang could be included here, but seven of the girls' gangs spent their time in such ways as practicing hobbies, discussing poems or books, writing secret reports, and talking about rival gangs.*

    c. Sport. *About the same proportion of both boys' and girls' gangs went hiking, fishing, rabbiting or playing competitive games. Swimming, always in the nude, was a very common activity of boys' gangs, but was not mentioned by the girls.*

    d. Social service. *This category is represented by four girls' gangs only. It included helping each other with school homework, spreading information about Health and Temperance, and helping disabled or disliked people. [Crane, 1952, p. 117]*

As we would expect, activities vary with age, sex, and other cultural influences. For instance, lower class children do not belong to Cub Scouts, Brownies, or Scouts as do their middle class age-mates.

Many activities center around combinations of competitive-cooperative endeavors. Team sports contain both elements. In some groups, joy riding and drag racing are predominant activities. Motion—whether running, chasing, bike riding, ball playing, or automotive—seems to be a basic activity of many peer groups.

In recent years the adult culture seems increasingly to have imposed its organizational pattern upon boys' activities. Before World War II the peer group was away from adult supervision in athletics and other activities, but Babe Ruth Leagues, Little Leagues, Boys' Clubs, and other organized recreation programs are now widespread. Many of these recreation programs were initiated to curb delinquency, but they serve to put the stamp of adult cultural values more firmly upon the child and to cut down the really free time he needs to explore on his own with his peers. The father could write such a book as *Where Did You Go? Out. What Did You Do? Nothing.*, but the son's activities are more controlled. Middle class youngsters, especially in suburbia, are deluged with planned and supervised activities—organized athletics, music lessons, dancing class. Parents force heterosexual activities at a time when children really want experiences with their own sex. Six-graders in some middle class schools have formal proms partly because their parents think it is "cute." In the middle and late 1960s, the electric guitar has helped the teenager reestablish some control over his own activities—what is noise to the adult is music to him.

Some older adolescents have counterattacked by developing crash-pad systems, moving out of the home, cruising as street people, and getting involved in the drug scene. There seems to be a reduction in the status of school-related organizations; this may be another symptom of resistance to adult control of peer life.

Cultural artifacts can lead to additional understanding of the peer society. In archeology, an artifact is anything manufactured and used by a society. Peer groups do not manufacture (except zip guns, perhaps, in certain antisocial gangs), but they use the manufactured objects of the adult society as means and symbols, and they put the peer stamp upon them.

Perhaps clothing is the best example of a cultural artifact, because it begins to be used for peer purposes in the primary grades. Each peer society develops its own uniform. It may be jeans (tight-fitting and low-waisted), tee-shirts, nondescript shoes, or black leather jackets studded with brass. Youngsters begin to dress for each other and to accentuate in their styles the current fad or fashion. In many ways, clothing manufacturers follow the peer lead, rather than create the style. Mod clothes, mini-skirts, work clothes, braless halters are recent examples.

Other artifacts are records, particularly in teenage groups, and, for older groups, the ultimate in tools—the automobile. In later chapters on adolescence we will discuss these last two in more detail. The point to be made here is that the peer society, like all societies, creates or borrows artifacts. These reveal the values, aspirations, and perceptions of the society in ways that are appropriate to it. In analyzing any peer group, the external observer can gain insights by seeing how these artifacts are used.

Values

Value systems can be inferred if we examine the factors that affect individual acceptance, the total organizational pattern, the codes and customs. Analysis of patterns of certain lower class delinquent groups showed:

> *For many youngsters the bases of prestige are to be found in toughness, physical prowess, skill, fearlessness, bravery, ability to con people, gaining money by wits, shrewdness, adroitness, smart repartee, seeking and finding thrills, risk, danger, freedom from external constraint, and freedom from superordinate authority.*
>
> *These are the explicit values of the most important and essential reference group of many delinquent youngsters. These are the things they respect and strive to attain. The lower-class youngster who engages in a long and recurrent series of delinquent behaviors that are sanctioned by his peer group is trying to achieve prestige within this reference system. [Kvaraceus, 1959, p. 16]*

Intermediate and junior high school youngsters in Denver ranked as their high goals interpersonal relationships and experiences, and developing those personal attitudes that contribute to group acceptance. (Cunningham, 1951, p. 71) Belonging, itself, was the chief value. It may be because of this value that the values of the children in a school seem to be set by the social class in the majority, whether it be middle or lower. (Wilson, 1959)

Other values that can be inferred from observation of the group are adequacy, as exemplified in athletics and social skills, and conformity, as exemplified in dress, common activities, language, and rituals. Indeed, conformity has been seen by some as the major problem of the peer culture. Riesman states: "The effort is to cut everyone down to size who stands up or out in any direction. . . . The peer group becomes the measure of all things; the individual has no defenses the group cannot batter down." (Riesman, 1950, pp. 71–83) The reason for this might be related to the reasons for the formation of the group and to its functions. It is the place in which status can be won, in which adults can be resisted. In order to be able to accomplish these functions, the group needs strength, and strength comes through order and the achievement of distinct peer patterns. Conformity, to some degree, is the result. The recognition of the rights of others is also a value learned in the group. Of course, "others" may be defined narrowly to include only group members, and this is often the case. New experiences, identification with "heroes," and becoming adult are other peer values.

All peer values are echoes of adult values. They may be conveyed in ways the adult world finds uncomfortable or inappropriate, but the value system of the peer world resembles the adult value system. The delinquent gang values toughness, loyalty, and bravery—the adult world awards medals to soldiers who distinguish themselves in combat and has "loyalty oaths" for many government employees; the peer group values good looks and social skills—the TV ads are full of such appeals to adults; the peer group values identification with status figures—the adult keeps up with the Joneses. The adult world experiences alienation and a breakdown in communication—the preadult world develops "counterculture." The difference lies not in the value but in the activities used to achieve these values.

DEVELOPMENTAL CHANGES

The peer age begins in childhood and lasts through adolescence. Since so many profound physiological and other developmental changes occur during these years, the peer culture changes too. Behavior that gained approval in first grade loses approval in the seventh grade. Attitudes toward the opposite sex change from preadolescence to adolescence.

We again suffer from a lack of data about developmental changes in group norms and activities. While it is clear that norms change and there are changes in organization, in the direction of increasing complexity, size, freedom from adults, and stability of structure, our research techniques are slim for detecting these at other than a gross level. There has been work on conformity and moral development that indicates an increasing degree of conformity with age and then a decrease in adolescence. However, since one of the purposes of a peer group is to have its own secrets, we have obviously not penetrated these. Sometimes one feels he knows as little of the real workings of real groups of children as he does of yet undiscovered tribes in remote areas of the globe!

Play activities also show the same trend toward complexity of organization. They "involve increasingly greater division of labor, differentiation of roles and status, teamwork, loyalty to a larger group, and breadth of leadership." (Ausubel, 1958, p. 468)

The principle of organizations moving toward greater complexity and, at the same time, higher levels of integration is thus seen to apply not only to the individual child but also to his groups. The group operates as a functioning whole, although each member—like each cell in the body—is individual. Although membership may change, the group as a whole survives, and the members become mutually dependent. In effect, the group develops a "self." We can find in group life the processes we found in the development of self in Chapters 5 and 6. The group has vital reasons for its existence and serves many valuable functions in the self-development of children. Groups cannot be destroyed; they must be lived with, understood, and aided to achieve socially acceptable goals.

FUNCTIONS OF THE PEER GROUP

We have stated many of the functions of peer groups. Here they are restated with a few additions. First, the reasons for the creation of such groups describe their functions—they provide for individual acceptance and belonging. They provide experiences with equals and give numerous opportunities to experiment with both objects and people. They provide a situation in which achievement needs can be met. They offer a safe haven from the pressures of the adult world, a home base from which the child can try to gain his independence from adults. They provide experiences for learning the skills and roles that will be needed in the adult society. They teach the child the appropriate sex-role behavior; no high school class would ever make the error of electing a male queen except as a deliberate put-down of homecoming or student activities.

Second, peer groups have become agents of the culture and teach the culture to the child. They reflect the adult cultural values, although in their own fashion. They are information centers for behavior, values, and skills.

What are the primary teaching procedures used by the group? We saw that rituals and activities are teaching methods in the school. They are also means used by the group. Campbell (1964) indicates that physical setting, activity, reward structure, group size, and clarity of the peer task all influence child behavior.

The group uses the needs of its members to motivate them—a highly successful educational practice. If these motives are not sufficiently strong, then external pressures are applied to keep a member in line. Peer groups do not operate on an acceptance of causality basis. They render punishment in keeping with the seriousness of the crime as they perceive it. Punishment may be simply ridicule, or it may be physical, or it may be the silent treatment, or expulsion. Punishments are often crude and sometimes cruel, but these groups are at the point in their development where group survival is perceived as all-important. If we again compare them to adult societies and view the latter's punishment for treason, we find the differences small indeed.

Rewards are used to reinforce acceptable group behavior. Since the individual joins the group to receive status, recognition, and belonging, the rewards offered are group symbols of these. It is no wonder that the group is often more effective than the school; it uses sound learning laws, such as a recognition that rewards must be perceived as valuable by the learner. The peer group always operates in terms of the self and personal meanings of its members; it provides the experiences its members seek, it teaches the facts (although often with misinformation) its members wish to know, it provides visible rewards by meeting the needs its members have. Altogether, it is a highly efficient educational institution.

Relations with Adults

The peer group is in constant transaction with the adult world. Like all such transactions between groups, the relationship can be peaceful coexistence, cold war, open warfare, or cooperation (either dominant-submissive or egalitarian). The relationship between peers and parents falls into all categories at different times.

Since one of the causes of peer-group formation is the independence-from-parents motive of the members, peer-parent transactions are sometimes struggles along the dominant-submissive axis. However, it is not always the parents who are dominant. Although we have seen that the peer groups' values are reflections of the adult values, it is sometimes the peer society that takes the lead. Peers teach adults, set expectations for adult conduct, and lead the way. We pointed out earlier in the chapter that the society is in such a state of flux that communication between generations is now more difficult. In such a situation, the peer group keeps parents up to date. TV advertisers often exploit this situation by telling the child to ask mother to buy super-duper, sugar-crusted wheat cereal.

In many other situations, it is the adult who is dominant, attempting to impose his will upon the child. The child reacts, depending upon his perceptions of the situation, either as submissive or aggressive. If he feels his peer values are in jeopardy, he will usually reject the parental message. A study of Jewish adolescents showed that they are more influenced by peers than parents in following certain dietary laws. (Rosen, 1955) Warner found that "an adolescent member of a boys' or girls' clique will sometimes defy his or her family to maintain the respect of clique-mates, should the interests of the two groups run counter to each other." (Warner and Lunt, 1941, p. 351)

Generally, each group attempts to learn about the other, to copy what it deems desirable, and to change the other to conform to its norms. Since the peer groups are subordinate in age, experience, and economic power, they adopt more guerrilla-like tactics. They have tremendous power on their side, however, in the form of the drives that created the group and the functions the group performs for its members. They also have on their side the uneasiness of the adult, who is not quite sure how to behave toward them and who often gives in to them because it is the easy way out. For example, on the collegiate level, administrations declare football holidays and lengthened vacations to appease the students. Homecoming becomes more important than homework, and teachers are evaluated by what their students say about them. In 1966–1969, student power, based upon tactics learned in civil rights activities and, to some degree, modeled after the sit-down strikes of the 1930s, led to direct confrontations between students and university and government administrators throughout the world.

Knowledge of the needs, functions, and organization of peer groups has sometimes been misinterpreted to mean that the adult society should just let the group be. The studies of modification of delinquent gang behavior show that these groups, with understanding and wisdom on the part of the adult, can change their behavior. Understanding behavior does not and should not imply condoning behavior. The adult still needs to come to terms with the group, but these terms need not be unconditional surrender.

SUMMARY

As we have indicated in previous chapters as well as here, there are many unanswered questions about human development. Hartup (1970) indicates, for example, that in the peer area, we lack a comprehensive theory, have used few methods (see later peer sections), and have not integrated data on peers into general developmental theory. This chapter has attempted, at least, to do the latter in one frame of reference. The peer group, created out of a combination of physical, social, and psychological pressures, becomes a powerful agent in the socialization of the child. The group develops its own culture, modeled upon the adult culture, and teaches this to its members. In the process of the development of the group, certain roles become differentiated that accord varying degrees of status, and certain codes and customs are adopted that give the group an integrity all its own. When it becomes such a force in its own right, it engages in transactions with the adult society. These transactions are part of the way in which the group helps its members meet their needs for independence, achievement, and status. Conflict between adult and peer society, even though the latter's values stem from the former, is probably inevitable. Each particular adult and peer group works out its own resolution of this struggle; both adults and children learn much from each other and act to modify each other's behavior.

The further development of self takes place in a transactional field in which the family, the school, the general culture, and peer culture are each presenting expectations and attempting to show the child how he should behave and what he should become. These agencies are sometimes cooperating and sometimes competing with each other in this situational field that surrounds the child. In the next chapters we shall see how the individual internalizes these external forces; how, in conjunction with the developmental processes within him and his already developed self, he continues to use these transactions to further develop his self.

REFERENCES AND ADDITIONAL READINGS

Ausubel, D. *Theory and problems of child development.* New York: Grune & Stratton, 1958.

Barker, R., & Wright, H. *Midwest and its children.* New York: Harper & Row, 1954.

Bonney, M., & Powell, J. Differences in social behavior between sociometrically high and sociometrically low children. *Journal of Educational Research,* 1953, *46,* 481–494.

Bronfenbrenner, U. Response to pressure from peers versus adults among Soviet and American school children. *International Journal of Psychology,* 1967, *2,* 199–207.

Bronfenbrenner, U. *Two worlds of childhood, U.S. and U.S.S.R.* New York: Russell Sage Foundation, 1970.

Campbell, J. Peer relations in childhood. In M. L. Hoffman & L. W. Hoffman (Eds.), *Review of child development research.* Vol. 1. New York: Russell Sage Foundation, 1964. Pp. 289–322.

Crane, A. R. Pre-adolescent gangs: A topological interpretation. *Journal of Genetic Psychology,* 1952, *81,* 113–123.

Cunningham, R. et al. *Understanding group behavior of boys and girls.* New York: Teachers College, 1951.

Davitz, J. Social perception and sociometric choice of children. *Journal of Abnormal and Social Psychology,* 1955, *50,* 173–176.

Dumphy, D. The social structure of urban adolescent peer groups. *Sociometry,* 1963, *26,* 230–245.

Feinberg, M. Relation of background of experience to social acceptance. *Journal of Abnormal and Social Psychology,* 1953, *48,* 206–214.

Glidewell, J. et al. Socialization and social structure in the classroom. In M. L. Hoffman & L. W. Hoffman (Eds.), *Review of child development research.* Vol. 2. New York: Russell Sage Foundation, 1966. Pp. 221–256.

Gordon, I. J. *The teacher as a guidance worker.* New York: Harper & Row, 1956.

Gordon, I. J., & Spears, W. D. Developmental patterns of peer relations as revealed by self-estimate data. Paper presented at Florida Psychological Association, 1961.

Gronlund, N. *Sociometry in the classroom.* New York: Harper & Row, 1959.

Harris, D., & Tseng, S. Children's attitudes toward peers and parents as revealed by sentence completions. *Child Development,* 1957, *28,* 401–411.

Hartup, W. Peer interaction and social organization. In P. H. Mussen (Ed.), *Carmichael's manual of child psychology.* (3rd ed.) Vol. 2. New York: Wiley, 1970. Pp. 361–456.

Havighurst, R., & Neugarten, D. *Society and education.* (3rd ed.) Boston: Allyn & Bacon, 1967.

Heber, R. The relation of intelligence and physical maturity to social status of children. *Journal of Educational Psychology, 1956, 47,* 158–162.

Kvaraceus, W. Culture and the delinquent. *National Educational Association Journal, 1959, 48,* 14–16.

Long, B., Henderson, E., & Ziller, R. Self-social correlates of originality in children. *Journal of Genetic Psychology, 1967, 111,* 47–57.

McGuire, C. Family and age-mates in personality formation. *Marriage and Family Living, 1953, 15,* 17–23.

Morrison, I., & Perry, J. Acceptance of average children by their classmates. *Elementary School Journal, 1956, 56,* 217–220.

Pitts, J. The family and peer groups. In N. Bell & E. Vogel (Eds.), *A modern introduction to the family.* New York: Free Press, 1960. Pp. 266–286.

Rapaport, D. The study of kibbutz education and its bearing on the theory of development. *American Journal of Orthopsychiatry, 1957, 28,* 587–596.

Renfroe, O. A study of the developmental sequence of the play behavior of children as revealed in the anecdotal records of teachers. Unpublished Ed.D. dissertation, University of Maryland, 1952.

Riesman, D. *The lonely crowd.* New Haven, Conn.: Yale University Press, 1950.

Rosen, B. Conflicting group membership: A study of parent-peer group cross pressures. *American Sociological Review, 1955, 20,* 155–161.

Sells, S., & Roff, M. *Peer acceptance-rejection and personality development.* Final Report, Project #OE–5–0417, U.S. Department of Health, Education, and Welfare, 1967.

Shapira, A., & Madsen, M. Cooperative and competitive behavior of kibbutz and urban children in Israel. In U. Bronfenbrenner (Ed.), *Influences on human development.* Hinsdale, Ill.: Dryden Press, 1972. Pp. 580–589.

Sherif, M., & Sherif, C. W. *Reference groups.* New York: Harper & Row, 1964.

Sowder, B. Socialization determinants in the development and modification of intergroup and intragroup attitudes and behaviors. In B. Sowder & J. Lazar, *Research problems and issues in the area of socialization.* Prepared for the Interagency Panel on Early Childhood Research and Development by Social Research Group, The George Washington University, Washington, D.C., 1972. Pp. 4–228.

Stendler, C. *Children of Brasstown.* Urbana, Ill.: Bureau of Research and Service, College of Education, University of Illinois, 1949.

Stodolsky, S., & Jensen, J. Ancona Montessori research project for culturally disadvantaged children. Final Report. Washington, D.C.: Office of Economic Opportunity, August 1969. P. 44.

Torrance, E. P. *Education and the creative potential.* Minneapolis: University of Minnesota Press, 1963.

Tryon, C. Evaluations of adolescent personality by adolescents. In R. Barker, J. Kounin, & H. Wright (Eds.), *Child behavior and development.* New York: McGraw-Hill, 1943. Pp. 545–566.

Warner, W., & Lunt, P. *The social life of a modern community.* New Haven, Conn.: Yale University Press, 1941.

Wilson, A. B. Residential segregation of social classes and aspirations of high school boys. *American Sociological Review, 1959, 24,* 836–845.

CHAPTER 10

THE YEARS OF MIDDLE CHILDHOOD

CHANGES IN BODILY FACTORS
Changes in Size and Rate of Growth

Throughout the years of middle childhood, the slow and steady growth that characterizes early childhood continues, and there is also an increasing range of individual differences. For boys, the spread between the tenth and ninetieth percentiles changes from 5.7 inches and 22 pounds at age 6 to 6.8 inches and 33.8 pounds at age 9. For girls, the spread changes from 4.8 inches and 22.6 pounds at age 6 to 7.2 inches and 40.2 pounds at age 9. At age 7, the girls catch up and go ahead of the boys in rate of gain in weight, whereas gains in height continue to be similar throughout this period of development. (See Tables 10.1 and 10.2, Figures 10.1 and 10.2.)

Increases in Coordination

Of great significance to the child during this period is his increasing ability to coordinate; this relates to his success both in school and his peer culture. Ability to read and write, to ride a bike, or to throw a ball with accuracy all occur during this age period.

The principle of the interrelatedness of structure and function, of heredity and environment, which was stated in Chapter 1, can be clearly seen in the middle childhood years. Ball throwing, in terms of cultural expectation, is a masculine activity. Thus, boys achieve a mature throwing pattern at 6½, whereas girls lag considerably in this activity. (Rarick, 1954) The boy who "throws like a girl" is a peer-group failure and object of much sarcasm. Boys seem to be favored in the motor learning of tasks involving accuracy. Since we know that girls mature more rapidly than boys, we can only attribute these differences in athletic tasks to cultural influences.

The changes in coordination during this time continue to follow the principle of movement toward increasing complexity. There are increases

TABLE 10.1 MEAN HEIGHTS, STANDARD DEVIATIONS FOR MEAN HEIGHTS, SELECTED PERCENTILES OF CHILDREN, 6–9 YEARS OF AGE, BY SEX AND AGE: UNITED STATES, 1963–1965.

SEX AND AGE	MEAN HEIGHT IN INCHES	STAN-DARD DEVIA-TION IN INCHES	PERCENTILES						
			5TH	10TH	25TH	50TH	75TH	90TH	95TH
Boys			*HEIGHT IN INCHES*						
6 years	46.7	2.07	43.4	43.9	45.7	46.7	48.3	49.6	50.6
7 years	49.0	2.13	45.4	46.1	47.6	49.0	50.6	52.2	53.0
8 years	51.2	2.23	47.3	48.2	49.7	51.2	52.8	54.3	54.9
9 years	53.3	2.64	49.0	49.9	51.7	53.5	55.2	56.7	57.4
Girls									
6 years	46.4	2.15	42.4	43.5	45.0	46.4	48.0	49.3	50.4
7 years	48.6	2.33	44.6	45.6	47.1	48.6	50.3	51.7	52.7
8 years	50.9	2.45	46.7	47.7	49.4	51.1	52.7	54.3	55.0
9 years	53.3	2.71	48.8	49.8	51.5	53.3	55.2	57.0	58.4

Source: Tables 10.1 and 10.2 adapted from Tables 2 and 4 in the National Center for Health Statistics, Public Health Service, USDHEW, *Height and Weight of Children,* United States: NC for HS, Series 11 (104), Rockville, Md., September 1970. Pp. 22 and 24.

TABLE 10.2 MEAN WEIGHTS, STANDARD DEVIATIONS FOR MEAN WEIGHTS, SELECTED PERCENTILES OF CHILDREN, 6–9 YEARS OF AGE, BY SEX AND AGE: UNITED STATES, 1963–1965

SEX AND AGE	MEAN WEIGHT IN POUNDS	STAN-DARD DEVIA-TION IN POUNDS	PERCENTILES						
			5TH	10TH	25TH	50TH	75TH	90TH	95TH
Boys			*WEIGHT IN POUNDS*						
6 years	48.4	7.65	35.0	37.0	43.1	48.4	53.0	59.0	63.4
7 years	54.3	8.94	40.3	44.4	47.7	53.0	60.3	65.3	71.7
8 years	61.1	10.68	45.1	47.1	52.8	59.6	65.6	75.0	81.6
9 years	68.6	15.00	48.0	52.4	58.3	65.3	74.8	86.2	97.2
Girls									
6 years	47.4	8.20	34.3	35.9	40.5	46.9	52.4	58.5	64.2
7 years	53.2	9.26	37.0	41.1	46.4	51.9	59.4	65.6	72.6
8 years	60.6	12.06	44.4	46.2	51.3	59.0	66.0	76.3	85.4
9 years	69.1	15.04	47.3	51.5	58.1	65.6	76.1	91.7	101.9

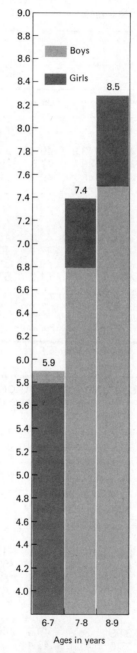

FIGURE 10.1

Expected mean increments in weight, 6–9 years. Created from data in National
Center for Health Statistics, Public Health Service, U.S. Dept. of HEW, *Height and
weight of children,* National Center for Health Statistics, Series 11, #104, Rockville, Md., September 1970.

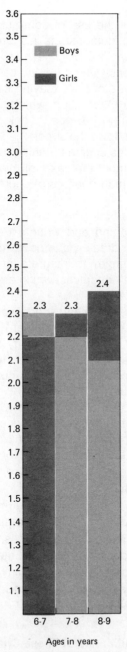

FIGURE 10.2

Expected mean increments in height, 6–9 years. Created from data in National Center for Health Statistics, Public Health Service, U.S. Dept. of HEW, *Height and weight of children,* National Center for Health Statistics, Series 11, #104, Rockville, Md., September 1970.

in speed and increases in the use of coordination ability for social purposes. The child likes to demonstrate his proficiency, to elaborate on basic skill, and to combine skills in new ways. It seems as though he never does anything the easy way if he can use a more complicated procedure. If we watch a group of boys playing catch or some girls jumping rope, we can observe this elaboration, which goes far beyond the simple throwing of a ball or turning of a rope. "Look, no hands!" is the exultant cry of the bike rider racing down the street.

Large-muscle activities such as running, chasing, climbing, and bike riding predominate throughout the years of middle childhood. Teams and group activities requiring high degrees of coordination appear toward the end of this period.

Many children in the first grade are not ready to make the fine coordination required in reading and writing. Reading is a complex skill, that requires the ability to create patterns, to make small discriminations (between *b* and *d,* for example), to integrate, and to categorize. It requires perceptual and conceptual readiness, which are functions of both maturation and experience.

Success in reading and other schoolwork depends upon, among other factors, perceptual-motor development, particularly the development of organization and control—the ability to create order out of the chaos of stimuli. We have, in this book, rejected the completely maturational view. Readiness for schoolwork does not depend solely on mental age (Tyler, 1964) but rather on the types of experience with self in an environment that relates to school-type tasks. Children enter middle childhood with a wide range of individual differences in their abilities to organize and integrate, differences growing out of both genetic and experiential factors. Requiring all children to learn to read and write at the same time imposes unreal standards on both those who are ready earlier and those who are not yet ready.

In general, the ages from 6 through 9 are years of high activity with slow but steady height-weight growth and rapid elaboration of coordination skills. The range of individuality increases, and the cultural impact of sex-role expectation produces differential interests, activities, and skill performance in boys and girls. The interplay of structure-function and heredity-environment shows up not only in peer activities but also in readiness for basic school tasks.

Significance of These Changes

What do these changes mean to the child? We know that both the school and peer cultures emphasize adequacy; we stated above that perceptual-motor coordination is one key to adequacy in both school and peer tasks. Children who are not ready for first grade and experience failure in their efforts to read may develop self-concepts about their ability to read that are detrimental to further growth. All the statistics on children who experience reading difficulties clearly indicate the heavy preponderance of boys over girls. At the same time, the evidence indicates that possession of a concept of self as adequate in kindergarten is predictive of later success in reading. (Wattenberg and Clifford, 1962; Lamy, 1962; Purkey, 1970)

For the well-coordinated child, for one who meets or exceeds the peer and school expectation, there are many opportunities to develop and extend positive self-concepts. The self is continuously influenced by evaluations of others as well as self-evaluation. As Havighurst (1953) points out, to an increasing degree the way the child sees himself is related to his skill. Self-acceptance, it seems, is connected to mastery of his world. With skill, the child contributes to his group, and his group's reaction adds to his self-concept. When the child perceives himself held in high esteem by teachers and peers, he tends to hold himself in high esteem. There is a positive correlation in the third grade, for example, between proficiency on motor tests and such behavior as calmness, cooperation, attentiveness, and resourcefulness. (Rarick and McKee, 1949) These attributes may be seen as indicative of high self-esteem.

Another significant aspect of physical factors during this period is that the children are becoming aware of their own bodies. The replacement of baby teeth, the increased meaning of being weighed and measured, and the increased capacity to make evaluative comparisons (not only of performance but also of appearance) lead each child into developing a body image. He sees this body image as "me," and this image remains fairly stable up to adolescence.

Even this view is influenced by cultural and sex factors. In general, for example, when first-grade children in Israel were asked to draw a human figure, sex differences of middle class Western children favored the girls, who articulated the body (detail, sex differentiation) more than the boys. There were no such differences between Israeli children from Arab lands. (Weller and Singer, 1971)

An American study (Lerner and Korn, 1972) showed that boys favored an average body build over either chubby or thin ones, especially the former. In conformity with the general view, their data show that chubby youngsters hold negative views of themselves. From our orientation, such views of self will affect further choice of activities and tend to perpetuate the child's self-picture.

Increasing motor control provides the child with additional avenues for the expression of self. Drawing, rhythmical activities, and wood and clay work become important to him. The manipulation of tools and the concern for accuracy and reality of detail are parts of his utilization of his body to relate himself to his world. In the last section of this chapter we shall develop this point further.

THE BROADENING OF HORIZONS
Concepts of the Interpersonal Field

Family. A second-grader in a Maryland school wrote: "Why I like Mother. I like Mother because she takes good care of me. I do not want to disobey her. I do some work for her." First- and second-graders, when called on to share experiences in school, talk about their parents and often reveal family secrets. Children of this age tend to conceive of their parents as admirable people and hold an ideal image of them. Parents are seen as good, powerful, and wise people. Children this age tend to perceive their relationships with parents as satisfactory. When asked to indicate "the person I would like to be like," children up to the age of 8 tended to choose parents. (Havighurst et al., 1946) They still seek parental approval and, like the second-grader who commented above, they see the parent as the giver of material satisfaction and the power figure. After age 8, the peers begin to possess some of these same qualities.

Children differentiate their views of father and mother. Fathers are consistently conceived of as being less friendly and more dominating than mothers, and there is a change in view of the parent of the same sex as the child grows from 6 to 10. The parent of the same sex presents a more threatening image as the child grows. (Kagan, 1956) We may infer that this is related to both the child's increasing efforts toward independence and acceptance by peers. It also may be closely related to concern over appropriate sex-role identification. The child is still clarifying his self-image, and since he perceives his parent more realistically than he did at 5 or 6, this may also create anxiety about his own ability to identify with his parent.

How do children conceive of siblings? How does the presence of siblings influence their attitudes toward parents? Koch reports the following comments of second-born boys with older brothers who were less than 2 years older: "Bill (older brother) does most of the good work. I never do and that's why I'd like to be Bill, if I could." " I would like to be Curt, then I could beat him up." "I would like to be Tom because he can read and write." These children not only expressed strong feelings of identification with their older sibling, but, when sibling quarrels arose, also conceived of mother as favoring the older sibling and father as being on their side. Boys with slightly younger sisters also conceived of mother as favoring the sibling. The older girl, on the other hand, saw mother and female teacher favorably as someone with whom they identified closely. (Koch, 1955, pp. 30–34)

Although the influence of the peer group has begun to be felt by the third grade, children are still essentially family oriented. In a study of third-graders' perceptions of interpersonal relationships, about two-thirds of the children ranked a parent first, sibling second, and then a friend. (Mensh and Glidewell, 1958)

We can conclude that children in middle childhood, although now exposed to many extrafamilial experiences, still see their families as the central group, the source of their identification and security. Their conceptions of parents change during this period and are influenced by the ordinal position and sex of the child.

School. As we would expect, children have many reactions to school. Virtually any parent can tell stories about his children's first day at school or of humorous events reported by the child. The child's perception of the school program, what he sees as good or bad in it, is fed back into the family circle during the primary years.

We have many studies on improving academic subjects and skills but little on how children perceive school. The difficulty of validating the reports of children is a part of the reason. How do we know that what the child says really reflects how he feels? Maybe he is merely reporting what he assumes we wish to hear. Attempts to infer the perceptions of children from their behavior, although perhaps a sound approach, is also fraught with difficulty. How can the researcher be sure he is not just projecting his own adult motivational patterns upon the child? Open-ended questions or interviews or play-therapy sessions used to assess children's perceptions are also subject to error. It is no wonder that most research on school children deals with the more tangible, measurable, external factors of physical growth, social behavior, and academic achievement. Our belief is that behavior reflects the self of the child and that analysis of this behavior (including self-reports) can yield valid inferences about how the child feels about school. For example, behavior protocol in a first-grade classroom illustrates a facet of children's concepts of ability.

> Carolyn asked Artie, "You thinkin' of that picture you're doin'?"
> Artie replied, "No. I was thinking of something else. I know what 3 and 3 is."
> Carolyn—"What?"
> He answered, "6."
> Susie said, "That's right."
> Carolyn asked her, "How do you know?"
> Susie held up 3 fingers in front of Carolyn. "See. Now I add 3 more and that's 6." She had the 5 fingers of her left hand and her forefinger of the right hand held up between them.
> "You're smart," Carolyn said.
> Artie was smiling at both girls.
> Susie said, "I ain't smart. Artie is. He didn'n' hold up any fingers at all."
> Artie continued to smile and said nothing.

We know that boys have far more reading problems than girls, even though they are equivalent in vocabulary at entry into school. Does it have to do with what teachers do, or how boys see school, or some combination of these? Good and Brophy (1969) examined both teacher and pupil behavior during reading instruction in first grade to see if boys and girls were receiving equal chances and were being responded to equally. They also observed child behavior and gathered children's self-reports about teachers. They found that the boys and girls were treated equally but that the teachers criticized the boys more, and the boys reported it. However, they state that this was due to the boys' behavior, not to teacher discrimination. It seems clear that boys behave differently than girls in school; teachers react to this, and boys then perceive teachers as more negative to them. While no one can say this explains differences in reading achievement, it does indicate the cyclical relationship between behavior, external response, and self-perception that influences further attitudes and behavior.

Depending upon the type of home atmosphere, the shift from home to school may be mild or radical. The child from a home that has provided numerous opportunities for self-expression, for individuality, and for relaxed play with parents may find himself in a classroom in which the very number of pupils precludes this type of atmosphere or in which the teacher, under pressure to have all her children read by the end of the year, makes few allowances for individuality. One report of a child's feelings about this type of situation states: " 'It's awful; all you do is sit and sit.' " (Murphy, Murphy, and Newcomb, 1937, p. 652) Schools have modified their programs since 1937, but there are still numerous places in which this report of first grade would be accurate.

Children may be expected to perform tasks at home that are not required in school and vice versa. Observation of behavior shows that children perceive school as different from home and teacher as different from mother (although some first-graders slip and call teacher "mommy") and that children behave differently in school than they do at home. Thus, the child may come home reporting proudly that he is on the cleaning committee, but his room at home is a shambles of jumbled toys, straightened out only occasionally under parental guidance and pressure. The disparity between middle class school and lower class home should not be overlooked. The same behavior-response-perception pattern may be occurring here, contributing to the widely reported achievement and behavior problems of lower class children, especially boys, in middle class schools.

Primary school children express liking for school and seek the approval of teachers. However, in Jersild's survey of children's wishes, in which children were "asked very simply, much as a teacher or a parent might ask, what they wish and what they like best or dislike most. . . . The children's wishes, as recorded, included a small number pertaining to school." (Jersild and Tasch, 1949, pp. 7, 12) Less than 4 percent refer to school at all. Primary children expressed more positive than negative wishes, but the most striking finding was that "there were relatively few [wishes] which bore upon the child's contemporary school life." (Jersild and Tasch, 1949, pp. 7, 12)

Does this mean school makes little impact upon the self-concept of the child? Stendler and Young's study, although the findings are based upon interviews with mothers rather than direct study of children, reveals that the phenomenon of beginning school has a profound impact on the child. They found (see Table 10.3) that children expected school to be academic. Further, the mothers reported on children's comments about how hard school was and how big the children felt about going to school. Mothers also reported changes (for the better) in child behavior. (Stendler and Young, 1950) The child in the primary grades has a positive conception of school and values the view of himself as big enough to be in school. He sees, as do his parents and teachers, academic learning as the major task of the school.

Peers. The end of middle childhood marks the transition period when the adult becomes replaced by the peer group as the primary anchorage point. As children mature during these years, their ability to empathize (that is, to put themselves in someone else's shoes) increases. They become better able to interpret the behavior of their friends and to express

TABLE 10.3 PERCENT OF CHILDREN ANTICIPATING FIRST-GRADE LEARNING

LEARNING	*PERCENT OF CHILDREN ANTICIPATING* (ACCORDING TO MOTHERS)
Reading	56
Writing	30
Creative activities	25
Social activities	16
Number	14
Discipline	5
Miscellaneous responses	25

Source: Reprinted from "The Impact of Beginning First Grade Upon Socialization as Reported by Mothers," Celia Burns Stendler and Norman Young, *Child Development,* 1950, *21,* 248. Used by permission of the Society for Research in Child Development, Inc., and of Celia Burns Stendler.

their own likes and dislikes. By the third grade, children are able to perceive their own and others' sociometric status. The child's changing awareness of his peers is indicated by studies of use of peers as reinforcers. Social-reinforcement studies, such as one by Hartup (1964), indicate that children do better in structured situations when they are reinforced by unpopular peers rather than by their friends, and Hartup (1970) infers that this may be due to the fact that such reinforcement was unexpected. We know that peers model their behavior on each other and tend to give high status to those they see as reinforcing them.

Laboratory studies also yield information on peer cultural values. Miller and Thomas (1972), for example, used a game technique in which group rewards were contrasted with individual rewards. They found that Blackfeet Indians continued to cooperate even under the individual reward system, whereas urban Canadian children's performance fell apart and became competitive (see Shapira and Madsen in Chapter 9 on Israeli children).

The use of reinforcement techniques for investigating peer relations in the above studies represents a move away from the more classical sociometric (peer choice of friend or work companion) studies. Since they measure actual task performance, they are more powerful means of assessing children's views of their peers. But, as we indicated in Chapter 9, we still have few methods for understanding all aspects of the peer situation.

Symbolic Concepts

General Conceptual Development.   The child, at the beginning of this period of development, is still oriented to concrete objects and to self. His concepts are still rather vague and simple. During middle childhood, several important changes occur that are not necessarily completed until later stages of development.

In Piagetian terms, these are the years the child moves from a preoperational stage of thought—characterized by (1) the here-and-now, (2) the centering upon the self, (3) the lack of ability to conserve (see Chapter 5), (4) the inability to do much in the way of classifying or grouping, and (5) the imputation of motive to nonanimate objects (it wants to rain)—to the concrete operational stage, which is characterized by mental operations, symbolic thought applied to the real world. An operation is an internal process; it takes place in the child. It is a mental activity by means of which he makes sense of his experience and organizes it in some fashion. Conservation is a main marker that indicates that the child is organizing his view of the external world in a way that corresponds to "reality." He sees that the world has some consistency and is not governed by his whim. He now has some understanding that the way things look depends upon where one is both psychologically and physically. He realizes that there are logical rules that can be applied to problem solution in at least some fields. (Inhelder and Piaget, 1958; Piaget and Inhelder, 1969) We shall explore this changeover in more detail below. During these years, the child is becoming more aware that the outside world is differentiated from the self. Of course, he still generalizes from his own experience, but now his experience is much broader because he can learn from abstract symbol systems (numbers, words) as well as from direct, concrete experience. Indeed, by the end of middle childhood, he seeks more often to learn from symbols, and he is able to deal with many abstractions. He can comprehend the meaning of words through the use of other words; direct tactual or observational experience is not always necessary. If this were not the case, formal education would be impossible.

Language Development.   The development of language and the development of concepts are closely related. Through words, the child can manipulate ideas. The child's vocabulary consists not only of the words he uses in speech or can recognize on a printed page but also those words he comprehends. It is through this understanding of vocabulary that he gains knowledge and mastery of his world.

The school years are characterized by tremendous growth in the use of words. Vocabulary development is influenced by motivation, opportunities to learn, social class position, and sex. There are wide individual differences in vocabulary, and any estimate of an average size should allow for wide range. On the average, the child doubles his vocabulary from first grade (20,000–24,000 words) to sixth grade (50,000 words). (Hurlock, 1956, p. 188)

Since understanding what teachers say is obviously important to school success, Jester (1970) investigated the vocabulary usage of both black and white teachers and of pupils in kindergarten and first grade and found that there was greater common language between middle class teachers and pupils than between these teachers and lower class pupils, regardless of the race of the teacher. Lower class black children, for example, knew the words used by white teachers as well as they did the black teachers, but all lower class children knew fewer teacher words than did middle class children.

But vocabulary is not all there is to language or understanding. How do we get at language understanding beyond vocabulary? How do we know children comprehend a sentence in both its semantic and syntactic meanings? McNeill (1970) indicates that it is not until about age 8 that children recall full grammatical sentences rather than strings of words and that they make grammatically consistent word associations.

A key Piagetian concept is *reversibility;* that is, the mental operation by means of which the child understands, without having to carry it out in action, that something done can be undone, such as changing the shape of plasticene. Slobin (1966) used the same term, reversibility, in several studies to see if children thought words in sentences were reversible when they looked at pictures to which the sentences applied. For example, a cat chasing a dog could be just as grammatically and realistically accurate as a dog chasing a cat, but a girl riding a pony could not be. When defined this way, several studies indicate that learning nonreversibility, the more mature response to the semantic content of the sentence, is accomplished by the middle childhood years.

Since thought, action, and language are all interrelated at this time, the child's knowledge of language and his ability to interpret a request or direction are important, especially in school learning. Experiments in which children had to connect action with a verbal instruction showed that they have more trouble (take longer) carrying out a direction in which the passive case is used (for example, the green truck is pulling the red truck is easier than the red truck is pulled by the green truck), and that *push* is more easily understood than *pull.* (Huttenlocher, Eisenberg, and Strauss, 1968; Huttenberg and Strauss, 1968) The problem here was not reversibility, but the passive case.

Another way to see language development related to concept development is the procedure used by Saltz, Soller, and Sigel (1972). They showed children (kindergarten, third, and sixth grades) a set of 72 picture cards that could be grouped under such natural concepts as food, clothing, and animal. The older children not only used functional and abstract qualities but also saw more pictures as belonging to correct groups. The kindergarten children, for example, did not necessarily see apparel worn on hands, head, or feet as clothing, nor did they all see such things as ice cream cones as food.

What does all this mean? Language development, especially as it relates to both action and concept attainment or classification, is still going on during these years. Further, the usual standardized tests used in schools, which tend to treat language only in terms of vocabulary, may provide considerable misinformation about both the language competence and language performance of children. Indeed, some may not even answer the vocabulary items correctly, although they may "know" the words, because of the way the instructions are framed.

Two anecdotes illustrate children's difficulties in getting correct answers because of their lack of understanding of the words in context rather than their lack of knowledge of operation. In one case, the child brought home a math assignment, and his father watched without intruding for about 15 minutes or so. He saw his son diligently and busily at work, erasing as hard as he could. Finally, his curiosity got the better of him and he asked his son what he was doing. His son replied, "It says here to take away 3, and that's what I'm trying to do!" In the other case, a child brought a paper home with all his columns correct but with three errors in the three cases where the problem had been stated, "What is 4 from 7?" After looking the paper over, the mother asked, "Do you know what 4 from 7 means?" The child said, "No, so I guessed." *From* had not been perceived as a synonym for *take away* and the *minus sign* with which he was familiar. Thus, lack of understanding of the meaning of words contributes to error. These "middle class" examples are cited so that one will not assume that learning difficulties are class-bound.

In addition, grammars appropriate within one social class or ethnic group may not be understood or accepted by others. Black English is structurally different from standard English at the phonological (speech sound) level and at the syntactic level. (Osser, 1971, p. 184) Some examples of the former are past-pass, help-hep, mend-men (pp. 184–185); examples of the latter are listed below.

VARIABLE	STANDARD ENGLISH	NEGRO NONSTANDARD
Linking verb	He *is* going.	He . . . going.
Subject expression	John . . . lives in New York.	John *he* live in New York.
Verb agreement	She *has* a bicycle.	She *have* a bicycle.
If construction	I asked *if he did it.*	I ask *did he do it.*
Preposition	He is over *at* his friend's house.	He over *to* his friend house.
Be	He *is here all the time.*	He *be here.*

Adapted from Joan Baratz, "Teaching reading in an urban Negro school system" in Baratz and Shuy (Eds.), *Teaching Black Children to Read.* Washington, D.C.: Center for Applied Linguistics, 1969. Pp. 90–100.

As Baratz indicates, there is general agreement that although black nonstandard English is a systematic language with rules, the differences between it and standard English can interfere with a child's learning of the latter in school. Since further development depends upon the transactions of the child with the world and since implications of language differences for school learning and teacher attitude are manifold, in this area, as in so many others, we have more issues and questions than answers.

The child's world becomes a verbal one, more abstract and symbolic, throughout the years of middle childhood. Although by age 10 the child will have acquired grammatical competence, there are many applications of language that will be faulty along the way. Words reflect experience, and the ability to classify by means of them is not simply a function of maturation. Jahoda (1964) showed that such words as *city* and *nation* are misunderstood not because of inability to classify but because under-standing these words required a large background of experience. A child's confusion over geography is apparent to any sensitive parent who has taken his family on long car trips. Let's look at a hypothetical conversa-tion:

Child: *Where are we, Daddy?*
Father: *We're in Gainesville.*
Child: *When do we get to Florida?*
Father: *We are in Florida; Gainesville is a city in Florida.*
   Florida is a state. Understand?
Child: *Oh . . . Yes.*
Child: *(two minutes later) Are we in Florida yet, Daddy?*

The confusion of city and state boundaries is evident in the child's ques-tions. Ability to conceptualize meanings is shaped by experience, and when experience is inadequate, the child may make errors in understand-ing because he can use a symbol without comprehending its real mean-ing. (For comprehensive reviews, see Sigel [1964] and Flavell [1970].)

Cognitive Development.   We mentioned above that the middle child-hood years are the ones in which the child moves from preoperational to concrete operational thought. Considerable research energy has been devoted in the past decade to testing many of Piaget's ideas about these stages of development, the timing of arrival at a new stage, and the pro-cess by means of which the child develops his understandings. The issue is far from decided, but there is no question that Piaget's insights have served one of the major functions of any scientific theory—they have provoked empirical investigations to test them out from a variety of ap-proaches. Even psychologists who rely primarily on conditioning ap-proaches have used such ideas as conservation and have designed learn-ing experiments around them. To some degree, what is happening in the quest for knowledge about children's cognitive development parallels an earlier amalgamation of Freudian ideas, such as identification and psycho-sexual and ego development, with conditioning orientations that led to social learning theory. Many of the investigations on the family cited in Chapter 3 grew out of that synthesis. We are beginning to get another synthesis, although there are still many unresolved disputes. The student is faced with many conflicting research reports, myth and rhetoric, and exhortations for application. Here we can only begin to indicate where we are.

   All schools of thought agree that experience—that is, contact with the world—is essential to development. Differences of opinion result from how one views the way in which the child organizes these encoun-

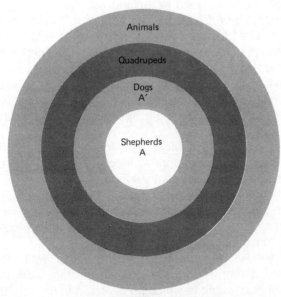

FIGURE 10.3

A demonstration of class inclusion. There are dogs that are not shepherds (A'), but the boundary around dogs includes them all. Arrival at class inclusion means understanding that a shepherd falls into both shepherd and dog categories at the same time.

ters, the role that direct instruction plays, and the child's behavior—does it merely reflect learned skill or is it an organizing process by means of which he takes the bits and pieces and comes up with new ways of thinking? Our assumption stems from Piaget. Just as we have said that the child's view of self is an organizational process, so his view of the world, which means not only the facts he holds but also his interpretation of the facts—his concepts—reflects his own way of putting things together.

Regardless of how the child got there, what can a child this age comprehend? What does the term *concrete operational level* mean? Central to Piagetian theory is the concept of *grouping*—the theory that objects and events can be arranged, or ordered, or categorized in ways that, although discovered anew by each child, match the regularities of the external world in logical fashion. For example, by the third grade (remember—ages are indicators, not absolutes!) the child can understand that something can belong to more than one group at a time and that one group can be included inside the other (class inclusion) (see Figure 10.3). Further, he has notions of *seriation;* that is, the arrangement of objects in order of size. By about age 7 he understands that if A > B (A is greater than B) and B > C, then he knows that A > C without having to see A and C together. He has moved to dealing with the problem symbolically rather than perceptually. Third, he can *conserve;* that is, he can hold in mind that perceptual clues or changes do not mean that basic characteristics have changed. He is able to *reverse;* that is, perform the mental operation of undoing what has been done. The order seems to be conservation of substance (changing the shape of a lump of clay does not change its mass), weight, and then volume. These seem to take place about a year or so apart, beginning about age 7. (Piaget and Inhelder, 1969)

The understanding of number concepts requires a combination of seriation and class inclusion. Merely being able to count does not mean understanding numbers. The child really does not have an operational grasp of number until he is not overwhelmed by perceptual clues, until he can conserve quantity in the face of physical appearance (see Figure 10.4). The teaching of mathematics from this orientation looks quite different from the rote memorization of number facts.

The child's views of causality, so essential to scientific thinking, also undergo change during these years. He moves from what Piaget called egocentric thought, thought in which he centered upon himself, to decen-

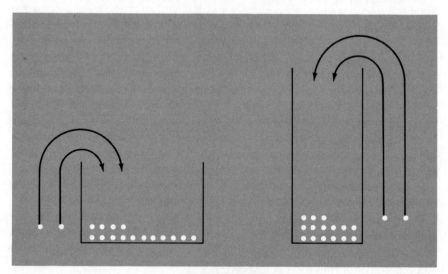

FIGURE 10.4

Conservation of quantity. Question: Will the number in the two containers stay even as I keep adding marbles all afternoon (after covering glasses with a cardboard box with a hole for the marble to be added)? Reply by conserving child: "Once you know, you know forever!" Created from J. Flavell's (1970) translation of an Inhelder and Piaget study. J. Flavell, Concept development, in P. Mussen (ed.), *Carmichael's manual of child psychology,* 3rd ed., Wiley, New York, 1970, Vol. 1, pp. 1003–1004.

tered, or more objective, thought. He comes to recognize that events are governed by physical laws (gravity, for example) and that other people see things from a different perspective than his own. This insight, or discovery, is a significant one not only for his understanding of the physical world but also, and maybe more important, for his comprehension of human relationships. An example of the measurement of decentering in the physical world is shown in Figure 10.5.

Another way to look at how the child puts it all together is to study the way he solves problems. All of us have played Twenty Questions and know that the trick is not to ask many specific questions but to narrow the field down by ruling out (or in) broad categories—"Is it alive?" Mosher and Hornsby (1966) used variations of the game and reported that there

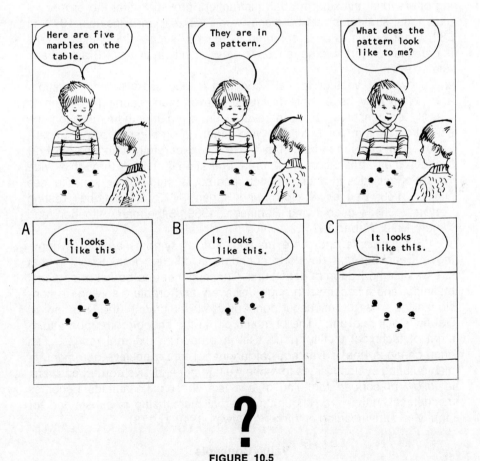

FIGURE 10.5

An example of decentering. Used with permission of the Boulder Valley Public Schools, Boulder, Colorado.

was a progression from age 6 to 11 from the specific to the categoric. Clue, a board detective game, becomes fun for children by the end of middle childhood, because it involves hypothesis making with classification. In it, one finds who killed whom with what and where.

"Teaching" for Cognitive Development. Obviously, for psychologists concerned with the application of their science to education, a crucial question is whether we can teach children to think, whether we can influence the rate and course of development. The answers are unclear, although there are many laboratory and school studies that have been and are being done (see, for example, Sigel and Hooper, 1968; Kohnstamm, 1970). In their review, Glaser and Resnick (1972) state that there are "grounds for considerable optimism concerning the possibility of developing operational thinking through instruction, providing that the proper instructional strategies can be discovered." (Glaser and Resnick, 1972, p. 233) What seems to be a common element in successful training efforts is practical, concrete experience with reversibility activities. (Brainerd and Allen, 1971)

However, whether formal schooling is necessary seems questionable. What may be a more fruitful endeavor than teaching children to classify or conserve, or even reverse, is to enable them, through the school curriculum, to (1) have a wide variety of precursor types of experiences with many materials that have been carefully chosen, and (2) broaden their application of concrete operational abilities through a wide variety of activities in math, science, and social studies (for example, see Duvall, 1969; Renner, Stafford, and Ragan, 1973; Educational Testing Service, 1965; Ausubel and Robinson, 1969; Silberman, Allender, and Yanoff, 1972; Weber, 1971).

But concepts and mere manipulation of symbols are not synonymous. Teaching that develops concepts is different from teaching that stresses memorization of definitions. Concepts need to be full of personal meaning, and this comes through discovery and problem solving. In considering efforts to influence conceptual development, the warning of Dewey is still relevant: "The premium put in the schoolroom upon attainment of technical facility, upon skill in producing external results, . . . often changes [the] advantage [of language] into a positive detriment. In manipulating symbols so as to recite well, to get and give correct answers, to follow prescribed formulae of analysis, the pupil's attitude becomes mechanical, rather than thoughtful; verbal memorizing is substituted for inquiry into the meaning of things." (Dewey, 1910, p. 178)

Value Concepts

Children are also developing their beliefs about right and wrong and good and bad during these primary school years. During these years the child's concepts of fairness and justice grow and change, and his recognition of rules becomes more abstract as it becomes more removed from immediate perceptual experience. Strauss's study of children's changing conceptions of rules (about buying items in a store) and the role-relations of people demonstrates a sequence of development:

> At initial levels, rules are definitional, consequences are few or envisaged by fiat, action is linked closely with immediate situations and activities, and so on. Rules come increasingly to cover more extensive activities of increasing numbers of related roleplayers. To comprehend such rules the child must learn to take into account simultaneously and systematically increasing numbers of perspectives. As he does this he learns to discount his own immediate perspective and perception. [Strauss, 1954, p. 204]

Basing their work upon Piaget (1926), several investigators have explored children's moral development (for example, Boehm, 1962; Johnson, 1962). The usual approach has been through open-ended stories in which some act is committed and the child has to say what ought to be done, how the various people feel, and why. Two examples are shown here.

FIGHT STORY

Two boys, Louis and George, very good friends, want to find out whether one of them is stronger than the other. So they decide to have a match, a fun fight, to see who is stronger. The next morning they meet early in the school yard for their fight. While they are fighting, by accident Louis hits George on the nose, which begins to bleed badly.

How do you think George felt about Louis?
How did Louis feel?

Because Louis felt sorry (or whichever term the child used), he wanted to do something about it and wondered what to do. He could ask his teacher. Louis thought the teacher might tell him to write "I should not fight" 100 times. Or he could ask some of his friends. One of them might say, "Why don't you bring George your favorite toy to play with?" Another one might say, "Buy him a gift." A third might say, "Just go to George and tell him you're sorry."

What do you think Louis did?
Why?

Louis went to George to tell him he was sorry (using the child's term), and he also brought him his toy. But George said, "You don't need to give me anything. You didn't mean to hurt me. It was an accident. I could have hurt you just as easily."

Do you think Louis left the toy or took it home?
Why?

Do you think George forgave Louis when he said he was sorry
    or when he gave him the toy?
Would the toy make George be a better friend?
Do you think it would make Louis feel better to write "I should
    not fight" 100 times to give his toy to George, or to hear
    George say that everything was all right?

SCOUT STORY

*A group of children X years old (the subject's age) want to give a
surprise birthday party for their scout leader. One boy, Charles, is to
decorate the room. He has never done this before and wonders
whom he should ask for advice. He could ask his homeroom teacher.
This teacher does not teach arts and crafts because he is not good
in it, but he is very good in English, social studies, mathematics, etc.
Or Charles could ask a boy in his classroom who takes lessons in
arts and crafts at the museum once a week and is excellent. He is so
talented that he has won a prize at the museum.*

Whom do you think he asked?
If he asked both and they gave him different ideas, whose advice
    would he follow?
If he thought both ideas were equally good, whose would he
    use?
A friend told him he liked the classmate's plan much better than
    the teacher's. Would Charles still rather use the teacher's?
If he follows the friend's advice and uses the boy's plan, will the
    teacher be hurt or angry?

Adapted from L. Boehm, The development of conscience: A comparison of American children of different mental and socioeconomic levels, *Child Development*, 1962, *33*, 577–578.

The most recent attempt to conceptualize the area of moral development from a cognitive point of view has been done by Kohlberg (1969)
and Kohlberg and Turiel (1971). He developed a stage theory based upon
Piaget that seems to be less age-bound than Piaget's. Although most of
his and his colleague's (Turiel, 1966) work was done by interviewing 10-
to 16-year-olds, the first stages he found are indicative of middle childhood beliefs:

I. STAGE O: PREMORAL STAGE

*Neither understands rules nor judges good or bad in terms of rules
and authority. Good is what is pleasant or exciting, bad is what is
painful or fearful. Has no idea of obligation, should, or have to, even
in terms of external authority, but is guided only by can do, and want
to do.*

II. PRECONVENTIONAL LEVEL

*At this level the child is responsive to cultural rules and labels of
good and bad, right or wrong, but interprets these labels in terms of*

*either the physical or the hedonistic consequences of action (punish-
ment, reward, exchange of favors) or in terms of the physical power
of those who enunciate the rules and labels. The level is divided into
two stages:*

Stage 1: *The punishment and obedience orientation. The physical
consequences of action determine its goodness or badness regardless of the human meaning or value of these consequences. Avoidance of punishment and unquestioning deference to power are
valued in their own right, not in terms of respect for an underlying
moral order supported by punishment and authority (the latter being
Stage 4).*

Stage 2: *The instrumental relativist orientation. Right action
consists of that which instrumentally satisfies one's own needs and
occasionally the needs of others. Human relations are viewed in
terms like those of the market place. Elements of fairness, reciprocity, and equal sharing are present, but they are always interpreted in a physical or pragmatic way. Reciprocity is a matter of "you
scratch my back and I'll scratch yours," not of loyalty, gratitude, or
justice.*

III. CONVENTIONAL LEVEL

*At this level, maintaining the expectations of the individual's family,
group, or nation is perceived as valuable in its own right, regardless
of immediate and obvious consequences. The attitude is not only one
of conformity to personal expectations and social order, but of loyalty
to it, of actively maintaining, supporting, and justifying the order
and of identifying with the persons or group involved in it. At this
level, there are two stages:*

Stage 3: *The interpersonal concordance or "good boy—nice
girl" orientation. Good behavior is that which pleases or helps others
and is approved by them. There is much conformity to stereotypical
images of what is majority or "natural" behavior. Behavior is frequently judged by intention: "He means well" becomes important
for the first time. One earns approval by being "nice."*

Stage 4: *The law and order orientation. There is orientation toward
authority, fixed rules, and the maintenance of the social order. Right
behavior consists of doing one's duty, showing respect for authority
and maintaining the given social order for its own sake.*

IV. POST-CONVENTIONAL, AUTONOMOUS, OR
PRINCIPLED LEVEL

*At this level, there is a clear effort to define moral values and princi-
ples which have validity and application apart from the authority of
the groups or persons holding these principles and apart from the
individual's own identification with these groups. This level has two
stages:*

Stage 5: The social-contract legalistic orientation. Generally with utilitarian overtones. Right action tends to be defined in terms of general individual rights and in terms of standards which have been critically examined and agreed upon by the whole society. There is a clear awareness of the relativism of personal values and opinions and a corresponding emphasis upon procedural rules for reaching consensus. Aside from what is constitutionally and democratically agreed upon, the right is a matter of personal values and opinion. The result is an emphasis upon the legal point of view, but with an emphasis upon the possibility of changing law in terms of rational considerations of social utility (rather than rigidly maintaining it in terms of Stage 4 law and order). Outside the legal realm, free agreement and contract is the binding element of obligation. This is the "official" morality of the American government and Constitution.

Stage 6: The universal ethical principle orientation. Right is defined by the decision of conscience in accord with self-chosen ethical principles appealing to logical comprehensiveness, universality, and consistency. These principles are abstract and ethical (the Golden Rule, the categorical imperative) and are not concrete moral rules like the Ten Commandments. At heart, these are universal principles of justice, of the reciprocity and equality of the human rights, and of respect for the dignity of human beings as individual persons.

In both Piaget's and Kohlberg's schemes, social interaction and social experience are major determinants of level of thought. A basic problem, however, is that there are few evidences that what a child says ought to be done corresponds with his actual behavior in a given situation. As Dewey long ago taught us, knowing and doing are two different things.

The child's behavior in the story above uses intent, but many moral judgments are made because of accidental events. Can a child comprehend the difference? To do so would be some evidence of *decentering* —the ability to go beyond the self. It seems clear that during these years children develop this ability. (King, 1971) Moreover, King (1971) and Kohlberg and Turiel (1971) believe that moral development can be influenced directly by instruction, and Kohlberg and Turiel propose such an effort in a systematic fashion.

The child in these years is constantly exposed to a hidden curriculum of moral judgments. These judgments and behaviors that reflect them surround him in school all day. Such classic teacher statements as "wait your turn," "do your own work," "raise your hand if you want to speak," "don't disturb your neighbor," "line up," "those who are finished may

. . ." surround him. The difference between this situation and Kohlberg's theory is that most of what occurs in classrooms keeps children at or below stage 4, and mostly at stage 1, whereas Kohlberg proposes to enable children to move up the ladder. Indeed, if Hoffman is right that "techniques which are predominantly power assertive are least effective in promoting development of moral standards and internalization of controls because they elicit intense hostility in the child and simultaneously provide him with a model for expressing that hostility outward" (Hoffman, 1970, p. 331), then we see what a bind the typical teacher is in. On the one hand, children need peer interaction, discussion, even conflict (at least in ideas) to develop morally; on the other, the school system, through its rules and regulations (including physical punishment in some places), often demonstrates the lower levels of moral development.

In general the development of language, logical reasoning, and moral judgment are intertwined. All reflect the transactions between a growing, maturing body, a self with already formulated ideas and skills, and a changing social situation. Each child, of course, makes his own integration.

Cognitive Style

One way to examine part of the personal contribution to the transaction is through the concept of *cognitive style*. The concept, like so many in human development, has been given different meanings and measured in different ways by different researchers. For some, it refers to degrees of reflection or impulsivity (Kagan, Moss, & Sigel, 1963); for others, the degree to which a person was analytic (field-independent) or global (field-dependent) in the way he looked at materials. (Witkin et al., 1962) In spite of these differences, the question is to what extent is the way a child tackles a task a consistent part of him, even though it may have been learned (not temperament—see Chapter 2), and to what degree does it depend upon the situation? If it is more the former, then it becomes an important element in understanding the person and even in the way we organize to teach him. Olmsted's review (1972) led her to suggest that educators need to attend to the concept, because behaviors that might be mislabeled, such as mental retardation or diffuse brain damage, might really be a function of testing a child without attention to his preferred style. A study by Ridberg, Parke, and Hetherington, however, indicated that "cognitive style does not appear to be a fixed unmodifiable dimension of behavior." (Ridberg, Parke, & Hetherington, 1971, p. 377) This does not negate the utility of the idea, because they deliberately set out to modify reflection-impulsivity. From our transactional view, we don't see any trait or pattern of behavior as unchangeable if it was learned in the first place. Nevertheless, it is clear that children (and adults) are disposed to organize their worlds and to relate to them in individually characteristic ways that, in the normal course of events, remain fairly consistent over time. Witkin, Goodenough, and Karp (1967), for example, show that, in a longitudinal study made over fourteen years, individuals remained relatively consistent in their styles. They are a part of their self-systems. (For procedures for assessing cognitive style in school, see I. J. Gordon's *Studying the child in school*.)

THE DEVELOPING SELF
Identifying and Role Taking

The processes of identifying and role taking begun during earlier stages of self-development continue throughout this period of growth. The child is extending his concept of self as "male" or "female" and is doing this primarily through his relationships with his peers. For girls, this seems to be a time of culturally created difficulty in acceptance of sex role, whereas the boys have clearly emerged from the protection of mother and are "all male." Brown, for example, found that girls in the first through the fourth grades showed a stronger preference for the masculine than for the feminine role (Brown, 1957), and Swensen and Newton (1955) found that, while sex differentiation on drawings increased with age, elementary school girls differentiated significantly better than the boys did.

We have seen earlier in this chapter that teachers respond differentially by the sex of a child and that boys are more often in trouble in school. This might, however, serve to enhance a boy's male image. It fits into the cultural stereotype and gives him peer status. The girl, on the other hand, while doing better in school, has become aware because of her cognitive development that this is still in many ways a man's world. She sees that the boys have greater freedom—both in deeds and words—and she needs to play the male role both in order to understand it and to solve her problem of basic acceptance of her own sex. Although hypothetical, this is one question we need to ask: How does the world appear to the primary school girl? Why might she perceive being masculine as more valuable than being feminine?

The peer group is the locus of much of the role taking that occurs during these years. Understanding the role of the "other," which previously involved the parents, now involves the peers. Through organized games, the child learns the rules and also the specific roles that must be played. In Chapter 9 we saw that these roles were essential for the survival of group life; but they have another result in the development of the self of the child. Through role taking in peer group life, the child forms an image of what G. H. Mead called the *generalized other*. The way a child behaves in a game situation is controlled by the fact that he projects himself into all his teammates and opponents. Each action is based upon his estimate of how all the others should and will behave. As pitcher, he has to have an idea as to how batter, catcher, fielders, and umpire behave. He cannot play pitcher all alone.

Even if he were to be playing alone in his yard, his imaginative game still includes the roles of these other players. Through this process of identifying with the generalized other, the organized social group, he not only takes over self-regarding attitudes, not only develops attitudes toward others, but also takes over and internalizes the value system and activities of his group. "Only in so far as he takes the attitudes of the organized social group to which he belongs toward the organized, cooperative social activity or set of such activities in which that group as such is engaged, does he develop a complete self or possess the sort of complete self he has developed." (Mead, 1934, p. 233)

In this area of self-development, then, we see still another link with the Piagetian concept of decentering and with the cognitive-developmental view of moral development.

Self-Evaluation

The primary school child becomes much more aware of his own body. He develops modesty about going to the toilet. Previously he either may have been unconcerned about this or may have wished to be observed, but now he seeks privacy. At the same time, he is curious about the physical makeup of the opposite sex and often engages in exploratory play. All the bathroom jokes and giggling over seeing underclothing reflect this new awareness of his body.

Along with this new recognition of his body comes a more complex evaluation of self. Previous self-evaluation was highly influenced by the evaluation of others, but now the child's own evaluations become more realistic and more critical. He is concerned with achievement and adequacy; both school and peer group demand it. He looks at his own efforts in a more deprecating manner; he can judge them against the efforts of many children around him rather than simply against the evaluations of his parents. An evaluation with insight into this phenomenon of self-depreciation is found in Biber's study of 7- and 8-year-olds:

> Sometimes the child's irritation with his own product seemed almost like impatience at being a child, as if the techniques of adults were perfect while his own were halting and inadequate. Certainly from the child's point of view this picture is not overdrawn. At seven, when the child's language is so fluent and his motor development so advanced, techniques such as reading, writing, and drawing are often in a stage of progress which makes complete mastery of them look like nothing short of omnipotence. Some awareness of these phenomena seems to be behind his frequently unduly harsh comments as to his work, on which he has perhaps put long and earnest effort, almost as if he said, "This is a child's work, and it's no good." Certainly this

consciousness of one's self as a child who has grown up from babyhood, but who is a long way from adulthood, is a real and rather recent acquisition at seven. The nursery age-child may have words about when he is grown up, but it is often fantasy pure and simple, like the often-heard remark, "When I get big and you get little." The seven-year-old has a much firmer hold on reality, and is gradually placing himself in the world about him. [Biber et al., 1942, pp. 184– 185. Reprinted by permission]

One way to examine a child's view of his work has been through experiments based on social-reinforcement theory. The question is this: Will a child work harder and reward himself less when he uses his own standard or when his behavior is, to some degree, influenced by an external observer who rewards him by an external standard? Bandura and Perloff (1971), for instance, found that 7- to 10-year-olds set high performance standards for themselves, and the girls seemed to exercise more self-control. Sometimes these standards seemed unusually high, but the researchers explain it as protective of self-esteem; a too-low standard is derogatory to the self.

More typical ways of finding out a child's evaluation of himself are (1) observing his behavior and then making inferences as to what it might mean (Combs and Soper, 1963; Gordon, 1966), (2) asking the child to evaluate himself (self-report) through responding to pictures that show smiling-to-sad faces in different situations (Yeatts and Bentley, 1970), (3) administering self-rating scales (see Chapter 11), (4) utilizing teacher observation and judgment (Purkey and Cage, 1971), (5) using items that require children to organize pictures of self, parent, teacher, and peers in ways in which the child does not have to use words or make ratings (Long, Henderson and Ziller, 1967), and (6) conducting structured interviews in which children respond to Piaget-type questions to determine self-identity. (Guardo and Bohan, 1971)

Coller (1971) reviewed the variety of techniques and scales and concluded that most were inadequate if the task was to measure a fairly stable aspect of the child that was still subject to modification through an educational program. In spite of such a pessimistic view, which is one we share, it still seems clear that children are aware and do make estimates. It also seems clear that these estimates are based upon their experience and are somewhat related to reality. The Guardo and Bohan study is especially noteworthy, because they demonstrate that the child's "self" can be seen as an identity and handled by the child according to Piagetian principles of cognitive development. What this means is that, just as in the case of the shepherd in the class inclusion problem (Figure 10.3) or in the case of conservation, although there are external changes, the child sees himself as a "class" and sees his continuity over time. Sex-role identity is an example of class-inclusion in this case.

We can infer, then, that the cognitive processes and the self-developmental processes of differentiation—integration, perception, and evaluation—are commingled. Ideas of self and ideas of world are learned in similar fashion and are all organized into a common structure used by the child to continue his development.

Since we hold a transactional view, we believe that children's attitudes as well as concepts can be modified by how we relate to them and teach them in the primary years. Although school programs tend to stress the intellectual phase of the child's life, our present understandings of self-concept should indicate to us that the affective domain, the domain of feelings, cannot be overlooked or bypassed. The development of positive feelings should continue to be an educational goal just as much as the development of knowledge and skill.

Creating and Imagining

Studies of children's drawing reveal a movement toward re-creating reality. The child draws what he knows or has seen, and attempts to reproduce it accurately. Perhaps this concern for reality and accuracy stems from his school experience and perhaps from his own increasing awareness of the objective world. In either case, the whirls and free-form shapes of the nursery-kindergarten period give way to the houses, trees, airplanes, rockets, and people of the period of middle childhood. Drawing, painting, and sculpting are used not only for free expression of how the child feels but also for depiction and interpretation of what he can see. With ability to conceptualize objects and space relations, and with increased motor control, the child now uses art both symbolically and representationally, deriving pleasure from the product as well as the activity. His art work is often accompanied by storytelling or by the acting out of an event.

Imagination is revealed not only through art work but also through play. The cowboy and Indian chase game carries over from the previous period and becomes more complex. Elaborate plots are evolved, roles are assigned even among the good guys and bad guys, and leaders emerge to run the game. Imaginative play using toy soldiers, blocks, and trucks are still pursued, but these games, too, become highly elaborate and complex. Imaginative play serves to enable the child to increase his understanding of the world, to depict reality, to play roles of the "other," and, thereby, enhance his self.

Various efforts have been made to assess the creativity of primary grade children, such as asking them how many uses they can think of for a common object such as a brick. (Torrance, 1963) Wallach and

Kogan (1965) also used such questions as the following: Name all the things you can think of that will make a noise; name all the square things you can think of; name all the things you can think of that move on wheels. (Wallach and Kogan, 1965, pp. 29–30)

The basic problem is that such scales, while yielding scores on uniqueness of response, amount of answers, etc., do not yet tell us in any predictive way that the child who scores well on them will be creative or be seen as creative when he is an adolescent or an adult. It is not clear (see Chapter 16) whether creativity is a dimension of cognitive ability or a personality variable, although most studies tend to indicate that whatever is measured by creativity tests is independent of what is measured by standard intelligence tests. (Tyler, 1972) In any case, we can see the range of responses children make, and we can go beyond the more mundane measures of achievement to tap the child's unique way of responding to stimuli. Such efforts broaden our own perceptions of childhood and thus make it possible for us to extend the range of activities and experiences we provide for children.

SUMMARY

The years of middle childhood are years of emergence from home, years of broadening horizons to include the school, the peers, and the world at large. This is a time of slow, steady physical growth but rapid and significant growth of self. The self-system constructed within the family is modified and extended by the new experiences that occur during this period. Increased motor development and conceptual development, in conjunction with new cultural demands, contribute to the increased complexity, integration, and organization of the child's self.

REFERENCES AND ADDITIONAL READINGS

Ausubel, D., & Robinson, F. *School learning*. New York: Holt, Rinehart, & Winston, 1969.

Ausubel, D., Schiff, H., & Gasser, E. Preliminary study of developmental trends in socioempathy: Accuracy of perception of own and others' sociometric status. *Child Development*, 1952, *23*, 111–128.

Bandura, A., & Perloff, B. Relative efficacy of self-monitored and externally imposed reinforcement systems. In I. J. Gordon (Ed.), *Readings in research in developmental psychology*. Glenview, Ill.: Scott, Foresman, 1971. Pp. 290–296.

Bereiter, C., & Engelmann, S. *Teaching disadvantaged children in the preschool*. Englewood Cliffs, N.J.: Prentice-Hall, 1966.

Berlyne, D. Children's reasoning and thinking. In P. Mussen (Ed.), *Carmichael's manual of child psychology*. (3rd ed.) Vol. 1. New York: Wiley, 1970. Pp. 939–982.

Biber, B. et al. *Child life in school*. New York: Dutton, 1942.

Boehm, L. The development of conscience: A comparison of American children of different mental and socioeconomic levels. *Child Development,* 1962, *33,* 575–590. Reprinted in I. J. Gordon (Ed.), *Human development: Readings in research.* Glenview, Ill.: Scott, Foresman, 1965.

Borke, H. Interpersonal perception of young children: Egocentrism or empathy? *Developmental Psychology,* 1971, *5,* 263–269.

Brainerd, C., & Allen, T. Experimental inductions of the conservation of "first order" quantitative invariants. *Psychological Bulletin,* 1971, *75,* 128–144.

Brown, D. G. Masculinity-femininity development in children. *Journal of Consulting Psychology,* 1957, *21,* 197–202.

Clarke, H. H., & Clarke, D. H. Relationship between level of aspiration and selected physical factors of boys aged nine years. *The Research Quarterly,* 1961, *32,* 12–19. Reprinted in I. J. Gordon (Ed.), *Human development: Readings in research.* Glenview, Ill.: Scott, Foresman, 1965.

Coller, A. *The assessment of "self-concept" in early childhood education.* Urbana, Ill.: ERIC Clearinghouse on Early Childhood Education, 1971.

Combs, A. W., & Soper, D. W. *The relationship of child perceptions to achievement and behavior in the early school years.* Cooperative Research Project No. 814, U.S. Office of Education, University of Florida, 1963.

DeHirsch, K. Tests designed to discover potential reading difficulties at the six-year-old level. *American Journal of Orthopsychiatry,* 1957, *27,* 566–576.

Dewey, J. *How we think.* Boston: Heath, 1910.

Durkin, D. Children's concepts of justice: A comparison with the Piaget data. *Child Development,* 1959, *30,* 59–67.

Duvall, A. *The TABA social studies curriculum.* Menlo Park, Calif. & Reading, Mass.: Addison-Wesley, 1969.

Educational Testing Service. *Instructional and assessment materials for first graders, manual of directions.* New York: Board of Education of the City of New York, 1965.

Elkind, D. The development of quantitative thinking: A systematic replication of Piaget's studies. *Journal of Genetic Psychology,* 1961, *98,* 37–46. Reprinted in I. J. Gordon (Ed.), *Human development: Readings in research.* Glenview, Ill.: Scott, Foresman, 1965.

Estes, B. Some mathematical and logical concepts in children. *Journal of Genetic Psychology,* 1956, *88,* 219–222.

Feifel, H., & Lorge, I. Qualitative differences in the vocabulary responses of children. *Journal of Educational Psychology,* 1950, *41,* 1–18.

Flavell, J. Concept development. In P. Mussen (Ed.), *Carmichael's manual of child psychology.* (3rd ed.) Vol. 1. New York: Wiley, 1970. Pp. 983–1060.

Gesell, A., & Ilg, F. *The child from five to ten.* New York: Harper & Row, 1946.

Glaser, R., & Resnick, L. Instructional psychology. In P. Mussen & M. Rosenzweig (Eds.), *Annual review of psychology.* Vol. 23. Palo Alto, Calif.: Annual Reviews, Inc., 1972. Pp. 207–276.

Goldschmid, M., & Bentler, P. The dimensions and measurement of conservation. *Child Development,* 1968, *39,* 787–802.

Gollin, E., & Moody, M. Developmental psychology. In P. Mussen and M. Rosenzweig (Eds.), *Annual review of psychology.* Vol. 24. Palo Alto, Calif.: Annual Reviews, Inc., 1973. Pp. 1–52.

Good, T., & Brophy, J. *Do boys and girls receive equal opportunity in first grade reading instruction?* Austin: University of Texas, The Research and Development Center for Teacher Education, Report Series No. 24, September 1969.

Gordon, I. J. *Studying the child in school.* New York: Wiley, 1966.

Gordon, I. J. (Ed.) *Readings in research in developmental psychology.* Glenview, Ill.: Scott, Foresman, 1971. Section on middle childhood.

Gordon, I. J., & Spears, W. D. Developmental patterns of peer relations as revealed by self-estimate data. Paper presented at the Florida Psychological Association, 1961.

Guardo, C., & Bohan, J. Development of a sense of self-identity in children. *Child Development,* 1971, *42,* 1909–1921.

Hartup, W. Friendship status and the effectiveness of peers as reinforcing agents. *Journal of Experimental Child Psychology,* 1964, *1,* 154–162.

Hartup, W. Peer interaction and social organization. In P. Mussen (Ed.), *Carmichael's manual of child psychology.* (3rd ed.) Vol. 2. New York: Wiley, 1970. Pp. 361–456.

Havighurst, R. *Human development and education.* New York: Longmans, 1953.

Havighurst, R., Robinson, M., & Dorr, M. The development of the ideal self in childhood and adolescence. *Journal of Educational Research,* 1946, *40,* 241–257.

Hawkes, G., Burchinal, L., & Gardner, B. Pre-adolescents' views of some of their relations with their parents. *Child Development,* 1957, *28,* 393–399.

Hoffman, M. Moral development. In P. Mussen (Ed.), *Carmichael's manual of child psychology.* (3rd ed.) New York: Wiley, 1970. Pp. 261–360.

Hurlock, E. *Child development.* (3rd ed.) New York: McGraw-Hill, 1956.

Huttenlocher, J., Eisenberg, K., & Strauss, S. Comprehension: Relation between perceived actor and logical subject. *Journal of Verbal Learning and Verbal Behavior,* 1968, *7*(2), 527–530.

Huttenlocher, J., & Strauss, S. Comprehension and a statement's relation to a situation it describes. *Journal of Verbal Learning and Verbal Behavior,* 1968, *7*(2), 300–304.

Inhelder, B., & Piaget, J. *The growth of logical thinking from childhood to adolescence.* New York: Basic Books, 1958.

Jahoda, G. Children's concepts of nationality: A critical study of Piaget's stages. *Child Development,* 1964, *35,* 1081–1092.

Jersild, A. T., & Tasch, R. *Children's interest and what they suggest for education.* New York: Teachers College, 1949.

Jester, R. E. *Relationship between teacher vocabulary usage and the vocabulary of kindergarten and first grade students.* Final Report, Project No. 8–D–056, 1970, University of Florida, Institute of Development of Human Resources, to the Office of Education, Bureau of Research.

Johnson, R. C. A study of children's moral judgments. *Child Development,* 1962, *33,* 327–354. Reprinted in I. J. Gordon (Ed.), *Human development: Readings in research.* Glenview, Ill.: Scott, Foresman, 1965.

Kagan, J. The child's perception of the parent. *Journal of Abnormal and Social Psychology,* 1956, *53,* 257–258.

Kagan, J., & Henlar, B. Developmental psychology. In P. R. Farnsworth (Ed.), *Annual review of psychology.* Stanford, Calif.: Stanford University Press, 1966. Pp. 1–50.

Kagan, J., & Moss, H. *Birth to maturity.* New York: Wiley, 1962.

Kagan, J., Moss, H., & Sigel, I. Psychological significance of styles of conceptualization. In J. C. Wright & J. Kagan (Eds.), Basic cognitive process in children. *Monograph Society for Research in Child Development,* 1963, *28,* 73–112.

Kaufman, A., & Kaufman, N. Tests built from Piaget's and Gesell's tasks as predictors of first grade achievement. *Child Development*, 1972, *43*, 521–535.

King, M. The development of some intention concepts in young children. *Child Development*, 1971, *42*, 1145–1152.

King, W. H. The development of scientific concepts in children. *British Journal of Educational Psychology*, 1960, *31*, 1–20. Reprinted in I. J. Gordon (Ed.), *Human development: Readings in research*. Glenview, Ill.: Scott, Foresman, 1965.

Koch, H. The relation of certain family constellation characteristics and the attitudes of children toward adults. *Child Development*, 1955, *26*, 13–40.

Kohlberg, L. Development of moral character and moral ideology. In M. L. Hoffman & L. W. Hoffman (Eds.), *Review of child development research*, Vol. 1. New York: Russell Sage Foundation, 1964. Pp. 383–431.

Kohlberg, L. Stage and sequence: The cognitive-developmental approach to socialization. In D. Goslin (Ed.), *Handbook of socialization: Theory and research*. Chicago: Rand McNally, 1969.

Kohlberg, L., & Turiel, E. Moral development and moral education. In G. Lesser (Ed.), *Psychological and educational practice*. Glenview, Ill.: Scott, Foresman, 1971. Pp. 410–465.

Kohnstamm, G. Experiments on teaching Piagetian thought operations. In J. Hellmuth, *Cognitive studies*. Vol. 1. New York: Brunner/Mazel, 1970. Pp. 370–382.

Lamy, M. W. Relationship of self-perceptions of early primary children to achievement in reading. Abstract of unpublished doctoral dissertation, University of Florida, 1962. Reprinted in I. J. Gordon (Ed.), *Human development: Readings in research*. Glenview, Ill.: Scott, Foresman, 1965.

Lerner, R., & Korn, S. The development of body-build stereotypes in males. *Child Development*, 1972, *43*, 908–920.

Long, B., Henderson, E., & Ziller, R. Developmental changes in the self-concept during middle-childhood. *Merrill-Palmer Quarterly*, 1967, *13*, 201–216.

McNeill, D. The development of language. In P. Mussen (Ed.), *Carmichael's manual of child psychology*. (3rd ed.) Vol. 1. New York: Wiley, 1970. Pp. 1061–1161.

Mead, G. H. *Mind, self and society*. Chicago: University of Chicago Press, 1934.

Mensh, J., & Glidewell, J. Children's perception of relationships among their family and friends. *Journal of Experimental Education*, 1958, *27*, 65–71.

Meyerowitz, J. H. Self-derogations in young retardates and special class placement. *Child Development*, 1962, *33*, 443–451. Reprinted in I. J. Gordon (Ed.), *Human development: Readings in research*. Glenview, Ill.: Scott, Foresman, 1965.

Meyers, C. E. et al. Primary abilities at mental age six. *Child Development Monographs*, 1962, *27*, 1.

Miller, A., & Thomas, R. Cooperation and competition among Blackfoot Indians and urban Canadian children. *Child Development*, 1972, *43*, 1104–1110.

Mosher, F., & Hornsby, J. On asking questions. In J. Bruner et al., *Studies in cognitive growth*. New York: Wiley, 1966.

Moustakas, C. *The teacher and the child*. New York: McGraw-Hill, 1956.

Murphy, G., Murphy, L., & Newcomb, T. *Experimental social psychology*. New York: Harper & Row, 1937.

Ojemann, R. H., Maxey, E. J., & Snider, B. C. The effect of a program of guided learning experiences in developing probability concepts at the third-grade level. *Journal of Experimental Education,* 1965, *33,* 321–330.

Ojemann, R. H., & Pritchett, K. Piaget and the role of guided experience in human development. *Perceptual and Motor Skills,* 1963, *17,* 927–940. Reprinted in I. J. Gordon (Ed.), *Human development: Readings in research.* Glenview, Ill.: Scott, Foresman, 1965.

Olmsted, P. Cognitive style in children: A review of the research. Unpublished manuscript, University of Florida: Institute for Development of Human Resources, 1972.

Osler, S. F., & Weiss, S. R. Studies in concept attainment: III. Effect of instructions at two levels of intelligence. *Journal of Experimental Psychology,* 1962, *63,* 528–533. Reprinted in I. J. Gordon (Ed.), *Human development: Readings in research.* Glenview, Ill.: Scott, Foresman, 1965.

Osser, H. Language development in children. In G. Lesser (Ed.), *Psychology and educational practice.* Glenview, Ill.: Scott, Foresman, 1971. Pp. 156–190.

Piaget, J. *The language and thought of the child.* New York: Harcourt Brace, 1926.

Piaget, J. *The moral judgment of the child.* London: Routledge & Kegan Paul, 1932.

Piaget, J., & Inhelder, B. *The psychology of the child.* New York: Basic Books, 1969.

Purkey, W. *Self concept and school achievement.* Englewood Cliffs, N.J.: Prentice-Hall, 1970.

Purkey, W. W., & Cage, B. N. The Florida key: An instrument to assess learning self-concept. (Unpublished experimental instrument) January 1971.

Rarick, G. L., & McKee, R. A study of twenty third-grade children exhibiting extreme levels of achievement on tests of motor proficiency. *Research Quarterly, American Association of Health,* 1949, *20,* 142–152.

Rarick, L. Maturity indicators and the development of strength and skill. *Education,* 1954, *75,* 69–73.

Renner, J., Stafford, D., & Ragan, W. *Teaching science in the elementary school.* (2nd ed.) New York: Harper & Row, 1973.

Ridberg, E., Parke, R., & Hetherington, M. Modification of impulsive and reflective cognitive styles through observation of film-mediated models. *Developmental Psychology,* 1971, *5,* 369–377.

Rosenbloom, P. C. What is coming in elementary mathematics. *Educational Leadership,* 1960, *18,* 96–100.

Saltz, E., Soller, E., & Sigel, I. The development of natural language concepts. *Child Development,* 1972, *43,* 1191–1202.

Schulman, R. Disrupted schools: Who's at fault? *Menninger Perspective,* 1971, *2(3),* 13–17.

Shapiro, D. Perceptions of significant family and environmental relationships in aggressive and withdrawn children. *Journal of Consulting Psychology,* 1957, *21,* 381–385.

Sigel, I. E. How intelligence tests limit understanding of intelligence. *Merrill-Palmer Quarterly,* 1963, *9,* 39–56. Reprinted in I. J. Gordon (Ed.), *Human development: Readings in research.* Glenview, Ill.: Scott, Foresman, 1965.

Sigel, I. E. The attainment of concepts. In M. L. Hoffman & L. W. Hoffman (Eds.), *Review of child development research.* Vol. 1. New York: Russell Sage Foundation, 1964. Pp. 209–248.

Sigel, I., & Hooper, F. (Eds.) *Logical thinking in children.* New York: Holt, Rinehart & Winston, 1968.

Silberman, M., Alexander, J., & Yanoff, J. *The psychology of open teaching and learning.* Boston: Little, Brown, 1972.

Slobin, D. Grammatical transformations and sentence comprehension in childhood and adulthood. *Journal of Verbal Learning and Verbal Behavior,* 1966, *5,* 219–227.

Smith, J. Relation of certain physical traits and abilities to motor learning in elementary school children. *Research Quarterly,* 1956, *27,* 220–228.

Stendler, C., & Young, N. The impact of beginning first grade upon socialization as reported by mothers. *Child Development,* 1950, *21,* 241–260.

Stern, C. Labeling and variety in concept identification with young children. *Journal of Educational Psychology,* 1965, *56,* 235–240.

Stevenson, H. Developmental psychology. In P. R. Farnsworth (Ed.), *Annual review of psychology, 1967.* Stanford, Calif.: Stanford University Press, 1967. Pp. 87–128.

Strauss, A. The development of conceptions of rules in children. *Child Development,* 1954, *25,* 193–208.

Sullivan, E. Transition problems in conservation research. *Journal of Genetic Psychology,* 1969, *115,* 41–54.

Swenson, C., Jr., & Newton, K. The development of sexual differentiation on the draw-a-person test. *Journal of Clinical Psychology,* 1955, *11,* 417–419.

Torrance, P. *Education and the creative potential.* Minneapolis: University of Minnesota Press, 1963.

Turiel, E. An experimental test of the sequentiality of developmental stages in the child's moral judgments. *Journal of Personality and Social Psychology,* 1966, *3,* 611–618.

Tyler, F. Issues related to readiness to learn. In NSSE, *Theories of learning and instruction.* 63rd Yearbook, Part I. Chicago: University of Chicago Press, 1964. Pp. 87–128.

Tyler, L. Human abilities. In P. Mussen & M. Rosenzweig (Eds.), *Annual review of psychology.* Vol. 23. Palo Alto, Calif.: Annual Reviews Inc., 1972. Pp. 177–206.

Vernon, M. D. The development of perception in children. *Educational Research,* 1960, *3,* 2–11. Reprinted in I. J. Gordon (Ed.), *Human development: Readings in research.* Glenview, Ill.: Scott, Foresman, 1965.

Vinacke, E. Concept formation in children of school ages. *Education,* 1954, *74,* 527–534.

Wallach, M., & Kogan, N. *Modes of thinking in young children.* New York: Holt, Rinehart & Winston, 1965.

Ward, W. Rate and uniqueness of children's creative responding. *Child Development,* 1969, *40,* 869–878.

Watson, E., & Lowrey, G. *Growth and development of children.* (4th ed.) Chicago: Year Book Publishers, 1962.

Wattenberg, W. W., & Clifford, C. *Relationship of self-concept to beginning achievement in reading.* U.S. Office of Education Cooperative Research Project No. 377, Wayne State University, Detroit, Michigan, 1962.

Weber, L. *The English infant school and informal education.* Englewood Cliffs, N.J.: Prentice-Hall, 1971.

Weener, P. Language structures and the free recall of verbal messages by children. *Developmental Psychology,* 1971, *5,* 237–243.

Weir, M., & Stevenson, H. The effect of verbalization in children's learning as a function of chronological age. *Child Development,* 1959, *30,* 143–149.

Weller, L., & Singer, S. Articulation of the body concept among first-grade Is-
    raeli children. *Child Development*, 1971, *42*, 1553–1559.
Witkin, H. et al. *Psychological differentiation.* New York: Wiley, 1962.
Witkin, H., Goodenough, D., & Karp, S. Stability of cognitive style from childhood
    to young adulthood. *Journal of Personality and Social Psychology*, 1967, *7*,
    291–300.
Wohlwill, J. F., & Lowe, R. C. Experimental analysis of the development of the
    conservation of number. *Child Development*, 1962, *33*, 153–167. Reprinted
    in I. J. Gordon (Ed.), *Human development: Readings in research.* Glen-
    view, Ill.: Scott, Foresman, 1965.
Yeatts, P. P., & Bentley, E. L., Jr. I feel, me feel; self concept appraisal. Athens,
    Ga., 1970.

FOUR
PREADOLESCENCE

CHAPTER 11

THE GREAT UNKNOWN

The years of preadolescence have been characterized as the mysterious years, the unknown years. The voluminous body of research on infancy and adolescence dwindles down to a small quantity of articles on the preadolescent. Redl's article, although written in 1943, still appears fresh and to the point. He says:

> The reason why we know so little about this phase of development is simple but significant: it is a phase which is especially disappointing for the adult, and especially so for the adult who loves youth and is interested in it. These youngsters are hard to live with even where there is the most ideal child-parent relationship. They are not as much fun to love as when they were younger, for they don't seem to appreciate what they get at all. And they certainly aren't much to brag about, academically or otherwise. You can't play the "friendly helper" toward them either—they think you are plain dumb if you try it; nor can you play the role of the proud shaper of youthful wax— they stick to your fingers like putty and things become messier and messier the more you try to "shape" that age. Nor can you play the role of the proud and sacerdotal warden of the values of society to be pointed out to eager youth. They think you are plain funny in that role. [Redl, 1943, p. 44]

The dominance of the peer group begins its period of ascendancy during this time. This adds to the difficulties of the adult in both knowing and working with the preadolescent. His group actively works to keep adults in the dark. The young child lives on the surface, is open and honest, and we can understand what he feels; the adolescent often tells us in no uncertain terms what he thinks of us, of life in general, and himself. The preadolescent tends to conceal from our direct view the "why" of his existence. His peers know him well, but the parent, teacher, and researcher are on the outside looking in. We have weighed and measured

TABLE 11.1 HEIGHT AND WEIGHT, AGES 10–11

	BOYS		GIRLS	
AGE	10 PERCENTILE	90 PERCENTILE	10 PERCENTILE	90 PERCENTILE
	HEIGHT IN INCHES			
10	51.7	58.7	51.8	59.2
11	53.8	60.9	54.4	62.2
	WEIGHT IN POUNDS			
10	57.9	92.6	57.0	100.5
11	66.0	108.5	65.3	116.8

Source: Table adapted from Tables 2 and 4 in the National Center for Health Statistics, Public Health Service, USDHEW, *Height and Weight of Children.* United States: NC for HS, Series 11 (104), Rockville, Md., September 1970. Pp. 2 and 4.

the child, tested him and scored him, praised him and punished him—but still we know him not.

From a perceptual, self-oriented point of view, these are truly the unknown years. We must say that we know little and emphasize that much remains to be learned about the life of the preadolescent as he perceives it. We can start readily enough by weighing and measuring. This we can do well; external data are plentiful!

CHANGES IN BODILY FACTORS
Changes in Size and Rate of Growth

The years of preadolescence are marked by the change from the slow, steady growth of childhood to the beginning of the spurt in growth that continues into adolescence. The range within the group widens, and we are easily able to observe the differences among youngsters in the same classroom. Table 11.1 clearly illustrates this. Some girls begin to mature sexually even in fourth grade. Figures 11.1 and 11.2 are graphic representations of the changes begun during a period formerly seen as one of little sexual interest, awareness, or bodily change. By the end of the preadolescent period, girls are about two years ahead of boys in development, a factor of much importance in the affairs of childhood and youth.

Increases in Coordination, Strength, and Health

The preadolescent is a healthier child than his younger brother. He has, largely, passed through the measles, mumps, and chicken pox stage. He shows more resistance to both disease and fatigue.

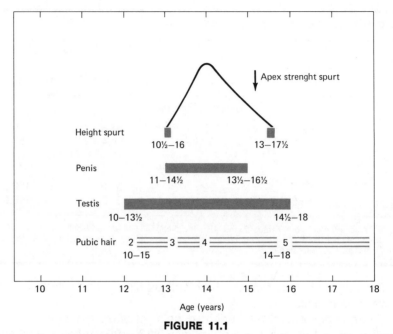

FIGURE 11.1

Diagram of sequence of events at adolescence in boys. An average boy is represented; the range of ages within which each event charted may begin and end is
given by the figures placed directly below its start and finish. From Tanner, 1962.

A major source of information about the physical growth of preadolescents and early adolescents is the California Growth Study. This longitudinal study of the same group of children assembled data on many types
of growth. Information from the California Study shows the following trends:
(1) A high steady increase in strength for both boys and girls occurs, with
the degree of variability both within and between the sexes increasing
with age. Thus, not only the range of performance but also the differences
between children in performance increases. (2) Early and late maturity
influences the individual's growth in strength. There is a significant relationship between other measures of physiological maturing and increase
in strength. The earlier average maturing of girls is reflected in their attainment of almost adult levels in thrusting (one measure of strength) at about
age 13½ or 14. (3) At about the age of 13 "boys have reached about 45
percent of their terminal strength, both in pull and thrust, while girls have
reached about 75 percent of their terminal strength in pull and over 90
percent in thrusting strength." (Jones, 1949, p. 48) This does not mean
that girls are stronger than the boys (except in thrusting), but that they are
closer to mature functioning. (4) The rise in strength is accompanied by
increased manual dexterity. The preadolescent can handle and use his

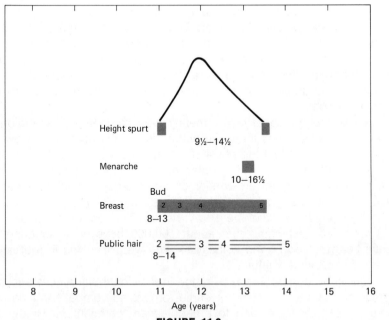

FIGURE 11.2

Diagram of sequence of events at adolescence in girls. An average girl is represented; the range of ages within which some of the events may occur is given by the figures placed directly below them. From Tanner, 1962.

body more efficiently and for longer periods of time (thus resisting fatigue) than he could have done a few years before.

Another study of skill revealed that with each year of growth during the intermediate grades (4 to 6), the youngster becomes significantly better able to throw, bat, or kick softballs, volleyballs, and basketballs at targets. (Latchaw, 1954)

In summary, the years of preadolescence are vigorous, active years with emphasis placed on skill and strength.

Personal Meanings of Bodily Factors

The child, perceiving his increasing ability and being concerned with adequacy and peer acceptance, seeks ways to utilize his new physical resources for self-enhancement. Games of skill become important for the boys. Girls are in their last period of high activity and at the last stage of their successful competition with boys. There is greater differentiation at this time into boy groups and girl groups.

Team play of a competitive nature has great personal meaning to the preadolescent boy. In such play he can gain status through his skill, can gain identity with his peers, and can use and enjoy his new abilities and vitality. He needs vigorous play, both for psychological satisfaction and for optimal functioning of his body. This is the age of the Midget League and the Little League. The adult world, seeking its own satisfactions, has created a highly organized competitive situation for these youngsters. Although children need to test themselves, to compete as well as cooperate, the question of the desirable extent of such efforts has often been overlooked.

What does personal failure mean? What does lack of selection to a team mean? What does the great outpouring of energy mean? How does competitive sport affect the physical development of the child? Krogman, one of the outstanding physical anthropologists in the United States, notes that in relation to organized, varsity, or midget league football games during this period (early and preadolescence), the child is most vulnerable to bodily injury because of the growth needs of the body. (Krogman, 1954) In 1972 it was estimated that about 100,000 boys were suffering from "Little League elbow" and virtually all who were involved in football had received some kind of injury.

Our knowledge of the wide range in individual differences and of the increasing cultural demands for earlier organized competition lead to the same conclusion in relation to preadolescent competition: Highly competitive, organized football and other contact sports are damaging, both in terms of personal meaning and physical processes. Boys of this age can and should play football, but it should be in the neighborhood or playground, where the intense emotional pressure is limited and where each child can find a group with which to play.

As a result of his analysis of the California growth data, and other data on youth of these ages, Jones concluded: "In the case of boys who are temporarily retarded in growth, informed guidance implies an understanding of their individual growth patterns and potentialities. Especially among these boys and among others of subaverage physical talents, the efforts should not be relaxed to provide adequate encouragement and a program of well-balanced training." (Jones, 1944, p. 119)

In what other ways do the physical forces in operation during preadolescence influence personal meaning? We can infer from their appearance (the dirty, disheveled look) and their behavior with their peers (strenuous play and lots of noise) that their bodies have taken on increased personal meaning. Preadolescents are much more aware of themselves and less concerned with such adult standards as neatness and quietness.

They are aware that the youngsters somewhat older than themselves are changing rapidly and growing away from them. They do not wish to be thought of as "babies." This increased consciousness of their own age level finds expression in their life with their peers and in their choice of activities.

The coordination required for success in school, since school deals with more abstract learning, is easily met by all except those at the bottom of the curve. The relationship between ability to do schoolwork and to coordinate has diminished greatly. The high energy level and the need for movement that formerly found outlets in primary school activities may now be frustrated in the intermediate grades. Attitudes toward teacher and school may be influenced by the conflict between bodily needs and the cultural demands of the school. But the situation created by his maturing body and the increasingly rigid demands of the school create discipline problems that he must face and resolve. For example, a fourth-grade boy (constantly in minor trouble) wrote the following comments in a composition about school: "It is hard not to talk for six and a half hours. I like lunch, play period, sharing, snack because you can talk. I like projects because you can talk quietly."

In summary, the child enters preadolescence continuing the slow, steady growth of childhood. He finishes this period at the beginning of the growth spurt. He gains in strength, health, and coordination, and these changes manifest themselves in behavior. The preadolescent has begun to mature sexually. His view of himself and his interpersonal world is influenced by his changing body. His concern with athletic prowess is partially attributable to his increased skill. His difficulties in school (boys have more troubles than girls) are partially attributable to his need for activity, which can no longer find acceptable outlets within the average school program. The growth in body is complemented by and exceeded by the conceptual development of the child during this time. He enlarges, clarifies, and sharpens his definition of self and world.

THE INTERPERSONAL WORLD
Family Relationships

A major task of the preadolescent is to sever his close, dependent relationships with his parents and move out into the world of peers and other adults. This process, begun with entrance into school, assumes more personal significance during the preadolescent years. Going to school was an adult, cultural decision over which the child had no control. Emancipation from the home and defining a new relationship with his parents is the child's decision. This movement away from the parents is not completed until the end of adolescence. The child still perceives his parents favorably and is very involved in family affairs. A large majority of the 730 rural and small-town midwestern youngsters in one study, for example, reported that they discussed their plans with their mothers (at least sometimes) and that their mothers were much more likely than not to tell them the reason for punishment. Eighty-four percent reported that they helped decide what clothes to buy, at least sometimes, and 75 percent played a role in choosing things at stores. These activities suggest a trend toward independence. (Hawkes et al., 1957, pp. 394–395)

Parents' views of what children need reveal the differences between their perceptions of boys and girls and support the boys' reports that parents are harder on them than they are on girls. A group of parents of sixth-graders attending the Ohio State University Laboratory School stated the following as the needs of their children:

> *Boys need help in: controlling temper, remembering chores, completing jobs started, becoming more detail-minded, being more cooperative, being willing to share, building more mature interests, becoming more mature in decisions. They need help in emotional development, in choice of values, overcoming dawdling, being prompt at mealtime and bedtime, improving cleanliness of body and clothing, getting imagination and achievement more in line, improving mechanical ability, improving skills, having more direct arts experiences.*
>
> *Girls need help in: working with tools, learning to concentrate, learning to budget time, overcoming nervousness. [Loomis, 1959, p. 28]*

It will be noted that these parents showed little understanding or acceptance of the youngster's perceptions of what is important and little awareness of the child's own private world. There is no mention of standing on one's own. They are concerned with getting a child to conform, to do something, to behave in an adult, socially acceptable fashion. Parents are dedicated to making their children responsible—a worthy dedication, but one that leads boys to feel that the peer group is the safest haven and that it is sometimes hard to live with parents.

In spite of the parents' long list of needs, and in spite of the efforts made by parents to teach youngsters responsibility by involving them in household chores, the evidence suggests the futility of this. Harris compiled answers to a questionnaire called "What Are My Jobs" as well as a rating of responsibility by teachers and an attitude scale toward citizenship in relation to 3,000 children between the ages of 6 and 14. He found that there is "little evidence that the routine tasks are associated with an attitude of responsibility." (Harris et al., 1954, p. 32) Although these tasks are worthwhile and parents may legitimately seek the child's help, they do not build character. The Ohio State parents placed "chores" and "completing jobs started" high in terms of their perception of need. We thus have parental pressure to perform and evidence that performance does not lead to incorporation of the concept of responsibility into the self of the preadolescent. The stronger demand for performance seems to be made upon the boys. The conflicting views between parents and male preadolescents of what is valuable has resulted in the discovery, in one study, for example, that "girls perceived themselves as significantly more accepted and intrinsically valued by parents than did boys." (Ausubel et al., 1954, p. 179)

Most children, in spite of their occasional difficulties with parents, view them in a positive light. They do not see their parents as the idols of early childhood, but they still respect, love, and obey them. They feel their parents love them but do not necessarily understand them. They still identify with them. Long and her colleagues, for example, have developed a nonverbal method for assessing a child's self-concept that includes an estimate of relative identification with parents, peers, and teachers. They found, in a study of white, semirural Maryland elementary school children in one school, that boys' peak of identification with father was in the sixth grade, that children identified more with parents than peers (except for sixth-grade girls who rated peers over father), and that generally parents ranked over teachers. (Long et al., 1967)

A midwestern study of black and white children in integrated class-rooms in rural, suburban, and small-town settings used sentence-completion items like the following to assess self-esteem, attitudes toward school, and perceptions of parents: "When I talk about school, my father ————" and "My family treats me like ————." (Schmuck and Luszki, 1969, p. 204) The investigators found that less than half the children perceived their parents as supportive of schoolwork. Black boys saw their parents as more supportive than white boys did (44 to 31 percent), but white girls saw their parents as more supportive than the black girls did (52 to 27 percent). There were other race and sex differences, the major ones being that "black boys spoke of their families in significantly more positive terms than did the white boys" (72 to 42 percent) (p. 210) and that white boys felt more achievement pressure than white girls; the reverse was true for the black children.

Of special note, even for this small sample from nonurban midwest settings, is the degree to which these children had varying perceptions of parental support and pressure and the degree to which many (about one-third) expressed alienation from parents. The trend is thus toward seeing parents less globally and less favorably than in the earlier years.

School Life

Children change from the fairly easy acceptance of the teacher in the primary grades to a more differentiated view during the intermediate and later school years. They can define the behavior of teachers they like and dislike. They tend to like behavior that shows the teacher is interested in their growth, is impartial and fair, is warm and human, and is interested in her own appearance. (Jersild, 1940) They respond favorably to a democratic classroom and a group climate in which they feel they have a voice in their own affairs.

They are also influenced by the teacher's behavior in terms of their own selves. Their self-understanding is affected by the way the teacher behaves toward them in the classroom. A study by Staines in Australia tested the hypothesis that specific changes can be made in the self-pictures of children in the classroom by teaching in a particular way. His study demonstrated that the self-picture is influenced by statements made by teachers about children. He first explored the type and amount of self-reference statements made by teachers to and about children. Teachers gave children such evaluations as "You're better at sums than you are at spelling" or "Jim, you're the tallest in the class," all alluding to physique and performance. In some classes, teachers made few such statements; in others, many.

Staines examined two classrooms. In the classroom of the teacher who was not aware of the self-picture of his pupils and who used normal methods of teaching to produce academic improvement in English and arithmetic, the pupils "showed significant decreases in certainty about Self and in differentiation." In the classroom of the teacher who "studied the Self-ratings of his class and tried to teach so that certain Self-ratings were changed . . . significant differences were found in two dimensions of the Self, certainty and differentiation." (Staines, 1958, p. 97) What do these findings mean? The experimenter defined certainty as the ability of the person to evaluate himself and differentiation as the ability to distinguish various levels and categories within the self.

This study also clearly revealed "that changes in the Self-picture are an inevitable part of both outcomes and conditions of learning in every classroom, whether or not the teacher is aware of them or aiming for them. . . . The Self can be deliberately produced by suitable teaching methods." (Staines, 1958, p. 109) This can be effectively done without sacrificing academic goals; in fact, the students in the experimental class did a little better than those in the control class.

Spaulding's study also indicates the effect of the teacher on pupil self-concept. He found that when teachers provided private individualized instruction, showed a concern for the divergent child, used appropriate techniques and material for a given task, and were calm and acceptant in their transactions, children in their rooms had higher self-concepts. (Spaulding, 1963)

Classroom life and teacher behavior influence the growing self of the child in ways other than those of differentiation and certainly about self. We have stressed the integrating process as concomitant with the differentiating process. When teachers are integrated their students' behavior becomes more spontaneous and constructive, more integrated, and reveals more initiative. The fluidity of the child's self is also evident in that his behavior changes in accordance with how like his present teacher his next teacher will be. Anderson and Brewer, 1946, a, b)

Since the middle of the 1950s, a number of highly sophisticated approaches to the study of teacher-pupil behavior in the classroom have been developed. (Rosenshine and Furst, 1972) These various forms of systematic observation have been used to look at social and emotional variables as well as cognitive variables. Some of these studies are summarized by Glidewell (1964) under the telling heading of "teacher power." He indicates that generally the teacher affects not only a wide range of immediate behavior but also the moral and academic values of his pupils. Soar (1967) shows that the way the teacher behaves can be looked at in terms of two dimensions: autonomy-control and warm-cold. It is interesting to note here how closely his model resembles Schaeffer's circumplex model of maternal behavior pictured in Chapter 3. According to Soar, placement of the teacher on both these dimensions is related to differential pupil achievement. For example, vocabulary gains seem to occur most under warm, autonomy-granting teachers. Straight reading achievement seems to occur at a higher level in those classes where teachers are warm and controlling or cold and autonomy-granting. In any event, Soar's work indicates the danger of making simple "commonsense" assumptions about "good" teachers.

Kounin (1970) has indicated that classroom management techniques are highly influential in affecting pupil behavior. His approach might be called ecological; that is, he examined the totality of the classroom and found overall management procedures, not keyed to any one child, that influenced class discipline. The way a teacher handled transitions from one activity to another, for example, was related to disruption. Perkins (1964) shows that the same behavior on the part of the teacher leads to quite different behaviors on the part of pupils. This effect, from our view of transaction, is easily understood. Perhaps the best summary is that of Sears and Hilgard, who state, "A classroom is a social situation, with a power structure, including peer relationships, and adult-child relationships; hence the most favorable motivational conditions need to take all of these factors into account, recognizing that the teacher is both model and reinforcer and, in ways not fully understood, a releaser of intrinsic motives." (Sears and Hilgard, 1964, p. 209)

Lipe and Jung (1971) reviewed the variety of studies, based mostly on operant conditioning or social-reinforcement models, that explored the relationships between incentive systems and child learning. From our perspective, their findings echo Perkins and Sears and Hilgard. They found that the student was the best judge of when he needed information on his performance and that systems of self-reward and self-managed learning were the more effective. The studies demonstrated not only the need to attend to the individual child's own value system ("If a student likes math the opportunity to study math may be employed as an incentive. . . ." Lipe and Jung, 1971, p. 262) but also that classrooms can be organized to enhance learning performance in a systematic fashion. Meeting individual needs does not mean chaos or laissez faire.

The classic study of boys' preadolescent group life by Lewin, Lippitt, and White (1939) demonstrated in still another way that behavior is transactional in nature, a function of the self in a given situation. Leadership technique, rather than any other personality variable, influenced the boys' behavior. When the situation was restrictive in nature, the behavior of the boys became aggressive, less sociable, etc.; when the situation was encouraging, free, accepted, and clearly defined the boys moved toward group cohesion and their behavior became more spontaneous, productive, and integrated. The absence of any guidance or help in the laissez-faire situation was not enhancing to the self. There was much frustration, low morale, and mutual interference. (Lippitt and White, 1943)

More recent studies of adult leadership (Hartup, 1970) show that adult personality, the nature of the situation, the social class background of the leader and peer members, and the leadership style all influence peer behavior.

All these studies illustrate the importance of the behavior of others (in these cases adult authority figures) in shaping and modifying the self of the child. As the situation changes, the behavior changes of others reflect the child's perception of what is permissible and possible. Even though preadolescence is a time of peer orientation, the role of the adult is still a vital and important one. When adults operate in ways that enable the child to perceive that they are seeking to understand him, to know him, and to aid him, the child responds by becoming more integrated and differentiated. By clarifying his view of himself, his behavior becomes more positive.

To balance our picture, let us again move to within the child. It is not the situation per se that modifies his behavior; it is his perception of it. This perception is influenced not only by the present situation but also by the already developed self. The teacher may behave in the same fashion toward two children with quite different results.

The preadolescent years are, for many boys, the time they begin to get into difficulty at school. They fall behind in their work and resist school standards; they perceive school as threatening or of little positive value. When asked to describe school experiences, they often reply in negative terms. They are concerned with how the class sees them and with the teacher's perception of their worth. For example, Mark, a sixth-grader of average intelligence but poor coordination, evaluated school as follows:

SCHOOL DAYS

4th grade first part of year in Mrs. Lewis room starting to—learn something how to write and hold a pencel then the latter part of the year I was transferred into a young teachers room Miss Smith. She had a rough time with a guy named Johnny he didn't know or do anything while I was in Miss Smiths room I learned nothing.

5th grade knowing nothing from following year had a tough time tring to chach up with the class could not chach up because I cound't hold the pencel right and it took me a long time to finesh the kids had no time for me you might say. Didn't learn much in grade 5 eather.

6th grade didn't know to much when I cam in I found out that the kids were real nice during the past year I feel I have learned much.

Sears and Sherman (1964) present a series of case studies of fifth- and sixth-graders that provide additional insight into the complex interrelationships of teacher-peer and family variables on the child's self-concept and perception of school. For example, when Harry was asked about an ideal classroom he said, "There would be lots of science and we'd eliminate a lot of talking," (p. 170) whereas Frances, a classmate, said, "I hate science." (p. 226) As teachers well know, you can't win them all.

Schmuck and Luszki (1969) found that black boys felt more positive toward school than white boys (59 to 39 percent) but that there were no race differences for girls. The great majority of youngsters do not feel negative about school; some feel neutral and most enjoy it. Jackson and Lahaderne (1967) investigated the relationship between achievement and feeling of satisfaction toward school and found there wasn't such a relationship. They said that it may be that students are rather neutral toward school instead of either hating or loving it.

An investigation using self-report techniques indicates children's views. Yeatts (1967), using Gordon's (1966, 1968) "How I See Myself" scale, analyzed the self-reports of more than 9000 children in a middle-sized Florida county. One part of the scale yields a score on self related to teachers and school. Although generally children in grades 3 to 6 reported a little on the positive side of the scale, she found, as has been so often indicated or hypothesized, that girls view school more favorably than do boys. Though there is no difference by race for the boys, the white girls reported the most positive attitudes. Yeatts's data also indicated that children of professionals, regardless of sex and race, had more favorable perceptions of school than did children of unskilled or unemployed parents.

Given our basic assumption that self-concept and perception of school influences learning and behavior, the teacher needs to find ways to learn how his pupils see themselves in relation to school. With this knowledge, he can provide opportunities and experiences in his room to enable children to modify negative concepts and to see themselves as worthwhile, able people and the school as an exciting place for discovering new things about themselves and their world.

Peer Perceptions

Chapter 9 presented a general view of peer group life. How do preadolescents perceive their relationships with peers? How do they evaluate peer behavior?

First, behavior toward the opposite sex is teasing, pushing, shoving, which may be aggression or may be likened to the first phases of courtship. Boys wouldn't be caught dead showing affection toward girls, although the girls do not behave so negatively toward the boys. Since sex identification is a major concern of the preadolescent, he perceives his same-sex gang as an essential force in enabling him to meet this concern. An attempt to see how preadolescents perceived their peers utilized an incomplete sentence technique in which 3000 children in a Minnesota county (grades 3 to 12) completed such statements as the following "Most boys ————," and "Most girls ————." An analysis of the content of the replies showed that most preadolescent youngsters were more favorably disposed to their same-sex peers and that the girls made increasingly unfavorable comments about boys through the sixth grade and then modified their position. (Harris and Tseng, 1957, pp. 401–411)

However, when we go below surface behavior, the picture changes somewhat. It is expected that there will be sex antagonism shown in behavior, but Reese (1966) found that reactions to the opposite sex cannot be so easily stereotyped. Generally, boys were more favorably disposed to girls than girls were to boys. Further, Yeatts (1967) and Gordon (1968) found that the peer group may be a more consistent idea for boys than for girls. For example, when boys answered the How I See Myself scale, an analysis of their items showed they could be grouped into an attitude-toward-boys and an attitude-toward-girls set. That is, the way they answered such an item as "I want the boys to like me" related highly to such other items as "The boys like me" and "I have lots of energy" but did not relate to the other set, including such items as "The girls like me," "I like teachers," and "I want the girls to like me," which in turn related to each other. No such patterns existed in the girls' answers. Generally, the boys held somewhat positive attitudes toward both sexes, but the white boys in the mid-Florida sample were more favorably disposed to girls than to boys.

Second, adequacy is of great importance in the peer group. Some insight into *why* this is so, into what the preadolescent seeks from his peers (and is willing to give to his peers), has been achieved through a longitudinal study conducted at Harvard. Sanford reports:

*What can be stated with some definiteness, on the basis of our
results, is that gravitation toward other children which appears to be
especially pronounced in the middle child [in this study an age group
9 to 13]—his tendency to be with other children . . . is not an
expression of his greater capacity for genuine social feeling. . . .
By joining with other children a subject at this age is better able to
carry out his practical aims. For some of his projects he requires
the cooperation of the group, and for satisfying some of his positive
needs, chiefly the need for "Dominance" and "Recognition" [as
measured by projective techniques] the response of the group is
necessary. Furthermore, it seems that the middle class [in age] child
derives necessary support from this group; he is better able to
master his childish fears if he has his "Gang" around him, and
problems of guilt and anxiety are solved by "doing what others do."*
[Sanford et al., 1943, p. 167]

Zelen tested the relationship between peer acceptance, self-acceptance, and acceptance of others among 145 fifth-grade boys and
girls in Iowa. These youngsters filled out self-rating scales and took a
sociometric test. He found a substantial relationship between acceptance
of others and peer acceptance, between acceptance of self and peer
status, but not between acceptance of self and acceptance of others. He
suggests that external, behavioral factors are perceived by peers of this
age, but little attention is paid to understanding others. (Zelen, 1954) In
other words, peers are judged on performance and utility. Belonging to
the gang enables the youngster to work on his adequacy needs. He
judges his peers in the same terms, looking at their adequacy and at
their roles in the group.

Each youngster establishes a reputation, and his peers evaluate
his standing in the group in terms of this reputation. In an interracial
camp setting, Yarrow and Campbell (1963) found that children assessed
each other on the basis of personal meaning. Their perceptions of each
other and the reputations they assigned were not related to behavior the
adults were able to observe and evaluate. These were low-income children, and the authors suggest that differences in meaning systems
(both age and class) might account for the lack of relationship between
the reputation the child established and adult observation of their behavior. This discrepancy is particularly pertinent for teachers and other
professionals who work with children's groups. Children's "realities" are
not necessarily ours.

Class differences affect both reputation and standing. Pope (1953)
used the California "guess who" technique, in which a child was asked
to identify children who were restless, talkative, fighters, etc., with 400
sixth-grade boys and girls in Oakland drawn from predominantly white
schools. About half the youngsters were in the lower class, and half were

in the highest social class in school. He found that high-prestige boys, regardless of class, were perceived by their peers as being active in games, possessing older friends, and being leaders. Lower class boys did not value "taking a joke" as highly as the higher class boys, and the latter did not find "fighting" so acceptable.

The class differences between the girls seemed to center about their definition of sexual role. For example, Pope reports: "The tomboy is an unpopular figure with the High Girls. She is placed very close to the rejected grouping of noisy, fighting, bossy and attention-getting traits. . . . In the low group, she has a good deal more prestige, personifying a status producing pattern which contrasts with the 'little lady.' She is known as the tough, fighting tomboy, who is more advanced in heterosexual interests than her lady-like contemporaries. The High Girls have no such well-defined, acceptable, directly aggressive type." (Pope, 1953, p. 205)

The preadolescent peer group, through its conformist pressures, its emphasis on the need of children to be accepted, its stereotypes of "good" and "bad" behavior, shapes the external behavior of its members. Even though children may resist inwardly or feel threatened, they attempt to produce the behavior they think the group expects of them. This is particularly true in ambiguous situations. Where what is right is clear, children can stick by their guns to some degree, but when it is unclear, the group attitude will affect the judgment of the individual child.

An example of the phenomenon of group pressure is contained in the study of Berenda. She set up judgmental situations in which the correct answer varied from clear to unclear and in which a single child or a small minority was placed in opposition to a prestige majority of peers. She found that even though the child in the minority thought the answer was wrong, he tended, if the situation was unclear, to change his judgment to conform with that of his peers. Even though he was disturbed, the child conformed. He followed, even when it was painful and obvious to him that he was changing to an incorrect answer. When the child was placed in opposition to the teacher, he more staunchly maintained the differences in his answers.

Berenda concludes: "Both the behavior during the test as well as the protocols obtained in personal interviews with each child point to the fact that the teacher is not viewed in the same way by a child as are his classmates. The position of the teacher really is one of an outsider who, although part of the school situation, is never judged as a member of the group. . . . The child's membership in the group is not threatened by the disagreement of the teacher." (Berenda, 1950, p. 77)

This situation is a matter of concern to adults. Teachers and parents do not like to find their power usurped by the child's age-mates. Conflicts between adults and peers become a part of the child's pattern and way of life in preadolescence. It is not that adults don't count, but that peers, under certain ambiguous conditions, count more. Two ideas should be stressed, however: (1) when the child has a clear-cut perception of right and wrong, he can resist peer pressure, and (2) clear-cut value perceptions are begun before this time. Peer pressures are strongest upon the child who has been taught to be dependent upon the judgment of others, to underevaluate his own self and his own knowledge, or who has not had clear models and images to identify with at earlier stages in his life.

SUMMARY

The preadolescent years are unique in the story of the self-development of the child. Bodily and social forces unite to present the child with new views of his interpersonal world and his own body. It is a time when growth in stature is slow, when coordination skill allows for team play, and when the culture provides numerous group experiences. It is the beginning of emancipation from the home and emergence into the life of the peer group. External control begins its great shift from adult to agemate. It is a time of high adequacy striving and evaluation of behavior of both self and others.

In this setting, the self continues its conceptual and evaluational development. Chapters 12 and 13 will focus upon self-development during these years.

REFERENCES AND ADDITIONAL READINGS

Anderson, H., & Brewer, J. Studies of teachers' classroom personalities, II. Effects of teachers' dominative and integrative contacts on children's classroom behavior. *Applied Psychology Monographs,* 1946, a, *8.*

Anderson, H., Brewer, J., & Reed, M. Studies of teachers' classroom personalities, III. Follow-up studies of the effects of dominative and integrative contacts on children's behaving. *Applied Psychology Monographs,* 1946, b, *11.*

Ausubel, D. et al. Perceived parent attitudes as determinants of children's ego structure. *Child Development,* 1954, *25,* 174–183.

Berenda, R. *The influence of the group on the judgments of children.* New York: King's Crown Press, 1950.

Campbell, J. Peer relations in childhood. In M. L. Hoffman & L. W. Hoffman (Eds.), *Review of child development research.* Vol 1. New York: Russell Sage Foundation, 1964. Pp. 289–322.

Glidewell, J. C. Unpublished data, reference file No. 884. St. Louis County Health Department, Clayton, Missouri, 1964.

Glidewell, J. C. et al. Socialization and social structure in the classroom. In L. W. Hoffman & M. L. Hoffman (Eds.), *Review of child development research.* Vol. 2. New York: Russell Sage Foundation, 1966. Pp. 221–256.

Gordon, I. J. *Human development: Readings in research.* Chicago: Scott, Foresman, 1965. Part IV.

Gordon, I. J. *Studying the child in school.* New York: Wiley, 1966.

Gordon, I. J. *A test manual for the "How I See Myself" scale.* Gainesville, Fla.: Florida Educational Research and Development Council, 1968.

Harris, D. B. et al. The relationship of children's home duties to an attitude of responsibility. *Child Development,* 1954, *25,* 29–33.

Harris, D. B., & Tseng, S. C. Children's attitudes toward peers and parents as revealed by sentence completions. *Child Development,* 1957, *28,* 401–411.

Hartup, W. Peer interaction and social organization. In P. Mussen (Ed.), *Carmichael's manual of child psychology.* (3rd ed.) Vol. 2. New York: Wiley, 1970. Pp. 361–456.

Hawkes, G., Burchinal, L., & Gardner, B. Pre-adolescents' view of some of their relations with their parents. *Child Development,* 1957, *28,* 393–399.

Iscoe, I., Williams, M., & Harvey, J. Age, intelligence and sex as variables in the conformity behavior of Negro and white children. *Child Development,* 1964, *35,* 451–460.

Jackson, P. W., & Lahaderne, H. M. Scholastic success and attitude toward school in a population of sixth graders. *Journal of Educational Psychology,* 1967, *58,* 15–18.

Jersild, A. T. Characteristics of teachers who are "liked best" and "disliked most." *Journal of Experimental Education,* 1940, *9,* 139–151.

Jones, H. The development of physical abilities. In N. Henry (Ed.), *Adolescence.* Forty-third Yearbook, NSSE. Chicago: University of Chicago Press, 1944. Pp. 100–122.

Jones, H. *Motor performance and growth.* Berkeley: University of California Press, 1949.

Kahn, S. B., & Weiss, J. The teaching of affective responses. In R. M. W. Travers (Ed.), *Second handbook of research on teaching.* (2nd ed.) Chicago: Rand McNally, 1973. Pp. 759–804.

Kounin, J. *Discipline and group management in classrooms.* New York: Holt, Rinehart & Winston, 1970.

Krogman, W. Some thoughts on football in pre- and early adolescence. (Mimeo) 1954.

Latchaw, M. Measuring selected motor skills in fourth, fifth, and sixth grades. *The Research Quarterly,* 1954, *25,* 439–449.

Lewin, K., Lippitt, R., & White, R. Patterns of aggressive behavior in experimentally created social climates. *Journal of Social Psychology,* 1939, *10,* 271–299.

Lipe, D., & Jung, S. Manipulating incentives to enhance school learning. *Review of Educational Research,* 1971, *41,* 249–280.

Lippitt, R., & White, R. K. The social climate of children's groups. In R. Barker, J. S. Kounin, & H. F. Wright (Eds.), *Child behavior and development.* New York: McGraw-Hill, 1943. Pp. 485–508.

Long, B., Henderson, E., & Ziller, R. Developmental changes in the self-concept during middle-childhood. *Merrill-Palmer Quarterly,* 1967, *13,* 201–216.

Loomis, M. *The preadolescent.* New York: Appleton-Century-Crofts, 1959.

Perkins, H. V. A procedure for assessing the classroom behavior of students and teachers. *American Educational Research Journal,* 1964, *1,* 249–260.

Pope, B. Socioeconomic contrasts in children's peer culture prestige values. *Genetic Psychology Monographs,* 1953, *48,* 157–220.

Redl, F. Pre-adolescents, what makes them tick? *Child Study,* 1943, *20,* 44–48.

Reese, H. W. Attitudes toward the opposite sex in late childhood. *Merrill-Palmer Quarterly,* 1966, *12,* 157–164.

Rosenshine, B., & Furst, N. The use of direct observation to study teaching. In R. M. W. Travers (Ed.), *Second handbook of research on teaching.* (2nd ed.) Chicago: Rand McNally, 1973. Pp. 122–183.

Sanford, R. et al. Physique, personality, and scholarship. *Child Development Monographs,* 1943, *8.*

Schmuck, R., & Luszki, M. Black and white students in several small communities. *The Journal of Applied Behavioral Science,* 1969, *5,* 203–220.

Schmuck, R. A., & Van Egmond, E. Sex difference in the relationship of interpersonal relations to academic performance. *Psychology in the Schools,* 1965, *2,* 32–40.

Sears, P. S., & Hilgard, E. R. The teacher's role in the motivation of the learner. In E. R. Hilgard (Ed.), *Theories of learning and instruction.* NSSE, 63rd Yearbook. Chicago: University of Chicago Press, 1964. Pp. 182–209.

Sears, P. S., & Sherman, V. S. *In pursuit of self-esteem.* Belmont, Calif.: Wadsworth, 1964.

Soar, R. S. Pupil growth over two years in relation to differences in classroom process. Paper presented at the meeting of the American Educational Research Association, New York, February 1967.

Spaulding, R. Achievement, creativity, and self-concept correlates of teacher-pupil transactions in elementary schools. (Mimeo) University of Illinois, Cooperative Research Project No. 1352, U.S. Office of Education, 1963.

Staines, J. The self-picture as a factor in the classroom. *British Journal of Educational Psychology,* 1958, *28,* 97–111.

Tanner, J. M. *Growth at adolescence.* (2nd ed.) Oxford: Blackwell Scientific Publications, 1962.

USPH, National Center for Health Statistics. *Height and weight of children, United States.* Washington, D.C.: U.S. Department of Health, Education, and Welfare, 1970.

Yarrow, M. R., & Campbell, J. D. Person perception in children. *Merrill-Palmer Quarterly,* 1963, *9,* 57–72.

Yeatts, P. *Developmental changes in the self-concept of children grades 3–12.* Gainesville, Fla.: Florida Educational Research and Development Council, 1967.

Zelen, S. The role of peer acceptance, acceptance of others and self-acceptance. *Proceedings, Iowa Academy of Science,* 1954, *61,* 446–449.

CHAPTER 12
CONCEPTUAL DEVELOPMENT

INCREASED UNDERSTANDING
OF THE WORLD
Concepts Held by Preadolescents

What does "zero" really mean? What does "being created in God's image" mean? How long ago was the American Revolution? What is meant by "behavior is caused"? What is "democracy"? Can preadolescents comprehend the answers to these questions? Are they able to conceptualize accurately about time, space, behavior, and society? Do they hold relatively clear pictures of their physical environment? How well can they deal with abstractions? Must they depend upon concrete experience in order to develop concepts?

The capabilities of this age group are of concern not only to the educator who is faced with the task of developing appropriate curriculums in this modern age but also to the parents and professionals who are trying to understand and help the child in his overall development. Parents lament their inability to "reason" with their children. Is this because the children are unable to understand or choose not to understand? What are the research data about the concepts held by preadolescents?

In our transactional framework, we know that particular concepts are functions of organism-environment transactions, so that age, intelligence, experience, socioeconomic status, and the *Zeitgeist* all influence the content and formation of concepts. We do not really know what children might conceptualize if we educated them differently. Some current studies of the subjects of mathematics and science suggest that a completely different sequence of curriculums might lead children to new and different concepts of the physical world. Thus, set theory, probabilities, and topology are being introduced much earlier than was previously thought possible.

Mathematical-scientific concepts held by children are subject to change. Children's scientific knowledge varies widely from generation to generation, from region to region, and also from child to child. Though these differences exist, the general trend is one in which knowledge grows as the child grows. Youngsters growing up in Florida's Cape Canaveral section discuss thrusts, gravity, etc., with much erudition, but 12-year-olds, on the average, discuss these terms and others with more knowledge than 9- or 10-year-olds.

Understanding of arithmetical concepts also shows a similar trend of development. The preadolescent seems able to comprehend the concept of zero at about the fifth-grade level. Concepts of indeterminates seem to come into focus in the sixth grade; then the child can use with accuracy such terms as *hardly, few,* and *several.* The movement from perceptual thinking during these years is also shown in the way distance is understood. Preadolescents and early adolescents do not have a general knowledge of distance, and they deal with distance by use of two frames of reference. For nearby locations, they use their own direct experience; for distant locations, they use maps. What is important is that they are able to use both; they are not dependent only on direct experience, although they use this where applicable, but can shift to a more conceptual, abstract approach when direct experience is insufficient. The child cannot develop a concept without experience, but the experience no longer need be direct.

The years of preadolescence, roughly grades 4 to 6, still fall within the "concrete operations" years of Piaget, but many children move into the logical operations stage by the time they are in sixth grade. *Logical operations* consists of such activities as hypothesizing, building abstract categories, and perceiving cause-effect relationships in the absence of concrete materials. Further, children can now come up with categories that really don't exist, except symbolically (see Chapter 16), and not be overwhelmed by perceptual reality. This may be why they can now handle zero or negative numbers. They can also solve problems that require handling more than two variables at the same time. We know that concept formation is a function of intelligence, direct experience, and instruction. (Osler and Weiss, 1962; Smedslund, 1964; Glaser and Resnick, 1972) For example, Inhelder and Piaget (1958) investigated children's responses to various situations that reflected scientific-mathematical principles. For example, they showed children an inclined plane (see Figure 12.1) and recorded children's responses to the problem of predicting movements of the wagon. Movement is a function of weight, counterweight, and inclination. The following response from a preadolescent indicates an understanding that more than weight is involved; he has a beginning concept of work.

JAN (10; 8): "To make it go up, you have to put a heavier weight here [*W*]."—*"What else could you do?"*—"Unload the wagon."—*"And*

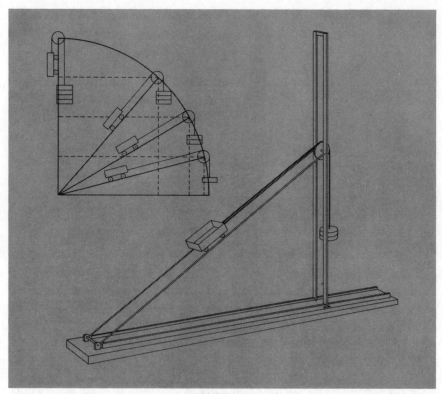

FIGURE 12.1

A toy dumping wagon, suspended by a cable, is hauled up the inclined plane by the counterweights at the other end of the cable. The counterweights can be varied and the angle of the plane is adjustable; weights placed in the wagon provide the third variable. Figure 10 from *The growth of logical thinking* by Barbel Inhelder and Jean Piaget, translated by Anne Parson and Stanley Milgram, © 1958 by Basic Books, Inc. British rights are owned by Routledge & Kegan Paul Ltd.

for the wagon to stay at the same point?"—He puts 4 units on the wagon and 4 at W. "The weights are equal. No, it doesn't move."— "*Can you do something with the rail?*"—"Maybe you could lower it; it's easier for the wagon to go forward because the track isn't as high."—"*If you lift the rail and add weight?*"—"It will stay poised because it's harder for it to go up." *Then he weighs the wagon and declares that it is equal to 4 weight units.—"So would it remain in equilibrium if you leave the wagon empty and put 4 weights here?* [W].—"No, it would go up" [*thus he understands that the equilibrium depends on inclination*].—"*And if you raise the rail?*"—"It's harder for it to go up."—"*Why?*"—"Because the wagon gets heavier." [*Inhelder and Piaget, 1958, p. 187*]

Jan's response is illustrative of only partial understanding. Inhelder and Piaget's problem was then used by Wiegand (1970), who took 12-year-olds through a series of steps that represented an orderly arrangement of the skills necessary to use logical thought to solve the inclined-plane problem. They were then able to do so. (Glaser and Resnick, 1972) Inhelder and Piaget demonstrated the usual child performance; Wiegand demonstrated the effect of instruction.

The child's *time* concepts are still in a state of development. The 10-year-old's concept of historical time is not yet accurate. We have numerous jokes about teachers being asked if they knew Lincoln or, worse still, Washington. Sunday School teachers have much difficulty in conveying the historical time of both the Old and the New Testament to preadolescent youngsters, who cannot conceive of the thousands of years between the times of Moses and Jesus and between the time of Jesus and now. Further, since history in the schools deals with yet other time periods and events (the exploration of America), the children have difficulty developing a sense of perspective from their experience. Thus, both age and experience combine to inhibit understanding. Children do comprehend how historical time is reckoned before they reach their teens; they can manipulate time lines (that is, locate dates on a line from 0 to 1974), but maturity is not reached until adolescence.

Social concepts, such as the meaning of democracy, also follow developmental patterns. For instance, Solomon et al. (1972) examined the development of ideas and behavior of Chicano children attending a Chicago Catholic school, using group discussion and individual interviews. They investigated such concepts as (1) equal representation, (2) equal participation, (3) equal resource distribution, (4) responsibility to state one's minority view, and (5) the art of compromise. They found from the interviews that by the fourth grade a large majority of children gave democratic responses, including a reason, for variables (2) and (4), but it wasn't until sixth grade or eighth grade that this happened for (1) and (5). It occurred early for (3). When they examined children's behavior in the group discussion, however, they found behavior occurring earlier than stated values. They also found that the sex of the adult in the group was a strong influence on behavior.

Torney and Hess (1971), who used a questionnaire to find out children's political attitudes, report that emotional attachment to America occurs in the early grades and stays unchanged, whereas recognition of the United States as being part of an international system does not come until after age 10. From our discussion of movement from concrete to logical thought, this rough timetable makes sense.

Preadolescents have the ability to conceptualize about *religion*. However, Goldman (1964) indicated that they operate, until roughly age 11 to 13, at a Piagetian concrete-operational level. They take Bible stories lit-

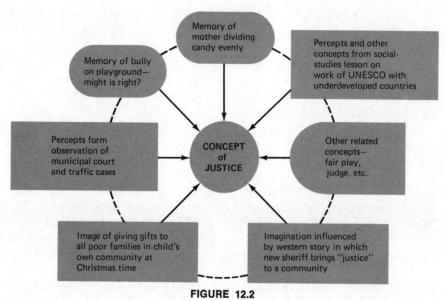

FIGURE 12.2

A few factors influencing a 12-year-old's concept of justice. Reprinted by permission of the publisher from *Children's thinking,* by D. Russell, © 1956 by Xerox Corporation, published by Xerox College Publishing.

erally and deal with the material about God anthropomorphically. For example, the dividing of the waters in Exodus is typically explained by preadolescents as intervention by God in natural forces, most often by directing the wind.

The ability to deal with abstractions is perhaps the great change that occurs during this age, though it is, of course, not an abrupt change. By fifth-grade most children seem able to handle some abstract ideas and relations.

Another aspect of the development of social concepts is the ability of children to understand the meaning of behavior. The work of Ojemann and his colleagues at the University of Iowa has contributed greatly to our understanding of the transactional nature of this ability. For about 20 years, they explored many ramifications of the problem of trying to improve mental hygiene in the elementary school. They trained teachers to use social studies materials to present the concept that behavior is caused. They found that such a concept could not be developed by merely introducing it as a subject for a part of the day while the rest of the program was unaffected.

One of their many research reports can serve as a guide to their program. Four teachers (one each from the fourth and fifth grade and two from the sixth grade) in a midwestern industrial town were given special training. The program covered developmental problems of normal children, teachers' personal problems, research techniques applicable to classroom use, the causal approach to behavior, techniques of meeting classroom problems, and preparation of special materials. In addition to the one-month intensive summer study of the above, 12 conferences were scheduled during the school year.

The materials that were developed included collections of problem stories, workbooks, an exposition of the causal approach, and revised social studies units. Two control teachers were selected for each experimental teacher, and the control teachers had access to the materials but not the training.

Two tests were administered, both before and after a semester of class experience. One test measured the punitiveness of the child; the other his understanding of causality of behavior.

> *The classes of the experimental teachers showed distinctly significant changes on the two measures when compared with classes of the control teachers. It thus appears that when we bring children of the upper elementary grade levels under the influence of causally oriented teachers teaching causal content we bring about significant differences in the child's growth in the aspects measured in this study. [Ojemann et al., 1955, p. 113]*

This study shows that scientific concepts about human behavior can be understood by preadolescents when they are fully exposed to them. Rather than leaving their development to chance experience, such concepts can be consciously built into the educational framework.

Psychologists and educators can make good use of Piaget's notions about the development of thought. The work cited above stresses the role of guided learning experiences in affecting the substantive concepts learned and the ability to conceptualize. Kohnstamm (1965, 1966) indicated the effect of explanations as a guide to thought; Soviet educators stress the importance of verbal behavior and of training orienting responses (Berlyne, 1963); Taba and her colleagues trained teachers to ask the kinds of questions that stimulated the cognitive processes of assimilation-accommodation (Taba, 1964); and Ojemann and his associates demonstrated not only learning social concepts but also probability (1965). Most of the new curricula in American schools are based upon the notion of learning to learn, although the authors are not necessarily clear or in agreement as to goals, tasks, the nature of the learner, or the learning process.

The research opens up many possibilities for exploring the role of guided experience in concept development. It offers support for the position that what children *are* does not necessarily control what children *may become*. It casts suspicion on procedures that utilize only current knowledge of children as the criterion for curriculum development. It emphasizes the vital influence of the transactional field in affecting future self-development. It removes from us the rigid, ontogenetic barrier to understanding behavior. Although, as we have stressed, age is an important condition in concept formation, we do not know the minimal age at which certain concepts could be learned if they were actively taught nor the possible effects this earlier acquisition might have on subsequent development.

The Increasing Ability to Conceptualize

Growth in intellectual ability is steady and continuous during these years. With each succeeding year, children become more intelligent as measured by intelligence tests. Two longitudinal studies demonstrate, however, the individuality of this growth. The Fels Research Center studied 140 children as they matured from age 3 to age 12 in an attempt to understand changes in their IQ scores. Sontag et al., 1958; Kagan et al., 1958) The California Growth Study data were analyzed for somewhat the same reasons. (Bayley, 1956) Both point out the continued development of idiosyncratic (individual) patterns of growth and change. Although there is individual fluctuation in score, there is at the same time a group trend of continued growth with age. (Bayley, 1970)

The changes of an individual's IQ seem to be related to personality factors within the individual. The changes in IQ scores during the school years are not due to the changing ratio between verbal and nonverbal items that occurs as the individual grows older (Baker, 1955)—that is, the composition of the test items themselves does not seem to make the difference. Rather, children's scores change for more complex reasons that lie within the children themselves. Intellectual functioning is but one aspect of total functioning and is compounded of maturational, experiential, and personal factors. Although we can safely predict that ability will increase with age for most children, some children will do less well because of their total life situation.

The role of age (seen as simply reflecting more time for experience) in increasing conceptual ability has been shown in many studies. A British study (Annett, 1959), for example, attempted to explore the development of concepts. Is there a sequence? When do "incorrect" responses change to "correct" ones? Annett had 303 children, ages 5 through 11, sort 16 cards (4 each having animals, plants, vehicles, and furniture) into any arrangement chosen by the child. She found that the errors (failure to sort into 4 equal piles) were systematic rather than random until such time as the correct responses occurred; for example, the young child placed a plant picture and a table together because plants go on tables. The sequence of development ran from the contiguity approach to the point where similarity was the criterion and finally to class name, such as *plant*. The latter was achieved by the 9- to 11-year-olds. Sigel (1953) also found this increasing use of conceptual grouping, in which an object is treated as a member of a class, as age increased from 7 to 9 to 11 years. In a later study, he questioned "stages" of conservation and suggested that, with age, there is increased ability to tolerate irrelevant cues. (Sigel, Salta, and Roskind, 1967)

Socioeconomic status, sex, and emotional factors also influence conceptual performance. Siller (1957) analyzed the performance of upper and lower class sixth-graders on conceptual items on intelligence tests. Because he concluded that upper class children do better, the question of the effects of experiential "deprivation" on conceptualization of preadolescents is raised.

The effects of emotions, which will be discussed in more detail in the next chapter, should not be overlooked here. If the child is disturbed, his ability to think is affected, for thinking and feeling are inextricably interwoven. An example of this may be found in a study of children's performance on the Stanford-Binet intelligence test in relation to their degree of emotional stability as measured both by tests and clinical judgments. The results indicated "that the children with personality dysfunctions do not perform intellectually in the same manner as those with more healthy personalities." (Granick, 1955, p. 656)

Cognitive style, as a learned pattern of behavior, probably influences learning and performance on concept attainment tasks for those children who are not able to adjust style to task. When style is classified as motoric or conceptual, it seems to be an independent and specific pattern distinct from the learning task (Singer and Brunk, 1967); when it is classified as impulsive-reflective, lower class children are more impulsive as well as poorer in verbal task performance. (Schwebel, 1966) If lower class children are more motoric, more impulsive, less conceptual, and less reflective, then one of the tasks of the school may be to so teach these children that they have a wider array of choices of behavior. This broader range of options might then allow them to maintain their own preferred pattern but use other behaviors at times and in situations where they may be more appropriate to the task.

Another aspect of cognitive style is the performance along a continuum from simple to complex. Kogan points out that cognitive complexity means the ability to move from simple labels such as good-bad to being able to see the shades of gray. Although Kogan indicates the many methodological problems still to be solved in investigating this continuum, the concept and Kogan's presentation of it relate to our earlier discussions of differentiation and to the Piagetian concept of decentering. They also relate to the Torney and Hess (1971) finding of the inability of young children to see the nation as one of many.

The effect of specific training techniques in concept development and on cognitive style needs much investigation. We still know relatively little about how children develop concepts, although we know factors that affect development. One study was concerned with the relative effect of different training methods for developing concepts about area in fifth-grade children. Three different methods were used; each involved differing amounts of laboratory materials. The conclusions reached were "that the laboratory approach where each student may actually use materials himself is more effective if we are interested not only in a child's success in solving problems familiar to him but also in his ability to transfer learning to new situations." It is also most effective "if we are interested not only in getting a general idea, but in developing an understanding." (Gibb and Van Engen, 1959, p. 37)

Blane (1967) varied the amount of feedback in a concept attainment task modeled after Bruner's (1956). In effect, she taught the children to become aware of their behavior; this approach was similar in some degree to the Russian emphasis on the orienting response. She found this enabled them to attain concepts faster than by a pure discovery approach. Lunda (1961) trained students in the use of algorithms through a guided discovery approach that reduced the frequency of error and aided in learning Russian grammar.

We have repeatedly stressed how much we still need to learn. However, the psychologist interested in application has to use what he knows. At the same time, research and evaluation of the effects of what is being done should continue. Thus, in spite of gaps in our knowledge, we do have to draw implications and use them.

Implications for Education

The increasing ability of preadolescents to conceptualize and to hold increasingly complex concepts is a function of age, previous general experience, intelligence, and direct, specific training. The role of experience in developing concepts suggests that schooling can be designed to facilitate both the acquisition of specific concepts and the time in which they are learned. All too often materials and information have been presented to children in school because of ideas held by adults about the sequence and ways in which facts and concepts should be learned. History has often been taught on a chronological basis when more exciting and conceptually fruitful ways might be found. The ability of intermediate grade pupils to abstract and to classify has often been ignored or undeveloped because of the emphasis on teaching masses of data rather than conceptual schemes for ordering these data. The need for laboratory experience has been recognized, but often this experience is not accompanied by the reflective thinking that is needed to help the child see the concrete experience in perspective so that he can achieve transfer.

Berlyne (1970) indicates that teaching for problem solving can be successful in preadolescence, but he also states that the type of experiences the child has had with question asking in his early years has lasting effects. Skill training is not enough. "Future research must pay at least as much attention to the motivational factors that govern readiness to embark on thinking, skillful choice between thinking and alternative epistemic activities (consultation, observation) and the ability to judge when epistemic efforts are worthwhile and how long they should continue." (Berlyne, 1970, p. 974)

An example of the application of cognitive developmental ideas is the Taba Social Studies Curriculum (Duvall, 1969). In relation to decentering, differentiation, and cognitive complexity, for example, they state:

> *Students need to be helped to identify with others in situations different from their own, to empathize with others' concerns, to "feel" as they do, and to see things from another's point of view. They may learn to do this by identifying how individuals in other cultures feel in a conflict situation, or by role-playing individuals who are trying to decide how to deal with a particular problem. . . .*
>
> *Students need to be helped to avoid using stereotypes as a means of classifying individuals (for example, by learning to recognize and analyze propaganda techniques; by learning to distinguish between factual reports, inferences, and value judgments; and by learning, as emphasized in the curriculum, that people in different cultures are individuals with unique perceptions and desires). [Duvall, 1969, p. A-5]*

Further, Taba pointed up the importance of questioning:

> *Inferring and generalizing, like the other cognitive tasks, requires that in classroom discussion the teacher and the children assume roles, one of which is the role of questioner. Initially, the teacher assumes this role, but his goal should be for the children to assume part of it; it is hoped that eventually they will question themselves, other children, the teacher, and their textbooks on their own.*
>
> *What can the teacher do to help children become questioners? Techniques such as pausing may encourage students to respond to or support another's point of view without having a question directed to them. [Duvall, 1969, p. A-9]*

In her investigations of elementary science teaching, Rowe (1973) found that wait-time, that is, a pause by the teacher before reasking a question or a pause before responding to a child's answer, was highly related to the level and amount of pupil questions. Increasing the length of pause to about 3 seconds from the characteristic less than 1 second improved the caliber and amount of pupil and teacher questions.

We need this kind of specific research into teaching science, social studies, and mathematics, and we need further research into the process by which concepts are developed. And we need to know much more about the way in which a child integrates his experiences, about the role of the emotions in concept development, and about the influence of self-concept upon other concepts.

VALUE CONCEPTS

What kinds of values do preadolescents hold? Are these children still essentially egocentric in their moral approach to the world? Do they perceive the adult mores more clearly than younger children, and do they attempt to identify with these mores? What are their ethical standards?

In this section we are concerned with children's concepts of "should" and "ought," "right" and "wrong." In earlier chapters, the development of value judgments through the identification process was discussed. There is general agreement that character development, or the development of conscience, is a result of the transactions between the organism and the cultural, interpersonal environment. The transactional nature of values needs to be emphasized, especially to parents who may feel that there is no point in reasoning with children or expecting them to make value judgments until they reach the "age of reason."

Turiel, a colleague of Kohlberg's, has examined the processes of movement from one stage of moral development to the next (see Chapter 10 for the Kohlberg stages). Preadolescents seem to be at stages 2 and 3. Turiel believes that individual movement is a natural one through all the stages in sequence and that "a stage is not learned but constructed by the individual himself." (Turiel, 1973, p. 742) This means that the process of moral development follows the same rules as that of Piagetian general cognitive development and our view of self-development. Further, the process of decentering, which requires peer clash of opinion, seems to hold here too. Turiel indicates that conflict of ideas is essential. However, the child has to see that the ideas *are* in conflict, so presenting him with reasons several stages above his own are not *perceived* as conflict. Thus, it is not that adults should not reason with children, it is that they have to create conflict between reasons in a way that the child sees and that requires, in Piaget's terms, accommodation.

We can see the developmental process. Ugurel-Semin's study of children in Istanbul, Johnson's study of midwestern American children, and Harrower's study of London children, among others, reveal a developmental pattern. In the Istanbul study, a child was faced with the problem of dividing 9 nuts with another child. He could be generous (divide them 5 to 4 in favor of the other child), selfish (divide 5 to 4 in his favor), or equalitarian (give the examiner, for example, the extra nut). The equalitarian pattern was found to be most characteristic of ages 9 to 11, replacing the generosity of 6- to 8-year-olds and the selfishness of the younger child. No sex differences were found. (Ugurel-Semin, 1952)

Harrower, who examined the sequence of development postulated by Piaget and then compared lower class children with upper class children by using stories involving punishment and cheating, found that the order of development (from retribution to understanding) in the lower class children was the same as that given by Piaget in his study of lower class children. (Piaget, 1932; Harrower, 1934)

The earlier discussion of Ojemann's work demonstrates training for thinking in causal terms. Ojemann did not simply describe how children behaved when presented with a situation; he attempted to manipulate the sequence of experiences in such a fashion that he led the children to learn something from the experience that put them far beyond the place they would have been if they had simply been asked to do a task in the fashion of Ugurel-Semin (for example, see pages 242–243).

A second look at two of these researches by Harrower and Ugurel-Semin illustrates the role of culture in conjunction with maturation. Harrower found that the upper class youngsters did not develop concepts at the same time as the lower class; many already had advanced concepts. There were class differences in Istanbul as well. The lower class children were mostly equalitarian, sometimes generous, and less frequently selfish. One can hypothesize about the role of "learning to do with little" in the Istanbul lower class home or the pressure to be adult in the London upper class home.

Anderson and Anderson (1961) used incomplete stories in a cross-cultural study of mental health. The results may be examined as reflective of values (democratic vs. authoritarian) in school children. They found that the way children answered did reflect their culture; the American and English samples were more "democratic"; the German and Mexican, more "authoritarian"; and, within the German group, Hamburg was more democratic than Karlsruhe and Munich.

Earlier we indicated that cross-cultural studies in North America show different patterns of cooperation and competition in Indian, Mexican, and Anglo subcultures. Most of the above studies deal with moral judgment or verbalized values. But does judgment or knowledge predict behavior?

Children not only know what behavior is expected of them; they also know how teachers and peers perceive this behavior. Boys and girls both know that teachers view the behavior of boys as more socially unacceptable, generally, than that of girls. They recognize clearly that more boys get into trouble with teachers. (Meyer and Thompson, 1956; Foshay et al.,

1954) This sex difference in school behavior shows aspects of behavior different from those shown in the studies cited earlier in this section. Mostly, it is aggressive behavior that triggers disapproval. The boys know teachers disapprove of aggression, but they continue to commit it. It could be, as Jones suggests, that "girls may be more submissive than boys and more influenced by what they think is expected of them by adult societies. Second, it seems that boys are more aggressive than girls." (Jones, 1954, pp. 797–798) Or is it, as Foshay believes, that "from the child's point of view, most aggression is counter-aggression"? (Foshay et al., 1954, p. 165) In Chapter 13 we will discuss the importance during these years of concepts of appropriate age-sex behavior. Whatever the conclusion may be, it is obvious to researchers and teachers that boys place a much higher value than girls on socially disapproved behavior during preadolescence.

A possible answer to the aggressive behavior of boys is that children value most highly the respect, admiration, and acceptance of their peers. Those values that they perceive as being peer values are implemented by action; behavior that is approved by adults but that does not lead to peer rewards is not executed. The child, in his judgments and values, now acknowledges the primary power of his peer group. His behavior becomes a function of his peer situation as he perceives it from moment to moment. It is in this situation that the discrepancy between *knowing* and *doing* lies. The preadolescent *knows* what is right and what he should do; however, he fails to do it when it conflicts with peer-group pressure.

Berkowitz (1962), in an excellent review of the development of moral values from the point of view of social learning theory (that is, that values are learned like behaviors), indicates that behavior is a function of self-esteem, ambiguity, and anonymity and that situational variables play a role. We saw in Chapters 9 and 11 the strong pull of the peer group. It may be that what is ambiguous is not the old code but its real acceptance by adults who demonstrate all modes of behavior. Anonymity may mean one's loss of identity within the group (as the outsider sees it). Self-esteem is not only a function of parental love early in life but of present acceptance by significant peers and adults. The cognitive-developmental view (Piaget, Kohlberg, Turiel) holds that the child synthesizes his experiences and generates his principles from them. From this perspective, there are two-way relationships between thought and action. The research summarized by Turiel (1973) also supports this view. While we lack convincing evidence about the relationships of thought and behavior in preadolescence, the two positions (Berkowitz and Turiel) are not irreconcilable. How a child behaves at a given moment may be based upon the actual situation and his interpretation of it, which includes his stage of moral development as well as self-esteem, identification with parental values, the degree of anonymity, and how ambiguous he thinks the situation is.

SUMMARY

Preadolescents are still thinking about behavior in stage 2 and 3 terms. That is, for example, that good behavior is that which is approved of by one's group (stage 3), and right action meets one's own needs (stage 2). They know what adults expect, even if they do not meet these expectations. They view aggression differently from adults, not always seeing it as bad, but sometimes seeing it as demanded by the situation. The discrepancy between boy and girl behavior is marked and is symptomatic, as we shall see in the next chapter, of a fundamental concern of these children.

What do these ideas mean to the student of behavior and to parents and teachers? They suggest that we look at the situation in which socially disapproved behavior occurs and, at the same time, attempt to see what values are important to children. These ideas indicate that verbal explanations, a favorite disciplinary technique, may not be comprehended by preadolescents if they are expressed at a stage too high for them. They suggest that values in action *can* be taught by utilization of group processes and laboratory means, provided we understand the viewpoint of the children. (Kohlberg and Turiel, 1971) Lastly, they indicate the need for careful research into both the concepts held by each generation of children and the processes by which concepts are developed and modified.

In our study of this period of development, we started by looking at external forces operating upon the child. In this chapter we have examined two important aspects of the child's self-system—his concepts of his world and his values. We will now focus, in the next chapter, upon those particular concepts that are central—his concepts of self as he continues his search for identity.

REFERENCES AND ADDITIONAL READINGS

Anderson, H. H., & Anderson, G. L. A cross-national study of children: A study in creativity and mental health. Paper presented at the Sixth International Congress on Mental Health, Technical Session, The Sorbonne, Paris, August 31, 1961. Reprinted in I. J. Gordon (Ed.), *Human development: Readings in research.* Glenview, Ill.: Scott, Foresman, 1965.

Annett, M. Classification of instances of four common class concepts by children and adults. *British Journal of Educational Psychology,* 1959, *29,* 223–236.

Baker, S. et al. Specific ability in IQ change. *Journal of Consulting Psychology,* 1955, *19,* 307–310.

Bayley, N. Individual patterns of development. *Child Development,* 1956, *27,* 45–75.

Bayley, N. Development of mental abilities. In P. Mussen (Ed.), *Carmichael's manual of child psychology.* (3rd ed.) Vol. 1. New York: Wiley, 1970. Pp. 1163–1210.

Berkowitz, L. *The development of motives and values in the child.* New York: Basic Books, 1962.

Berlyne, D. E. Soviet research on intellectual processes in children. In J. Wright & J. Kagan (Eds.), Basic cognitive processes in children. *Child Development Monographs,* 1963, *28(86),* 165–183.

Berlyne, D. Children's reasoning and thinking. In P. Mussen (Ed.), *Carmichael's manual of child psychology.* (3rd ed.) Vol. 1. New York: Wiley, 1970. Pp. 939–981.

Blane, L. The effects of thematic material and informational feedback on the ability of children to achieve concepts. Unpublished doctoral dissertation, University of Florida, 1967.

Bruner, J., Goodnow, J., & Austin, G. *A study of thinking.* New York: Wiley, 1956.

Duvall, A. *The TABA social studies curriculum.* Menlo Park, Calif.: Addison-Wesley, 1969.

Foshay, A. et al. *Children's social values: An action research study.* New York: Teachers College, 1954.

Gibb, E., & Van Engen, H. Structuring kinesthetic experiences to facilitate conceptual learning. *Educational Service Studies.* Cedar Falls, Iowa State Teachers College, 1959.

Glaser, R., & Resnick, L. Instructional psychology. In P. Mussen & M. Rosenzweig (Eds.), *Annual review of psychology.* Vol. 23. Palo Alto, Calif.: Annual Reviews, Inc., 1972. Pp. 207–276.

Goldman, R. *Religious thinking from childhood to adolescence.* London: Routledge & Kegan Paul, 1964.

Gordon, I. J. Guided learning experiences and the new curricula. In R. H. Ojemann & K. Pritchett (Eds.), *Giving emphasis to guided learning.* Cleveland: Educational Research Council of Greater Cleveland, 1966. Pp. 73–91.

Granick, S. Intellectual performance as related to emotional instability in children. *Journal of Abnormal and Social Psychology,* 1955, *51,* 653–656.

Harrower, M. Social status and the moral development of the child. *British Journal of Educational Psychology,* 1934, *1,* 75–94.

Inhelder, B., & Piaget, J. *The growth of logical thought in childhood and adolescence.* New York: Basic Books, 1958.

Jones, V. Character development in children—an objective approach. In L. Carmichael (Ed.), *Manual of child psychology,* (2nd ed.) New York: Wiley, 1954. Pp. 781–832.

Kagan, J. et al. Personality and IQ change. *Journal of Abnormal and Social Psychology,* 1958, *56,* 261–266.

Kogan, N. Educational implications of cognitive styles. In G. Lesser (Ed.), *Psychology and educational practice.* Glenview, Ill.: Scott, Foresman, 1971. Pp. 242–293.

Kohlberg, L., & Turiel, E. Moral development and moral education. In G. Lesser (Ed.), *Psychology and educational practice.* Glenview, Ill.: Scott, Foresman, 1971. Pp. 410–465.

Kohnstamm, G. A. Developmental psychology and the teaching of thought operation. *Paedagogica Europaea.* Vol. 1. New York: American Elsevier, 1965. Pp. 79–97.

Kohnstamm, G. A. The gap between the psychology of cognitive development and education as seen from Europe. Paper presented at Jennings lecture series, Educational Research Council of Greater Cleveland, January 22, 1966.

Lunda, L. Training pupils in the methods of rational thinking and problem of algorithms. *Voprosy Psikhologii,* 1961, *1,* 103–118.

Meyer, W., & Thompson, G. Sex differences in the distribution of teacher approval and disapproval among sixth-grade children. *Journal of Educational Psychology,* 1956, *47,* 385–396.

Ojemann, R. The human relations program at the State University of Iowa. *Personnel and Guidance Journal,* 1958, *37,* 199–206.

Ojemann, R. et al. The effects of a causal teacher-training program and certain curricula changes on grade school children. *Journal of Experimental Education,* 1955, *24,* 95–114.

Ojemann, R., Maxey, E., & Snider, B. The effect of a program of guided learning experiences in developing probability concepts at the third grade level. *Journal of Experimental Education,* 1965, *33,* 321–330.

Osler, S. F., & Weiss, S. R. Studies in concept attainment: III. Effect of instruction at two levels of intelligence. *Journal of Experimental Psychology,* 1962, *63,* 528–533. Reprinted in I. J. Gordon (Ed.), *Human development: Readings in research.* Glenview, Ill.: Scott, Foresman, 1965.

Piaget, J. *The moral judgment of the child.* New York: Harcourt, Brace, 1932.

Piaget, J., & Inhelder, B. *The psychology of the child.* New York: Basic Books, 1969.

Raths, L., Harmin, M., & Simon, S. *Values and teaching.* Columbus, Ohio: Merrill, 1966.

Rowe, M. B. *Teaching science as continuous inquiry.* New York: McGraw-Hill, 1973.

Russell, D. *Children's thinking.* Lexington, Mass.: Ginn, 1956.

Schwebel, A. Effects of impulsivity on performance of verbal tasks in middle- and lower-class children. *American Journal of Orthopsychiatry,* 1966, *36,* 13–21.

Shantz, D. W., & Pentz, T. Situational effects on justifiableness of aggression at three age levels. *Child Development,* 1972, *43,* 274–281.

Sigel, I. Developmental trends in the abstraction ability of children. *Child Development,* 1953, *24,* 131–144.

Sigel, I., Salta, E., & Roskind, W. Variables determining concept conservation in children. *Journal of Experimental Psychology,* 1967, *74,* 471–475.

Siller, J. Socioeconomic status and conceptual thinking. *Journal of Abnormal and Social Psychology,* 1957, *55,* 365–371.

Singer, R., & Brunk, J. Relation of perceptual-motor ability and intellectual ability in elementary school children. *Perceptual and Motor Skills,* 1967, *24,* 967–970.

Smedslund, J. Concrete reasoning: A study of intellectual development. *Child Development Monographs,* 1964, *29*(2).

Solomon, D. et al. The development of democratic values and behavior among Mexican-American children. *Child Development,* 1972, *43,* 625–638.

Sontag, L. et al. Mental growth and personality development: A longitudinal study. *Child Development Monographs,* 1958, *23.*

Taba, H., Levine, S., & Elzey, F. Thinking in elementary school children. Cooperative Research Project No. 1574. San Francisco: San Francisco State College, 1964.

Torney, J., & Hess, R. The development of political attitudes in children. In G. Lesser (Ed.), *Psychology and educational practice.* Chicago: Scott, Foresman, 1971. Pp. 466–501.

Turiel, E. Stage transition in moral development. In R. M. W. Travers (Ed.), *Second handbook of research on teaching.* Chicago: Rand McNally, 1973. Pp. 732–758.

Ugurel-Semin, R. Moral behavior and moral judgment of children. *Journal of Abnormal and Social Psychology,* 1952, *47,* 463–474.

Wiegand, V. A study of subordinate skills in science problem solving. Paper presented at the annual meeting of the American Educational Research Association, 1970.

CHAPTER 13

THE CONTINUING SEARCH FOR IDENTITY

DEVELOPING SEX-ROLE IDENTIFICATION

"Goodby to Oedipus," the title of an article that appeared in *Harper's Magazine*, describes the feelings of a mother as she watches preadolescent boys in action. It is a highly appropriate and clever title, because this is the time when boys say farewell to maternal and matriarchal ties and seek vigorous, rugged, self-sufficient maleness. To be a boy involves an all-out effort to dissociate oneself from any signs of female control or interest. To be a sissy is to be doomed. As one mother so aptly expresses it:

> As early as preadolescence, boys have begun to sense that society is going to make demands on them as men which it will not make on their sisters as women. Without being able to articulate what those demands are to be, boys still feel the evidence of them; out of that sense comes their surging need for whatever will help them grow strong enough to meet their futures. They seek the company of men, without which they can never learn to become men themselves; then, because the pattern of their culture forces them to live more than ever before in the company of women, even more than before they need to find a strength and firmness in their mothers which will support their own need to grow strong. . . .
> For me and mine, the end of the idyll is very much in view. He is on the turn now, like milk ready to curdle. His feet get longer and his shoulders broader every time I look at him; one day I will turn round to find that he has crossed the threshold of the mysterious cavern of adolescence, where, if I know what is good for both of us, I had better not try to follow him. [Eustis, 1959, pp. 229–230]

Of particular concern to boys is the changing conception of maleness in the general culture. They wish to be male, but what does being male mean? For the girls, the changing concepts of sex-role behavior also create difficulties. The girl's difficulties are different; she's not so sure she wishes to be female in the submissive way this was traditionally defined. Thus, both boys and girls are faced with the task of identifying themselves in appropriate ways while the cultural concept of appropriateness is changing. We can see the effects of this in several studies.

A basic technique for investigating sexual preference in preadolescence has been the use of play and game choices. This technique has been used in a series of researches by Rosenberg and Sutton-Smith (1960 and 1964). Between third and sixth grade, girls tend to increase, though only slightly, in their selection of masculine items and to decrease in their selection of feminine items. In effect, then, the girls move over into selecting boys' activities, which also change in nature from pastimes toward organized sports. By the sixth grade a pattern of girls' choices is similar to that of the boys, most of which has been brought about by a decrease in choice of formerly feminine items. (Sutton-Smith, Rosenberg, and Morgan, 1963) Walker (1964) suggests that this may occur earlier in his Connecticut sample than in the Midwestern sample studied by Rosenberg and Sutton-Smith. In examining dynamics, the latter indicate that the fourth grade may be seen as a time of highest anxiety in terms of sex role for girls and that this may be related to girls' seeing themselves as tomboys.

Another indication of a girl's tomboy trend can be found in studies using projective techniques. Brown used ambiguous photographs and asked children to identify them as either male or female. He found that boys expressed stronger preferences for the masculine role than girls did for the feminine role. Girls from 6 to 9 preferred the masculine, and even 10- and 11-year-olds had mixed reactions. He also reports the same reduction of male choice, saying, "Boys simply do not have the same freedom of choice as girls when it comes to sex-typed objects and activities." (Brown, 1958, p. 236) Girls can be boys (in dress and play), but boys can be only boys. (Although there are some current trends in grooming and attire that sometimes makes it difficult to tell male from female adolescents and young adults from the rear view, this pattern has not yet reached down into the middle childhood years.) Whether this exists because of the notion that the Western culture is male-oriented was investigated by Hartley and her colleagues (1962). They found no evidence for the notion that children perceive being male as being more desired and prized by adults. It may simply be that being a girl today allows a wider range of choice and activity and offers the girl inconsistent role patterns. Both the tomboy and the lady are part of the accepted feminine image. Hartley quotes a middle class mother, "There's no point to make an issue of it— when they need to be feminine they grow out of their tomboyish ways." (Hartley, 1963, p. 8) She also indicates that there are clear class distinctions in role preference and that there are sex-specific barriers to behavior for girls. The barriers seem related to work roles rather than play activities.

She concludes that sex-role differentiation comes about through a variety of processes rather than through any single dynamic.

In a comprehensive review of masculine development, Biller and Borstelmann (1967) indicate that masculine sex-role identification is also a highly complex learning. The importance of role modeling is indicated both in the female and male role. A pattern of high masculine orientation, high masculine preference, and high masculine role adoption seems to be positively related to the presence of a father or other significant adult male, the reception of positive feedback for male behavior, and the existence of a parental role appropriate for the male in the family. Biller also indicates that the father is important for girls. "When the father is not involved in the family, his daughter is likely to have sex-role development problems. . . . For girls the *optimal level* of paternal dominance may be moderate, allowing the mother to also be viewed as a salient controller of resources. It is important that the girl perceive her father as masculine and warmly appreciating her feminine behavior, even if she does not perceive him as the dominant parent." (Biller, 1971, pp. 108–109) Biller also points up the importance of the early years in setting the pattern.

The game studies seem to stress preference, whereas both Hartley and Biller indicate that sex-role identification goes far beyond the surface choices. If Biller is right in indicating that a culturally appropriate role structure must exist in the family, then the American society complicates the difficulties of children in their search for identity. As the women's liberation movement, changing economic and social conditions, and new advances in birth control continue to have impact, concepts of appropriate sex-role behavior will continue to change, and new identity crises may emerge.

The effort of children to be male or female does not take place without strain. Gray's study, using both social reputation and anxiety measures, found that in both boys and girls high sex-appropriate behavior was related to high anxiety. Since this was not expected of the boys, Gray hypothesized that "it is possible that striving to maintain a masculine role is, for the boys of this age group, stressful enough to be associated with manifest anxiety. Or one could argue contrariwise that only the boy who is secure in his masculine role is willing to admit to such unmanly characteristics." (Gray, 1957, p. 212)

Sears (1970), reporting on longitudinal data gathered in 1958, found relationships between children's views of gender role at age 12 and parent interview information collected when the children were 5 years old. His self-concept measure was a self-report scale developed by Pauline Sears (1963) and a femininity scale adapted from the California Psychological Inventory. Although he found no direct relationships between gender role at age 12 and maternal data at age 5, he reported that there were positive relationships between the latter and self-concept, especially for maternal and paternal warmth for both sexes and low paternal dominance for boys only. Of particular relevance, and somewhat in line with Gray's discussion of stress, he found that femininity (as measured!) was related to poor self-concept and aggression anxiety.

It is clear that the preadolescent period is not one of quiet acceptance of one's own sex. The obviously self-conscious peer grouping of boys with boys and girls with girls does not indicate that there is mutual disinterest. It indicates, perhaps, a heightened self-awareness and a seeking after models and support. Boys are confronted with many female models and increasingly restricted avenues for self-expression.

When we examine Sears' (1970) findings, they can be interpreted to mean that, in 1958, at least, these personality characteristics associated with the feminine role were not esteemed. But this picture, although there is a deplorable lack of careful investigation of the change in sex-role identity and its relationships to self-esteem, does not seem to be the same today. It would be important to see how 12-year-olds today view this.

Girls are not content to be girls in the conventional sense; they now feel they can be both girl and Little Leaguer simultaneously. This trend is not confined to preadolescence but is manifest in all areas of recreation, work, politics, and social settings. This does not imply that the differences between the sexes are being eliminated or that girls are becoming less feminine. It means that the preadolescent girl can be girlish, can learn her sex role, can see herself as feminine, but that she defines this more broadly.

In 1960, preadolescents perceived occupational choice along sex lines—boys envisioned themselves as doctors, scientists, baseball players, engineers, and soldiers, whereas girls looked forward to careers as teachers, nurses, secretaries, mothers and housewives, and airline hostesses. (Witty et al., 1960) There seem to be no current studies in this area, but one would hope the picture has changed.

Children are quite aware of their sex roles and activities; self-reports and choices reflect their search for acceptable patterns of sex-role behavior. For boys and girls, it is farewell to both Oedipus and Electra.

DEVELOPING INTERESTS
AND ASPIRATIONS
Recreational Interests

How do these busy, active preteenagers spend their time? The school day, of course, consumes about six hours, leaving another seven or so for recreation and the routines of daily living. By studying how children spend their time, we can increase our understanding of what life means to them, what interests them. Interests compel us to spend our time in certain ways. These are aspects of our concepts of self; they reveal what we deem to be important. Children's interests are of concern to adults because they point out pathways for education and guidance. These interests can serve as springboards into the deep pool of the preadolescent self.

The *mass media* demand a large share of the attention of children. Parents sometimes have the feeling that all their children do is watch TV. This may be because the favorite viewing times are during the late afternoon and early evening, when one can turn the dial and see only programs for children. Preadolescents spend about 20 hours a week in front of the television set. This seems to be the figure regardless of sex or geographic area. Boys and girls like to watch different programs. (Woe to the family with more than one child this age!)

The *reading* interests of youngsters have been intensively studied over the years. Witty's (1960) questionnaire of Chicago children disclosed that they read outside of school only about one hour a week in contrast to the 20 hours of TV. Again, boys and girls differ, the girls preferring science fiction to the boys' choice of adventure.

The child's keen interest in science makes this subject one of the top three choices across the country. Parents and teachers are well aware of the highly technical space-age vocabulary of children. Mystery, adventure, and animal stories are also popular with youngsters.

A careful study of what children read about, ask about, and look up in books yields interesting data. Several thousand children were asked about their reading interests, but Rudman (1955) found little difference in interest among rural, urban, and metropolitan children. In connection with what children ask about, he found a strong interest in ethics, values, religion, and, with the approach of puberty, a dramatically increasing concern with personal problems.

Reading for reference is different from reading for recreation or for general knowledge. Rudman reports that reference reading in science rates highest. However, children look up materials different from what they want to read about or ask about. School assignments influence choice more than the child's own urge to explore. The differences between the sexes may be more indicative of the actual interests of children. Boys seek out more information about physical sciences and sports; girls lean toward social sciences, biography, and mathematics.

Children's reading and TV watching seem to serve several functions: they provide opportunities for boys or girls to experience excitement vicariously; they broaden children's awareness of both the real and fictional world (30 percent of the children surveyed regarded TV as useful for schoolwork); and they allow boys and girls to move out of themselves and their immediate environments, both in time and space.

Active play dominates the rest of the children's time. Boys prefer more active pursuits, girls more sedentary ones. The group is the setting for this play, as we have noted in Chapter 9.

One way of finding out how children spend their time, as a way of uncovering their interests, is to ask them to keep logs of themselves. This "dear diary" approach, when carefully done on an objective time basis rather than through subjective recall, yields valuable data. McCullough (1957) used this technique in the San Francisco Bay area with about 400 fifth-graders drawn from waterfront (lower class), central (lower middle), and hill (upper middle and upper class) homes. These children kept records of their out-of-school activities over a five-day period. Again, TV led the list in terms of time. Active sports were second for all groups, with work third.

Parents and alarmists lament the irresponsibility of youth. However, these children were doing many household tasks. Of course, they may have been doing them under duress, but they spent many hours helping. Girls spent about half their time working, and waterfront boys spent a third of their time as mothers' helpers by doing dishes, running errands, and the like. Even hill boys did laundry, although this may have consisted in putting a load in the automatic washer-dryer. Work need not necessarily reflect interest, but it does reflect both the changing concept of sex roles and the sense of obligation to the family held by these youngsters.

One interesting class difference was shown: hill boys engaged in many more sociable and eventful activities, central boys were most sedentary—playing games was the high activity for them—and waterfront boys were their mothers' helpers. This may be because their mothers worked or needed their services more. Girls reported a wider variety of activities, thus again suggesting the diminution of choice open to boys.

Expressed Interests

A third technique, in addition to the specific questionnaire and the log for gathering data on interests, is the generalized interest inventory. This elicits information about the range of children's concerns. Instead of asking what children did, Amatora (1960) asked, "What are three of your greatest interests, in order of importance to you?" She grouped the responses, from a small sample of fourth-graders from all over the United States, and reported that approximately half of them named possession of objects first; this was followed by the "good life," pets, and vocation (with more boys than girls choosing the last item). In eighth and ninth position were school and education; travel, relatives, and money were fifth, sixth, and seventh, respectively. This corresponds to other studies which show that children regard school as just part of the daily scenery.

Kauffmann (1955) attempted to find a relationship between expressed interests and organismic age, socioeconomic status, and race membership in about 2000 Illinois children. He used an interest inventory and found no relationship with purely chronological age, as we would expect. He did find that children in the fourth through eighth grades were strongly concerned about their bodies. Developmentally, he found a trend toward a greater choice of games requiring higher levels of organization with increasing age. This can be seen as further support for the concept of development as a process whereby the organism moves to higher and higher levels of complexity.

A sentence-completion instrument that required the children to finish such sentences as "I wish I were ————" and "I wish my mother (or father or teacher) would ————" was used by Cobb to overcome the limitations he felt were involved in a too-open type inventory, such as the one Amatora used. Cobb's results revealed both age and sex differences. He concluded that "there are highly significant sex differences within the general similarity, boys' wishes exceeding those of girls in the direction of personal achievement and self aggrandizement, girls' exceeding boys' in the direction of social and family relations and personal characteristics. . . . There are also clear developmental differences, with a peak of concern about identity, family, possessions, living situation, and travel in the elementary grades (4–5–6)." (Cobb, 1954, p. 170)

Occupational Interests

Self-factors.   It should not be assumed that preadolescents' vocational interests are at all indicative of actual future vocational choices. The "when I grow up I want to be a fireman" refrain of the 6-year-old still finds its echo in the unrealistic choices of the child aged 9 to 12. Vocational-interest inventory results are invalid for individual counseling or educational guidance. But vocational interest inventories do serve a useful research purpose, for they help us see how vocational choice develops. They can be used by the skilled, perceptive investigator in the exploration of the child's general field of interests.

A perceptive application of the Strong Vocational Interest Blank may be found in Tyler's (1955) study. She had fourth-graders complete a blank like Strong. She did not use the occupational keys (in which a person's interests are compared to the interests of persons in a particular profession) because of their inappropriateness at this age level. She analyzed the results by use of statistical procedures that enabled her to detect the clusters or groupings of interests held by these preadolescents. This technique of factor analysis yielded several patterns of interests.

Tyler found that children liked many more things than they either disliked or were indifferent to. At this age they are still very open to wide choice, and development involves not the addition of choices but their diminution.

A second finding, "that there is no sort of polarity about these likes and dislikes" (Tyler, 1955, p. 36), has relevance for adults. We often hear parents and other adults talk in either-or terms about both ability and interest. The layman's view is that if a child isn't interested or can't do academic work, he should do manual work. Tyler's study refutes this common sense approach. There is no such neat dichotomy for the preadolescent.

Her main conclusion is that the clusters "look more like general attitudes toward the world and the role one is playing in it. . . . The suggestion that general attitudes may take precedence over experience with specific activities in organizing one's interests may be the most important outcome of this research." (Tyler, 1955, p. 38) The findings on sex differences may be seen as fitting into this category.

In general, children's choices are differentiated on the basis of their self-concepts. The importance to the child of his conception of masculinity-feminity can thus be seen as more pervasive than even Freud thought. This is not a latency period in the sense that interest in one's own sex identification and heterosexual concerns are absent. It is a stable, preadolescent establishment and acceptance of one's sex. Choices of vocations and interests are heavily involved with sexually appropriate symbols. Not physical sex, but cultural identification is significant.

Cultural Factors.   Cultural factors, as we would expect, are evident in the vocational interests of boys and girls. A comparison of English with American youngsters revealed a very great similarity of interest patterns. The main difference lay in the fact that English children listed more dislikes than their American cousins. (Tyler, 1956) The reasons for this have not yet been investigated.

When we turn to a non-Western society that has been exposed to American influence, we find some interesting differences. Goodman used a topic-essay technique in which children wrote on "What I want to be when I grow up, and why."

One of the most striking differences is in the area of politics. ". . . American boys are remarkably indifferent to politics and public office, while Japanese boys in comparatively large proportions [34 percent in grades five to eight to 4½ percent of Americans] aim toward careers in diplomacy, the Diet, as ministers of state or even prime minister, and— suggesting that the democratic concept has taken hold with a vengeance —one small boy aspires to be Emperor!" (Goodman, 1957, p. 982) For girls, the pattern is similar.

Another evidence of the effect of cultural experience is the difference in outlook toward military careers. In Japan, "there is resounding silence, and never so much as a passing mention of the military." (Goodman, 1957, p. 983) At the same time, about 8 percent of American boys choose this career and give patriotic reasons for so doing. There are many other differences in choice of business, professions, religious careers (virtually none for the Japanese), but in spite of the degree of American cultural influence, all add up to overall cultural differences. Goodman concludes:

> *American children exhibit strong inclinations suggesting such themes as may be identified by the labels scientific-technical, urban-sophisticate, pragmatic-humanistic, and individualistic. The inclinations of Japanese children suggest themes which we might label commercial, sentimental-humanistic, and others-oriented.*
>
> *We are impressed especially with the degree to which individualism —the "self-orientation" attitude as we have preferred to put it—is apparent in the statements from American children as contrasted with the Japanese. . . . American culture, with all its emphasis upon the autonomy of the individual and his rights with respect to self-expression, self-fulfillment, and self-satisfaction, finds unmistakable expression among the children of this study. Among the Japanese children there is expressed with equal clarity features repeatedly commented upon by observers of Japanese culture past and present, rural and urban, i.e., the Japanese individual does not think of himself as autonomous, and it is his duties and obligations rather than his rights which are stressed; his attention is deflected away from self and toward family, community, and the wider society. [Goodman, 1957, pp. 997–998]*

An investigation of differences between Vietnamese and American concepts of self and family again reveals the role of culture, particularly in attitudes toward parents, toward self-reliance, and toward authority. (Leichty, 1963)

To summarize, vocational interests, like all other interest patterns of preadolescents, are influenced by the forces of both the culture and the self interacting within the individual child. Studies of such interests show that children are still open to much change, that vocational patterns are not fixed, and that the children's vocational interest patterns mirror the adult world.

Although these studies of interests were conducted some time ago, there is a lack of new descriptive research. Child development, like all other fields, goes through fads and cycles. At this time, purely descriptive work is not "in"; experimental work and, to some degree, studies that relate sets of variables to each other, whether longitudinal (such as Sears) or occurring at the same time (such as the relationship between social class and achievement) are. While the change may reflect sophistication, it makes it harder to answer students' (and teachers' and parents') questions about what children are like at a particular age. The summary in the paragraph above is probably true; but the content of interests and the way these relate to general social change might be different; we just don't know.

SELF-CONCEPTUALIZING

How does the preadolescent conceive of himself? We have been able, to some degree, to infer his self-concepts by examining his peer groups, his behavior, and his expressed interests. Now we will look at the data that bears directly on self-concept. What do children say when asked to define themselves? How do they see their bodies? What effect does self-concept of ability have upon schoolwork?

Body Image

Because of the verbal skills and the greater maturity of preadolescents, more techniques become available to explore their self-conceptualizations. A major study by Jersild (1952) used unstructured compositions on the topics "What I Like about Myself" and "What I Dislike about Myself." Jersild categorized the responses into the following classifications:

CATEGORY

    I. Physical characteristics
      B. Size, weight
      D. Features of face and head

    II. Clothing and grooming
      A. Clothes

    VI. Home and family
      B. Own home behavior

   VIII. Recreation (Enjoyment of)
      B. Play and sports

    IX. Ability in sports, play

    X. School
      E. Study habits, industry, perseverance
      G. Ability in school work

    XII. Special talents

    XIII. Just me, myself

   XIIIx. Personality, character
      A. Moral character
      B. Inner resources

    E. Emotional tendencies
        1. Poise, control
        2. Inferiority feelings
        3. Fears
        4. Temper

XIV. Social attitudes and relationships
    A. Friendships, social activities
    B. Attitudes of others toward me
    C. My attitude toward others

Note: Only those items reported by over 10 percent of either elementary boys or girls are included. The category headings are much abbreviated, and readers interested in a fuller exposition of the categories should consult pages 135–141 in the original study. It should be noted that all responses specifically mentioning school were placed under category X, even though they refer to character traits that otherwise might fall under another heading.
Source: Adapted from Table 1 in A. T. Jersild, *In Search of Self,* Teachers College, Columbia University, 1952. Used by permission.

    He found that a substantial percentage of children in the upper grades of elementary school were sufficiently interested in their bodies to express both positive and negative feelings about them. For example, more fifth-grade girls commented favorably on their physical characteristics than on any other category, and only social relationships had a higher percentage for sixth-grade girls. For boys, a combination of the categories of athletic ability and physical characteristics indicates bodily interest.

    The major changes in physical development (growth spurt, puberty) take place primarily in the junior high school years. Of course, some children, particularly girls, have begun to develop secondary sex characteristics in the fifth and sixth grade. Jersild's data show that the greatest concern with one's body (both positive and negative) comes after the elementary school years. Preadolescents rarely (less than 5 percent of fourth- and fifth-graders) disliked their height and weight, but dislike increased with age, beginning with about 10 percent in the sixth grade and reaching its peak (about 18 percent) in the ninth grade.

    When children were presented with a structured self-report scale, with such items as "My hair is nice looking," "My face is pretty," "My skin is nice," "I'm good at athletics," and were asked to rate themselves on a 5-point scale with the above items at one end and items such as "I'm a poor athlete," "I wish I could do something about my skin," on the "How I See Myself" Scale (Gordon, 1966, 1968), Yeatts' (1967) study revealed a factor labeled "physical adequacy" present for junior and senior high school pupils (see Chapter 14), but not for third- to sixth-graders. A factor (that is, a group of items highly related to each other) called physical appearance was present for girls in grades 3 through 6 as well as for secondary pupils, but not for boys. The girls in grades 3 through 6 had the highest mean scores of any age group of girls on this factor, which indicates acceptance of their bodies.

The two types of measures, unstructured and structured, yield somewhat different evidence. A higher percentage of secondary school girls than of elementary reported favorably about their appearance in Jersild's study; the reverse is true on the "How I See Myself" Scale. The studies were of different populations, used different procedures, and were made fifteen years apart. Any interpretations must be made with these facts in mind, which illustrates one of the problems of such research.

Cohen, Money, and Uhlenhuth (1972) used an approach completely different from the verbal ones above. They had children draw two drawings of two persons, one of self-and-friend and another of self-and-examiner. The children were all middle class white suburbanites in one school. (Figure 13.1 is a typical drawing with scoring.) They found that children usually drew a friend of the same sex and drew him at their own height. They drew themselves as shorter—but not enough so—than the examiner (although Figure 13.1 does not reflect this). Each grade level drew itself taller than the preceding one, and girls saw themselves as taller than boys.

We can say that most children accept their bodies but do not single them out for special concern during preadolescence. We might hypothesize that those who do are either early or late maturers or differ significantly in some way (obesity, illness) from their peers.

Unfortunately, most body-image research has not been conducted on children. This is a relatively unexplored field, but one well worth investigating. In the next chapter we shall see the importance of maturity differences to the early adolescent. We need comparable data on earlier periods.

Self-definition

As we indicated in Chapter 6, there are many problems in the measurement of self. We have referred to self-report scales, inference from observation of behavior, incomplete sentences, drawings, etc. One way to conceptualize this is shown in Figure 13.2. We can infer from the model that there will not be much overlap; but even within the sector called self-report, there are various techniques that may yield different answers. For example, Perkins (1958), using the Jersild categories, constructed a *Q-sort,* a series of statements that the child can evaluate as being either representative or nonrepresentative of himself. The fourth- and sixth-grade children in his study sorted the cards twice—once for as they were and once for ideal. The child placed each statement along a continuum from most to least and was forced to place a certain number of items at each location so that the arrangement of items resembled the normal bell-

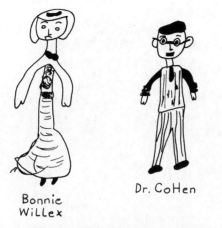

Bonnie
Willex

Dr. CoHen

Self-and-Examiner drawn by an 11-year-old 6th grade girl represents a typical drawing for her age and sex. Scoring as follows:

1. Self drawn: first
2. Height self actual: 62″
3. Height examiner actual: 77″
4. Height self drawn: 88 mm
5. Height examiner drawn: 75 mm
6. Position of drawing vertical: +1
7. Position of drawing horizontal: −1

8. Abnormal parts in drawing: −0
9. Multiple starts: −0
10. Secret erasures: −0
11. Shading: present
12. Line quality: normal
13. Background features: 0
14. Movement: 0

FIGURE 13.1

Reproduced from Stephen M. Cohen, John Money, and Eberhard H. Uhlenhuth, A computer study of selected features of self-and-other drawings by 385 children, *Journal of learning disabilities,* 1972, **5** (3), 146, where it appeared as Figure 2. Used with permission.

shaped curve. Figure 13.3 depicts a typical sort. This enables the researcher to compare, by means of correlation, the child's sort, or distribution, with other distributions; that is, he can compare the child with himself (self-ideal) or a group of children with other groups.

He found that the most representative item was "I like my parents." The most rejected items were "(1) I do not like animals, (2) I have a brother or sister that I don't like, (3) I have poor health, (4) I am weak, (5) I am unpopular." (Perkins, 1958, p. 83) His data show that boys and girls generally feel confident of scholastic ability, are happy or at least optimistic, are concerned about appearance (boys wishing to be taller, girls wishing to be good-looking). Perkins found that self-conceptualizing could be seen as related to development as well as to experience. He reports (Perkins, 1958) that girls have a higher correlation between self and ideal self than do boys and that such correlation becomes greater with time.

Another type of self-report is the *semantic differential.* Here the child

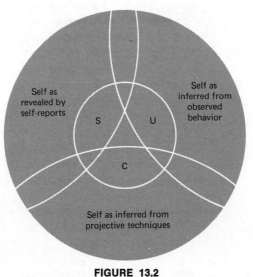

FIGURE 13.2

A tentative model depicting three facets of the self. Key: S-C is the Self-Concept, that highly organized, central core of the self. U is the part of the self unavailable to public study. From I. J. Gordon, *Studying the child in school,* Wiley, New York, 1966, p. 53. Used with permission.

is given a topic word such as boy and a series of adjectives arranged in two columns with space between them—for instance, happy-sad, strong-weak. The child indicates where, in that space, he would place his idea of the main word. He might, for example, place a mark on or near the adjective strong to go with the topic word boy.

Sherman (1965) used this technique and found that certain sets of adjectives grouped together into clusters that children saw were descriptive of themselves. She found that boys in fifth grade cluster a group of items around "liveliness" in contrast to girls' "niceness." In sixth grade, "straightforwardness" contrasts with "wholesomeness." It seems to this author that all four components might be seen by the cynical adolescent as "square," or whatever term currently conveys that image. Sherman's work illustrates another way to try to see how children evaluate what is important to them. It also reveals developmental trends.

Gordon used a 5-point rating scale "How I See Myself," which he based upon the Jersild categories. A study of its factor structure, partly designed to examine developmental trends, yielded, in addition to the school and peer factors mentioned in Chapter 11 and the physical factors mentioned above, several other factors when 9000 Florida school children (grades 3 through 12) completed the scale. (Yeatts, 1967) A rather general factor, interpersonal adequacy, containing 17 of the 40 items on the scale and an academic adequacy factor were present for both boys and

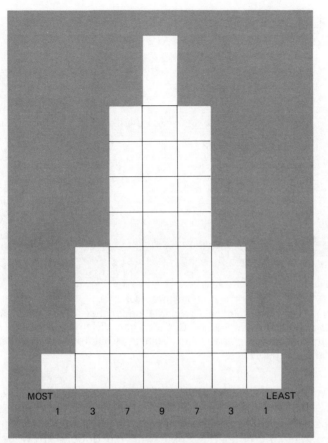

FIGURE 13.3

A Q-sort arrangement for a deck of 31 items. Adapted from Hugh V. Perkins, Factors influencing change in children's self-concepts. *Child Development,* 1958, **29,** 221–230. Copyright © 1958 by The Society for Research in Child Development, Inc.

girls in grades 3 through 6. Scores on these factors indicate that, in general, the average child, regardless of race and sex, tended to report himself a little on the positive side. Girls, however, gave themselves significantly better ratings on interpersonal adequacy than did the boys.

Long and her colleagues (1967) used a nonverbal self-report and investigated changes in self-concept in relation to other people. Although the sample was small, they concluded that children increase in self-esteem in third and fourth grade with a slight decline after that. Scores increased in individuation, which they defined as seeing self as a reflection of what Piaget called decentering; that is, a recognition that things look different to different people or from different places.

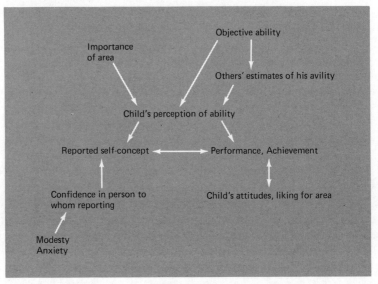

FIGURE 13.4

Factors relating children's self-concepts and school achievements. From *In Pursuit of Self-Esteem* by Pauline S. Sears and Vivian S. Sherman. © 1964 by Wadsworth Publishing Company, Inc., Belmont, California 94002. Reproduced by permission of the publisher.

How much faith can be placed in children's reports about themselves? Sears and Sherman (1963) present a model for describing the forces that might influence the accuracy of self-report (see Figure 13.4). We are particularly concerned here with the double arrow between reported self-report and performance achievement. In addition to the studies cited above, Lipsitt (1958), Bruce (1957), Horowitz (1962), and Coopersmith (1967) also used self-reporting instruments with children. All report them to be reliable. Reliability means that the child will report on himself consistently from time to time if the time gap is not too long. The question of accuracy still remains. Lipsitt, Bruce, and Horowitz found a high relationship between self-report and the Children's Manifest Anxiety Scale, an adaptation of the Minnesota Multiphasic Personality Inventory. This means that the way the children completed the self-report corresponded with the data on the objective personality test. In addition, Horowitz found a relation between high sociometric status and high self-concept. Simon (1972) found a high relationship between two self-reports—the Coopersmith Self-Esteem Inventory and a self-rating of peer popularity. All this may mean is that these sixth graders were consistent. We lack an external measure of their popularity.

Yeatts secured academic performance data on her population and placed each child at one of three points: above, at, or below grade average. Children's placement on this scale was highly related to the "How I See Myself" items that reflected children's feelings of academic adequacy. The study shows that these children's self-reports were related to their actual performances. The Sears and Sherman model contains "other's estimates." When the other is the teacher, how does this influence the child? We saw, in previous chapters, how observed teacher behavior and school practice affects self-concept.

In a Swedish study (Magnusson, 1965), self-rating was found to be influenced by school-class group, and Magnusson hypothesized that the critical factor was the teacher. A study by Gordon and Wood (1963) of 150 fifth- and sixth-grade children in a metropolitan Florida school showed that neither teachers nor pupils were very accurate in predicting pupil performance (rank in class) on standardized scholastic achievement tests. There was, however, agreement (at the 0.01 level of significance) between teacher and pupil on the nature of the error; that is, when one overestimated, the other was likely to overestimate. The pupils also evaluated themselves on a rating scale of attitudes toward school. Those who saw themselves as favorably disposed toward school were most likely to overestimate their achievement; those least favorable, to underestimate it. Very few were accurate. Since this study was conducted by a teacher in her own school, the question of the degree of threat is significant. Do children err more in estimation under threat? Self-concept theory and level-of aspiration studies would suggest that they do.

Hughes (1971), in addition to finding a reliable relationship between self-esteem as measured by the Piers-Harris Children's Self-Concept Scale (a self-report based on the 1952 Jersild items) and the Iowa Test of Basic Skills, found that school report card practices were also related to self-esteem: "The very traditional report card was associated with lowest pupil self-esteem, lowest pupil achievement and negative pupil attitudes toward the reporting process." (Hughes, 1971, p. 5106A) Most likely the report card is just a symptom that reflects the school organization and value system.

In an attempt to measure accuracy with threat removed, Brandt presented sixth- and eleventh-grade pupils with the opportunity to increase scientific knowledge. He also used carefully designed, very specific directions and tried to create a comfortable "climate." His subjects rated themselves on academic, physical, and social abilities. He reports:

No simple pattern emerged regarding accuracy of self-estimate. . . . Some students were highly accurate in assessing their abilities in all six areas. Other students were more consistent in their accuracy, from task to task, yet tended to be inaccurate on the average. Others tended to be consistently accurate on four self-estimates, but inaccurate on the other two. Almost every conceivable pattern of accuracy of self-estimate prevailed. Although there was a tendency for students to differ in a general sense with respect to accuracy of self-estimate, there was also a tendency among the majority of students (inconsistent group) for some area of the self-concept to be more sharply differentiated than other areas. With a particular student, spelling and arithmetic might have been more sharply differentiated than other assessment areas; with another student, baseball-throwing and grip strength. [Brandt, 1958, p. 77]

Sears (1960) found some interesting differences between boys and girls in respect to both level of self-esteem and degree of differentiation. She found that girls' self-reports on mental ability were highly inaccurate and that they differentiated less than boys. We may speculate that ability to differentiate, to look at one's self and see differences within the self, is related to the degree of comfort one has with one's self. In a study of English schoolchildren, Lunn (1972) found that girls had far more favorable attitudes toward school than boys but that boys had more favorable attitudes toward their personal and social relationships. She found social class and achievement were also involved; brighter children and those from middle class homes tended to be more positive.

This variation of estimate within the individual child seems to exist in all these studies. It suggests a developmental trend away from early childhood's global, unclear, undifferentiated image of self. Preadolescence seems to be the stage in between this and the reorganization and reintegration of self in adolescence. What we may have is a pattern of movement from a global view ("I'm a good boy") through the preadolescent differentiated view ("I'm good at sports, but I'm not good in arithmetic, and I don't think much about how I am overall") to the mature position ("I see myself as generally adequate, but I recognize differential abilities within myself"). This is, of course, speculative in terms of what we know but would be consistent with general development theory.

We must, therefore, consider the age, sex, and social situation in any attempt to use individual self-reports as predictive devices at this stage of our knowledge. This does not reduce the utility of such techniques. They do reveal how children perceive the way they should present themselves. Further, such techniques show the areas of interest and concern of children. Preadolescents make many more differential, specific comments about themselves than they do about themselves as an integrated totality—"Just me, myself." (Jersild, 1952)

Comparative studies indicate that adults are not very good at ascertaining how children see themselves. The discrepancy between the adult view of the child and the child's report on himself is large, and these techniques reveal the extent of this important perceptual difference.

As we have indicated before, measurement is a problem. Zirkel (1971), in addition to listing 15 definitions of self-concept, made a distinction between global and specific self-concepts and between self-definition and self-evaluation. Both of these distinctions are valuable, especially for understanding preadolescents and young adolescents. A child may be able to see himself as good in some areas of schoolwork, inadequate with peers, and able to relate to adults (all self-definition) and yet have high self-esteem (self-evaluation). He likes that self-organization. Another child with the same definition (assuming both views are in line with reality) may despair. For him, peer acceptance is crucial, and his success areas rate lower on his private totem pole. Further, we should include as a dimension of self-concept the view that the person has about the amount of control he has over his fate, a dimension labeled *locus of control.*

Self-concept and Performance

Our theoretical position is that the way one views himself is a significant variable in his performance. A basic problem in the research on this notion is that we can demonstrate a relationship between self-concept and performance, but relationships do not indicate cause. The studies cited earlier in Chapter 6 follow an antecedent-consequent pattern between kindergarten and first grade. Studies of upper elementary grade children are of the relationship type, in which we find that low achievement is accompanied by low self-concept. For example, Walsh (1956) used doll-play equipment to see whether bright boys with learning difficulties defined themselves differently from those who were achieving adequately. She concluded that low achievers perceived themselves as less free to pursue their own interests, to express their feelings, and to respond adequately to their environment. All three conclusions might be generalized into a single statement: Low achievers perceive themselves as more constricted in their communications with their world.

Bilby, Brookover, and Erickson (1972) demonstrated that not only do parental evaluations and expectations relate to the reported self-concepts of over 2000 fourth- through sixth-grade children but that a combination of parental variables and children's self-concepts are also related to the children's future school plans. But again, this is not prediction, nor is it surprising. A view of the future is part of the child's present self-concept, so we still are dealing with present-time relationships.

Purkey (1970) reviewed the literature on the self and academic achievement. Although most of the studies he cited are of secondary school pupils, he concludes that there is a strong relationship between attitudes toward self and achievement. Again, this cannot be verified as a causal relationship. The assumption has been that self-concept influences behavior. From our view, it is transactional; changes in behavior or performance itself should influence self-concept. The Sears (1970) study cited earlier provides some evidence. Children's self-concepts at age 12 were reliably related to their reading achievement three years before.

Experiments have been conducted as another approach to examining the relationships between self-concept and performance. For example, Friend and Neale (1972) gave fifth graders different types of feedback on a reading task to determine whether children saw ability and energy expended as more influential than chance or task difficulty. They reported that white children were more likely to assign the former; blacks, the latter. This fits in with a number of studies on children's locus of control, including Coleman's (1966) now classic educational survey. However, results always have to be interpreted in a real world, and for many poor black children, their view is a realistic one. The world has treated them as pawns.

Children who are anxious about themselves, regardless of whether this anxiety is "real" in the eyes of the outsider, reflect this anxiety in their approach to the world. Their perceptions become more rigid and more constricted. (Smock, 1958) They just do not see what others see.

Although we can only establish, at this time, a functional relationship between self-concept and external variables such as teacher and peer evaluation and actual performance, the pragmatic question is what to do to help children see themselves in growth-producing ways. Chances are that the attack can be made any place in the transactional field. We can work on skill, on self-concept, on changing teacher and peer perceptions, or on modifying family expectations. DeCharms (1971) developed a sixth-grade program designed to change children's motivation from what he called pawns to origins. Kahn and Weiss (1973) indicate that, although attempts have been made to add an affective component to the teaching of subject matter, this is a relatively new development. Much research remains to be done in exploring varieties of approaches to the question.

SUMMARY

In this chapter we have not only examined research findings but also have stressed the techniques used to discover children's concepts of self.

Four major procedures, each of which offers data on various aspects of self-development, have been used. First, observation and inference from behavior, a technique used on children from infancy, continues to be a constructive approach. Second, projective techniques, such as the TAT, Rorschach, and various sentence-completion devices, by which the researcher infers self-concept from test data, offer avenues to the self. Third, various "objective" tests, such as vocational-interest blanks and personality scales, have been utilized. Fourth, many self-reporting devices, which become operative during the preadolescent period because of the increased language development and reading and writing skills, require the child to state his own picture of self.

In our study of adolescents, we shall see that these same four basic approaches will apply. Devices may differ in sophistication but not in type. Although we perhaps tend to be concerned only with results, the student of human behavior must understand the procedures by which results are obtained. Only then can he accurately assess their merit and draw practical implications from them.

What can we conclude concerning the results of these various studies? First, we need to learn much more about the relationship between self-concept and achievement during childhood. Second, we can conclude that there is a relationship, and we can hypothesize, although it is difficult to demonstrate, that this relationship seems to follow a pattern of experience → reinforcing experience → self-concept → seeking experience. Third, it is clear that preadolescents do consciously evaluate themselves and that their evaluations are influential in their behavior. Their evaluations are related to activities more than to feelings and are related more to specifics than to overall estimates of self. Fourth, we can conclude that we have only begun to scratch the surface of the preadolescent's private world. We know very little about his inner life. We also know that parents and teachers are poor judges of the conceptual world of the child. In large measure, particularly in the realm of the self-concept, these are still the unknown years. On the positive side, we are beginning to learn how to look for self-concept data, and we can expect rapid gains in our knowledge. Fifth, self-conceptualizing is a developmental process. There is a movement toward a more stable image of self at the end of preadolescence. The child generally has a positive image and, perhaps, even a more optimistic view than is otherwise warranted. He seems to have reached a plateau somewhat comparable to the physical growth plateau just before the spurt.

The preadolescent holds many concepts, arranged in a hierarchy, even though the whole system is not a highly integrated one. He has tested himself against his world. He does not look back upon his past and does not hesitate to approach his future. He comes bounding into adolescence.

REFERENCES AND ADDITIONAL READINGS

Amatora, M. Developmental trends in pre-adolescence and early adolescence in self-evaluation. *Journal of Genetic Psychology,* 1957, *91,* 89–97.

Amatora, M. Expressed interests in later childhood. *Journal of Genetic Psychology,* 1960, *96,* 327–342.

Baldwin, A. Pride and shame in children. *Newsletter, Division of Developmental Psychology,* Fall 1959, 1–11.

Baldwin, A., & Levin, H. Effects of public and private success or failure on children's repetitive motor behavior. *Child Development,* 1958, *29,* 363–372.

Bilby, R., Brookover, W., & Erickson, E. Characterizations of self and student decision making. *Review of Educational Research,* 1972, *42,* 505–524.

Biller, H. *Father, child and sex role.* Lexington, Mass.: Heath Lexington, 1971.

Biller, H., & Borstelmann, L. Masculine development: An integrative review. *Merrill-Palmer Quarterly,* 1967, *13,* 253–294.

Bobroff, O. The stages of maturation in socialized thinking and in the ego development of two groups of children. *Child Development,* 1960, *31,* 321–339.

Brandt, R. The accuracy of self-estimate: A measure of self-concept reality. *Genetic Psychology Monographs,* 1958, *58,* 55–99.

Brown, D. Sex-role development in a changing culture. *Psychological Bulletin,* 1958, *55,* 232–242.

Bruce, P. A study of the self-concept in sixth grade children. Doctoral dissertation, State University of Iowa. Iowa City, Iowa: *Dissertation Abstracts,* 1957, *17,* 2915.

Cobb, H. Role-wishes and general wishes of children and adolescents. *Child Development,* 1954, *25,* 161–171.

Cohen, S., Money, J., & Uhlenhoth, E. A computer study of selected features of self-and-other drawings by 385 children. *Journal of Learning Disabilities,* 1972, *5(3),* 145–155.

Coleman, J. *Equality of educational opportunity.* Washington, D.C.: U.S. Office of Education, 1966.

Coopersmith, S. *The antecedents of self-esteem.* San Francisco: Freeman, 1967.

Crane, A. Pre-adolescent gangs: A socio-psychological interpretation. *Journal of Genetic Psychology,* 1955, *86,* 275–279.

DeCharms, R. From pawns to origins: Toward self-motivation. In G. Lesser (Ed.), *Psychology and educational practice.* Glenview, Ill.: Scott, Foresman, 1971. Pp. 380–407.

Eustis, H. Good-by to Oedipus. In H. Knowles (Ed.), *Gentlemen, scholars, and scoundrels.* New York: Harper & Row, 1959. Pp. 221–230.

Fisher, S., & Fisher, L. Developmental analysis of some body image and body reactivity dimensions. *Child Development,* 1959, *30,* 389–402.

Friend, R., & Neale, J. Children's perceptions of success and failure: An attributional analysis of the effects of race and social class. *Developmental Psychology,* 1972, *7,* 124–128.

Gardner, R., & Moriarty, A. *Personality development at preadolescence.* Seattle: University of Washington Press, 1968.

Goodman, M. Values, attitudes and social concepts of Japanese and American children. *American Anthropologist,* 1957, *59(6),* 979–999. Reproduced by permission of the American Anthropological Association.

Gordon, I. J. *Studying the child in school.* New York: Wiley, 1966.

Gordon, I. J., & Wood, P. The relationship between pupil self-evaluation, teacher evaluation of the pupil and scholastic achievement. *Journal of Educational Research,* 1963, *56,* 440–443. Reprinted in I. J. Gordon (Ed.), *Human development: Readings in research.* Glenview, Ill.: Scott, Foresman, 1965.

Gray, S. Masculinity-femininity in relation to anxiety and social acceptance. *Child Development,* 1957, *28,* 203–214.

Hartley, R. A developmental view of female sex-role definition and identification. (Mimeo) Paper presented at the meeting of the Society for Research in Child Development, 1963.

Hartley, R., Hardesty, R., & Gorfein, D. Children's perceptions and expressions of sex preference. *Child Development,* 1962, *33,* 221–227.

Horowitz, F. The relationship of anxiety, self-concept, and sociometric status among 4th, 5th, and 6th grade children. *Journal of Abnormal Social Psychology,* 1962, *165,* 212–214.

Hughes, C. Self-esteem and achievement as related to elementary school reporting instruments. *Dissertation Abstracts,* 1971, *32,* 5106A.

Jersild, A. T. *In search of self.* New York: Teachers College, 1952.

Kahn, S., & Weiss, J. The teaching of affective responses. In R. M. W. Travers (Ed.), *Second Handbook of Research on Teaching.* Chicago: Rand McNally, 1973. Pp. 759–804.

Kauffmann, M. Expressed interests of children in relation to a maturity-age index in grades four through eight. Unpublished doctoral dissertation, Northwestern University, 1955.

Leichty, M. Family attitudes and self-concepts in Vietnamese and U.S. children. *American Journal of Orthopsychiatry,* 1963, *33,* 38–50.

Levin, H., & Baldwin, A. The choice to exhibit. *Child Development,* 1958, *29,* 373–380.

Liebert, R. M., & Baron, R. A. Some immediate effects of televised violence on children's behavior. *Developmental Psychology,* 1972, *6,* 469–475.

Lipsitt, L. P. A self-concept scale for children and its relationship to the children's form of the manifest anxiety scale. *Child Development,* 1958, *29,* 463–474.

Long, B., Henderson, E., & Ziller, R. Developmental changes in the self-concept during middle-childhood. *Merrill-Palmer Quarterly,* 1967, *13,* 201–216.

Lunn, J. The influence of sex, achievement level and social class on junior school children's attitudes. *British Journal of Educational Psychology,* 1972, *42,* 70–74.

Magnusson, D. Class-bound factors as determiners of self-rating level in the school situation. *Reports from the Psychological Laboratories,* No. 185. University of Stockholm, 1965.

McCullough, C. A log of children's out-of-school activities. *Elementary School Journal,* 1957, *58,* 157–165.

Perkins, H. Factors influencing change in children's self-concepts. *Child Development,* 1958, *29,* 221–230.

Purkey, W. *Self concept and school achievement.* Englewood Cliffs, N.J.: Prentice-Hall, 1970.

Rosenberg, B., Sutton-Smith, B. A revised conception of masculine-feminine differences in play activities. *Journal of Genetic Psychology,* 1960, *96,* 165–170.

Rosenberg, B., & Sutton-Smith, B. The measurement of masculinity and femininity in children: An extension and revalidation. *Journal of Genetic Psychology,* 1964, *104,* 259–264.

Rudman, H. The informational needs and reading interests of children in grades IV through VIII. *Elementary School Journal,* 1955, *55,* 502–512.

Savonko, E. I. Appraisal and self-appraisal as motives of behavior of children. *Voprosy Psikhologii,* 1969, *4,* 107–116.

Sears, P. The pursuit of self-esteem: The middle childhood years. *Newsletter, Division of Developmental Psychology,* Fall 1960, 1–5.

Sears, P. The effect of classroom conditions on the strength of achievement motive and work output of elementary school children. Washington, D.C.: U.S.O.E. Cooperative Research Project No. 873, 1963.

Sears, P., & Sherman, V. *In pursuit of self-esteem.* Belmont, Calif.: Wadsworth, 1964.

Sears, R. Relation of early socialization experiences to self-concepts and gender role in middle childhood. *Child Development,* 1970, *41,* 267–290.

Sherman, V. Sex and grade differences in first principal components underlying children's self-descriptions. (Mimeo) Paper presented at the meeting of the American Psychological Association, 1965.

Simon, W. Some sociometric evidence for validity of Coopersmith's Self-Esteem Inventory. *Perceptual and Motor Skills,* 1972, *34,* 93–94.

Smock, C. Perceptual rigidity and closure phenomenon as a function of manifest anxiety in children. *Child Development,* 1958, *29,* 237–247.

Sutton-Smith, B., Rosenberg, B., & Morgan, E., Jr. Development of sex differences in play choices during preadolescence. *Child Development,* 1963, *34,* 119–126.

Tyler, L. The development of vocational interests, 1. The organization of likes and dislikes in ten-year-old children. *Journal of Genetic Psychology,* 1955, *86,* 33–44.

Tyler, L. A comparison of the interests of English and American school children. *Journal of Genetic Psychology,* 1956, *88,* 175–181.

Walker, R. Measuring masculinity and femininity by children's games choices. *Child Development,* 1964, *35,* 961–971.

Walsh, A. *Self concepts of bright boys with learning difficulties.* New York: Teachers College, 1956.

Witty, P. et al. A study of the interests of children and youth. (Mimeo) Evanston, Ill.: Northwestern University, 1959.

Yamamoto, K. (Ed.) *The child and his image.* Boston: Houghton Mifflin, 1972.

Yeatts, P. Developmental changes in the self-concept of children grades 3–12. *Florida Educational Research and Development Council Research Bulletin,* 1967, *3.*

Zirkel, P. Self-concept and the "disadvantage" of ethnic group membership and mixture. *Review of Educational Research,* 1971, *41,* 211–226.

FIVE
ADOLESCENCE

CHAPTER 14
METAMORPHOSIS

COMING OF AGE PHYSICALLY

The cultural anthropologist, exploring the customs of societies around the world, speaks of "rites of passage," during which a boy becomes a man and a girl becomes a woman in the eyes of the tribe or nation. In America, for example, the Jewish boy of 13 mounts to the altar, is permitted to pray over the Torah, and gives a speech that says, in effect," Today I am a man." He may be a man in his ritual life, but he is far from being a man in all other areas of his daily life. He may make his own peace with his God, but Mom still gets him up in the morning to go to school, his teachers still control that portion of his existence, Dad still controls the allowance, and the law says he's too young to drive, drink, or marry.

In American society, these rites of passage consume not a single instant or a few days' celebration but the several years that constitute the teens. There is no one time in which the child becomes a man. We label this nebulous period of growth *adolescence*.

When does it begin? How long does it last? When does it end? For these questions we have only the classical answer: it depends upon the individual. Some authorities include the years from 10 to 20; some .use puberty (a most indefinite time in boys) as the starting point. For our purposes, and we recognize the artificiality of the limits, the late middle-school or junior high school years (grades 7–9) will be considered as early adolescence and the senior high school as late adolescence.

Throughout these next two sections, "Adolescence" and "Becoming Adult," we will see that the principle of individual differences in growth and development, clearly perceived in early growth stages, becomes even more central to understanding behavior. Although school epochs are being used as rough limits, many youngsters are early adolescents in fifth and sixth grade, whereas others are not through the puberal growth spurt in senior high. With this limitation always in mind, we can talk about early or late adolescence.

Adolescence is not merely a period of achieving sexual maturity or one's final height. It cannot be defined in physical terms or purely in cultural terms. In adolescence, the child experiences a series of events, some of which are initiated by his own body, some initiated by the people who surround him, and some initiated by his own self-system.

The period can be seen as one in which the youngster undergoes a concurrent series of "agonizing reappraisals" of himself, his immediate interpersonal world, and his view of the world at large. Each of these reappraisals creates a period of instability at the end of which a more integrated plateau is attained. At the end of adolescence, a new image of self-as-adult has been evolved. When this occurs, regardless of chronological age, the metamorphosis from child to man or woman is completed.

One of the reappraisals, of course, centers around one's own body. The adolescent's body is his fundamental baseline. When he deviates from his peers or fails to meet his own idealized hopes, his self-concept is affected, and his generalized self-image becomes an adverse one. We shall therefore explore the physical changes and their meaning to the early adolescent as our first step in this chapter.

As Lewin so aptly stated, "One can view adolescence as a change in group-belongingness. The individual has been considered by himself and by others as a child. Now he does not wish to be treated as such." (Lewin, 1960, p. 33) The second reappraisal requires of the adolescent that he shift his view of himself and his parents. Previously, even with his preadolescent peer activity, he perceived his parents as powerful people. Now he must see them more clearly; he must see that they cannot remain this powerful if he is to grow. For many youngsters, this change of anchorage point from parent to self creates guilt. They equate moving away from parent with loving the parent less. Unfortunately, many parents see it this way, too. They create a situation in which the youngster is forced to rebel or submit, in which it becomes virtually impossible for the adolescent to love but not surrender.

Included in this shift, or alteration of the frame of reference, is the need to develop inner controls. The child cannot safely give up the external control of the parent unless he has, within himself, the controls or morality to function in a modern society. The third area of reappraisal, therefore, is in the area of values and relationships with others.

These three factors—changing body, changing parent-child relations, and changing values—all work together to create instability. They all force the child to shift from the known position of child to the unknown position of adult. Further, they cause him to give up a degree of reliability and predictability about himself, which he has painstakingly learned. He has accumulated roughly 12 years of experience in behaving in certain patterns and eliciting certain responses. Now, these behaviors bring new responses, and inner feelings create the need for new behaviors. For example, in as simple an act as sitting down at the table, the adolescent may now find that he knocks things flying. He finds that physical contact with the girl next door in a rough and tumble game, once pleasurable for the sheer sport (football, for instance), now arouses erotic feelings. He is literally in a new world, one which has impinged upon his awareness gradually but increasingly.

Erikson characterizes adolescence as a period fraught with the danger of role diffusion as youth seeks identity. He says adolescents "are now primarily concerned . . . with the question of how to connect the roles and skills cultivated earlier with the occupational prototypes of the day. In their search for a new sense of continuity and sameness, adolescents have to refight many battles of earlier years. . . ." (Erikson, 1954, p. 217) The 13-year-old thus occasionally resembles the 3-year-old in the way he relates to authority. He must reappraise his sense of identity.

A continuing task, carried over from preadolescence, is his search for identification with the appropriate sex role. This is heightened in adolescence by the hormonal changes that create genital sexual strivings. It is, of course, inseparable from the search for inner controls and the new look at parents. The task is now in a new setting. Formerly, Dad approved when Son displayed identification through mimicry; now Dad (and Mom) are concerned about how fast and how far Junior goes in his attempts to be a man.

In this ambiguous and ambivalent position, the youngster becomes what has been labeled a *marginal* person. He doesn't belong to the child world; he has not yet been admitted to the adult world. "Characteristic symptoms of behavior of the marginal man are emotional instability and sensitivity. They tend to unbalanced behavior, to either boisterousness or shyness, exhibiting too much tension, and a frequent shift between extremes of contradictory behavior. . . . To some extent behavior symptomatic of the marginal man can be found in the adolescent. He too is oversensitive, easily shifted from one extreme to the other, and particularly sensitive to the shortcomings of his younger fellows." (Lewin, 1960, p. 41) This phenomenon is probably more predominant in industrialized societies, where there is such a discontinuity of role between child and adult and a long period of dependency labeled schooling. In the United States, for example, there is virtually no economic role for the adolescent other than consumer; this contributes to marginality.

We saw in earlier chapters that the vocational aspirations of children are highly unrealistic. Their image of future time is vague and autistic. They live essentially in the present. One of the changes in adolescence is the widening of perception to include future time. Both vocational and educational planning shift from a position of unawareness to a much more central place in the adolescent's perceptual world. He begins to examine himself from a new perspective, that of his abilities to make a living. What the voca-

TABLE 14.1 HEIGHT GAINS, AGES 13–18

	BOYS		GIRLS	
AGE	10 PERCENTILE	90 PERCENTILE	10 PERCENTILE	90 PERCENTILE
13	57.7	65.1	58.7	64.9
13½	58.8	66.5	59.5	65.3
14	59.9	67.9	60.2	65.7
14½	61	68.7	60.7	66
15	62.1	69.6	61.1	66.2
15½	63.1	70.2	61.3	66.4
16	64.1	70.7	61.5	66.5
16½	64.6	71.1	61.5	66.6
17	65.2	71.5	61.5	66.7
17½	65.3	71.6	61.5	66.7
18	65.5	71.8	61.5	66.7

Source: Combined from Tables 4–4 and 4–5 in G. H. Lowrey, *Growth and Development of Children*, 6th ed., Year Book Publishers, 1973. Used by permission.

tional counselor calls the "world of work" becomes a part of the adolescent's world. The inclusion of future along with past and present in his perceptual scheme and in his self-system represents a major step toward adulthood. His views of his ability are important in this choice for the future, and those who work with adolescents need to understand the self-factors in vocational and educational choice. Chapters 15 and 17 will discuss this aspect as it relates to the junior and senior high school.

In general, the adolescent period is one in which the child redefines himself, discovers new aspects of himself, modifies previously held self-images, and emerges with a new sense of identity. The central problem of the adolescent is thus his self.

We turn now to a more detailed view of how the adolescent meets and solves this problem. In this chapter we will explore the bodily changes and in the two following chapters, we will focus on the changing situational field and on the adolescent's changing view of himself.

EXTERNAL CHANGES

The most visible signs of adolescence are the changes in height, weight, and body proportions. Growth throughout adolescence is asynchronous; that is, different organ systems and body parts do not keep pace with each other. Whatever awkwardness there is in adolescence may be attributed to this.

The order in which changes occur is fairly well established, although individuals may vary in this respect as well as in the actual time of occurrence. Figures 11.1 and 11.2 show the usual time of appearance of sexual

TABLE 14.2   WEIGHT GAINS, AGES 13–18

	BOYS		GIRLS	
AGE	10 PERCENTILE	90 PERCENTILE	10 PERCENTILE	90 PERCENTILE
13	77.1	123.2	79.9	124.5
13½	82.2	130.1	85.5	128.9
14	87.2	136.9	91	133.3
14½	93.3	142.4	94.2	135.7
15	99.4	147.8	97.4	138.1
15½	105.2	152.6	99.2	139.6
16	111	157.3	100.9	141.1
16½	114.3	161	101.9	142.2
17	117.5	164.6	102.8	143.3
17½	118.8	166.8	103.2	143.9
18	120	169	103.5	144.5

Source: Combined from Tables 4–4 and 4–5 in G. H. Lowrey, *Growth and Development of Children*, 6th ed., Yearbook Publishers, 1973. Used by permission.

characteristics. Even a quick glance at these shows the faster maturity rate of girls. For instance, pubic hair appears about two years earlier, and most other indices show up at least a year sooner in girls than in boys.

Growth Spurt

The adolescent growth spurt, in which children seem literally to outgrow their clothes right before their parents' eyes, also covers a period of years. The spread between early and late maturers becomes even more pronounced during this spurt (see Tables 14.1 and 14.2). Stolz and Stolz, reporting on the boys in the Adolescent Growth Study, give the following times for the onset of the puberal growth period for height from 10.40 years to 15.75 years, with the average at 12.88 years. The termination occurs between 13.10 years and 17.50 years, with the average at 15.33. If one looks at speed of growth, the apex of velocity takes place as early as 11.90 years and as late as 16.65 years, with the mean at 13.99. (Stolz and Stolz, 1951, p. 69) Thus, two boys, both 13 years of age, can be about five years apart in this particular phase of maturity.

Body Build

Body proportions, especially the stem: leg ratio, are greatly modified in the adolescent years. (The stem consists of the head and trunk.) In general, the stem grows less than the leg in prepubescence and halfway through pubescence, and more in the second half of pubescence and the postpubescent period. This gives the early adolescent an "all legs" appearance that disappears later on.

There is a wide range of variation among individuals in the stem: leg ratio. Stolz and Stolz (1951) found that stem growth moved toward greater variability during adolescence, whereas leg growth moved toward the average. As a result, even though two youngsters may be the same height, the relative contributions of stem and leg give them different appearances and affect their posture and movement.

The differences in body build between early and late maturers is summarized as follows:

> We find a number of differences in the patterns of growth and of build between boys and girls, and between individuals who show different rates of maturing. For both sexes the faster maturing children have more intense spurts of rapid growth, with the period of acceleration both starting and stopping abruptly, while the late maturers have less intense periods of acceleration and with a subsequent growth which is longer continued, more even, and gradual. Boys who mature early tend to be large at all ages, especially so during the accelerated phase; as previously noted they are also usually broad built with relatively wide hips. . . .
>
> Late maturing boys, on the other hand, are more likely to be long-legged and slender, to have a "linear" or "asthenic" build, and to be narrow-headed. The later maturers are relatively small around 13 and 14 years, when their spurt of rapid growth is not yet started, but they grow up to be average or tall adults. [Bayley and Tuddenham, 1944, pp. 46–47]

Our concern is not only with external appearance but also with the meanings and effects this has upon the growing boy or girl. The most impressive finding of the longitudinal studies is the individuality of growth pattern. This pattern of growth is uneven, as Figure 14.1 illustrates. Yet, there is a particular personal pattern to growth within the individual, a personal pattern that leaves its impact upon the self-concept of the child.

By and large, the culture makes little allowance in its institutions, especially the school, for this tremendous range of individual development; it makes even less allowance for the private meanings. The extent of individuality is emphasized in the conclusions of Stolz and Stolz:

> The systematic study of the process of growth as it occurs in a considerable sample of adolescent boys emphasizes not only the uniqueness of each individual's status at any chronological age but also the idiomatic nature of the process in each individual. In every aspect of development the manifestations of individuality multiply as

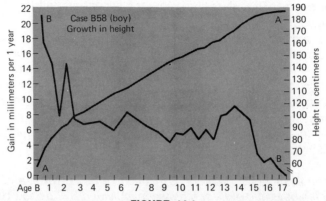

FIGURE 14.1

These profiles illustrate two ways in which the same growth data may be arranged and presented. Profile A shows how tall a boy was at successive chronological ages and the general trend of his growth. Profile B shows the changes in the same boy's growth rate during successive periods. Changes from acceleration to deceleration, or the reverse, and changes of gradients from one period to the next constitute the outstanding features of Profile B but are scarcely noticeable in Profile A. Even if they are magnified in A by increasing the value of the scale units, the variations in rate would be less obvious than in B because of the cumulative nature of the growth-achieved arrangement. Note particularly the distinctive features of this boy's sequential growth pattern for height as they are emphasized in Profile B. Reprinted from H. Stolz and L. Stolz, *Somatic development of adolescent boys.* Copyright 1951 by the Macmillan Company and used with their permission.

> *the frequency and variety phenomena* in the individual *becomes more impressive as evidence of differences in growth dynamics* among individuals *accumulates. The patterns of change in skeletal dimensions, subcutaneous tissue, muscular tissue, body hair, genitalia, muscular strength, and body weight show that whatever may be the similarities in growth achieved at the end of adolescence they do not mean identity or even similarity of growth experience.*
> [*Stolz and Stolz, 1951, p. 429*]

Adults who work with teenagers must become aware of the growth status of each youngster with whom they work. They need to be able to see where he fits into the general picture of development. Further, they need to become sensitive to the roles that his growth pattern and current growth status are playing in influencing his behavior.

The more speculative student, utilizing the transactional position in which mind and body are one and in which the individual is seen as functioning in keeping with his perceptual field, may well ask a difficult but important research question: If the evidence shows systematic uniqueness and there is a relationship between one's developmental status and his self-concept, could the self-concept be a factor in effecting growth? This would require a new type of longitudinal study but would certainly be well worth the effort. Why not the self affecting growth patterns as well as growth patterns affecting the self?

To test such a hypothesis, one would have to have a valid measure of maturity rate very early in the life of the child. He would have to be sure, therefore, of the mechanisms involved in maturity rate. This is beyond our abilities at the moment. Further, he would need valid and reliable measures of self-concept, especially concepts of independence-dependence, body image, and satisfaction fairly early in life. This we cannot as yet do. He would need to establish other than a response-response correlational design, so that he could demonstrate antecedent variables. There are other difficulties as well, but in time they may not be insurmountable. For example, we do have fairly good evidence of the effect of severe psychological stress on growth. Widdowson (1951) attempted to study the effect of increased food on orphanage children who were malnourished and found that these children's growth was more influenced by the behavior of a particular adult than by food. We also cited earlier the Powell et al. (1967) study.

PHYSIOLOGICAL CHANGES

Hormonal secretions, whether or not we speculate about the effect of self on the endocrine system, act as instigators of adolescent development. What triggers them off is still to be understood, but their effect is obvious.

The major physiological change is the beginning of the secretion of the gonads—the ovaries in the girl and the testes in the boy. These secretions are begun as a result of pituitary gland action. The pituitary secretes gonadotropic hormone, which activates the gonads. In turn, androgen and estrogen, the secretions of the gonads, influence growth. When their secretion is large, they cause the pituitary to slow down and cease its production of growth hormone.

There is a clear relationship between gonadal secretion and both the spurt of growth that takes place when hormone production is low and the tapering off of growth when hormonal secretion becomes substantial. Androgen, the major male secretion, in low amounts stimulates growth, whereas estrogen inhibits growth. Since estrogen secretion in girls begins to increase about age 8 or 9, this may account, to some degree, for the smaller final height of girls. Figure 14.2 illustrates the relationship between menarche and growth.

A variety of physiological measures have been made on adolescents —basal metabolism, temperature, pulse, and respiration. It has been found that with menarche there is a sudden fall in basal metabolism and an in-

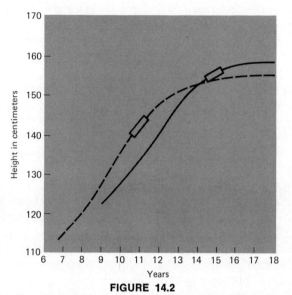

FIGURE 14.2

Relation of growth and onset of menarche. The blocks in the curves represent the time of menarche in two groups of girls. Girls with early menarche, and presumably reaching maturity early, have a more accelerated growth curve than girls with late menarche, but the duration of their growth is shorter. As a result of this growth pattern, girls with late maturation are taller, on the average, when final stature is attained. From Holt and McIntosh. *Holt Pediatrics,* 12th edition, 1953. Courtesy of Appleton-Century-Crofts, Publishing Division of Prentice-Hall, Inc., Englewood Cliffs, N.J.

crease in respiratory volume. (Shock, 1944) Unfortunately, there is no clear-cut indication of puberty for boys to parallel the menarche for girls.

The major question is whether or not the normal stability of body function is disrupted by all the changes that occur during adolescence. Is adolescence, physiologically, a period of upset? Is physiological instability a fact? If it is, some of the behavior of adolescents can probably be attributed to the state of their internal environments.

In Chapter 1 and in subsequent chapters, the concepts of the steady-state, differentiation-integration, and movement toward higher levels of organization have been discussed. If there is physiological instability in adolescence, this might suggest the need of the organism to reorganize, to modify its previous system, and to incorporate the changes into a new alignment. In other words, the physiological changes create a situation in which the body has to learn and establish new rhythms and patterns.

A review of the Adolescent Growth Study data, a major source for us in our knowledge and understanding of adolescence, leads to the conclusion that ''the data do not support the notion that there is a *generalized* physiological instability during adolescence. Rather they suggest that some functions become stable and others less." (Eichorn and McKee, 1958, p. 261)

Shock, using longitudinal data on 100 teenage boys and girls, found the same variability with respect to physiological function that we have already seen is characteristic of external physical appearance. He found that sex differences in certain measures, notably blood pressure and respiration, first appear in adolescence. From our point of view, his inference as to the meaning of the wide inter- and intra-individual variations is most intriguing. He states: "This information [that there exists wide variation from the average and that changes are often rapid and abrupt] is of considerable value in interpreting the results of physiological measurements in individual cases. The increased variability . . . may be taken as an indication that one of the important aspects of development is learning to maintain physiological equilibrium. . . . An example of such physiological learning is the regulation of menstrual periodicity. When menstruation first begins in adolescent girls it does not recur at uniform intervals." (Shock, 1960, p. 127) This irregularity decreases with length of time following menarche, with regularity becoming established no sooner than 2 years after first menses. The lag between menarche and the ability to conceive also lasts at least a year and often 4 to 6 years. The earlier the menarche, the longer the lag. (Stuart, 1960)

We therefore may say that, physiologically as well as psychologically, adolescence is a period of reorganization and reintegration. The girl, for example, as she grows toward womanhood, is faced with the task not only of comprehending her social role as woman but also of adapting herself to cyclic changes within her body system. Her concept of herself must encompass both the physiological and the social environment.

Health and Nutrition

The early adolescent years, like the years immediately preceding, are years of relative good health. Youth is relatively resistant to infection during this time. The "library of immunity" is fairly well stocked. The main cause of death is accident, especially for boys.

However, this is also a period of increased energy need. The importance of adequate diet cannot be overemphasized. The age of menarche, rather than being influenced by the factors assigned in folklore (for example, that girls from the tropics mature earlier than girls from the temperate zones), is affected by nutrition. Because of better nutrition and control of disease, the age of menarche has gone down (see Figure 14.3).

In a study of the possible connection between nutrition and menarche, for example, Frish and Revelle (1970) examined the height and weight of early and late arrivers at menarche at the time of menarche. They found that both groups, regardless of chronological age, weighed

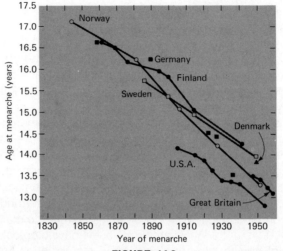

FIGURE 14.3
Secular trend in age at menarche, 1830–1960. Sources of data and method of plotting detailed in Tanner, 1962. From J. M. Tanner, Physical growth, in P. H. Mussen (ed.), *Carmichael's manual of child psychology,* 3d ed., Wiley, New York, 1970, Vol. 1, p. 146. Used with permission.

the same (106 pounds [48 kg.]) but that late maturers were taller. Further, weight for all groups was the same (about 68 pounds [31 kg.]) at the beginning of the growth spurt and at the maximum rate of weight gain (86 pounds [39 kg.]). They suggest that "the attainment of a critical weight may be essential for each of these events." (Frisch and Revelle, 1970, p. 398) They believe weight influences metabolic rate.

Another example of the role of nutrition is shown by charts of the caloric requirements of different age groups. The 8-year-old boy needs about 1700 calories; the 14-year-old needs almost double this amount. The 14-year-old girl, who is at the peak of her energy requirement, needs about 2800 calories as compared to the 1700 she needed when she was 8. Cokes and hamburgers just won't do. It is no wonder that adolescents are incessant refrigerator-raiders and snack-artists. They need the food, but the wise adult makes sure that high-protein foods are easily available.

BODY IMAGE AND THE SELF
If there is anything more individual than the way an adolescent follows the general path of development, it is the unique view he takes of his own progress. Although the interrelationships between one's body and one's self are extremely complex, they exist and are of vital concern to the adolescent.

As we take up this topic, we should be aware that the evidence is far from conclusive and that we are, in effect, "going beyond our data" to theorize about the relationships between the body and the self. We will use data where they exist, but much still remains to be learned.

A seventh-grade art teacher in a Virginia school, in seeking to help students use art as a means of self-expression and self-understanding, gave them several assignments. One was to draw yourself as you saw yourself 10 years later. The results were quite revealing. Many of the girls drew themselves as Hollywood sex symbols in long, slinky, décolleté gowns. Many of the boys portrayed themselves as jet pilots or athletic heroes. The picture that stays with this author, however, is that drawn by a late-maturing girl. Her drawing depicted, in her words, a championship Olympic swimmer. The interesting point about the picture was that all you could see was part of a face and part of an arm; the rest was hidden by the water. As we came to understand—and as this girl saw herself—she had rejected her body. She did not wish it to be seen, nor did she wish to see it herself. For her, it was submerged.

A postpolio boy in his teens wrote the following as part of a paper in school:

> For me, as a physically handicapped person, my two greatest fears and worries have been of falling in the presence of others or while others were watching; and of people not accepting me as an equal because of my disability. I am also afraid of meeting people without their knowing of my disability—at a table or in a car for instance—and then having to watch their display of emotions when they do see it.
>
> I think that it is possible that many of my fears—social acceptance, peer status and personal recognition—are often not well founded. All too often we find what we look for, be it "reality" or not. I think that the things a person looks for and finds depends on the individual and the circumstances.
>
> The physically handicapped, like everyone else, need to be shown that they are loved, that they are accepted. But for them, I think this need is even greater. I never forget for one moment that I am not "like" everyone else. Things that others aren't even conscious of are of importance to me as a handicapped person. This being the case, ordinary acceptance isn't enough—I must be really made to see that I am "ok"—accepted. This can be accomplished, not by a great display of sympathy, but by an attempt to treat me as an "equal" with the rest, but also at the same time seeing me as an individual, and keeping in mind my limitations.

The author and other adults who knew him were hardly aware of his very slight limp. What seemed to us a minor impairment loomed large in this boy's self-image.

These two instances are not isolated examples; they portray quite vividly the intense meaning the body has to the adolescent.

Physical Appearance

We all know the Snow White story, in which the beautiful but vain Queen implored her magic mirror to reassure her that she was the fairest one of all. Each child has his magic mirror, too. It consists of his idealized image of what he might look like when he grows up. Before the changes of adolescence, such an image is safe. As he sees himself assume his virtually final appearance, the rude awakening comes for many an adolescent. The magic mirror image retreats before the "real" one he sees each day.

We are aware of what seems—to the adult—the inordinate amount of time the early adolescent spends in front of the mirror. Could it be that he needs this time to attempt a reconciliation between the hoped-for and the emergent reality? He evaluates what he is becoming, and then must learn to live with it. He assesses his height, weight, general body build, and facial appearance (including the presence of acne) and modifies his self-concept in terms of what he perceives.

The tall girl perceives herself, perhaps, as facing unfair competition on the dance floor. She shudders at the vision of dancing with a boy a head shorter. She may slump as she walks, wear clothes that give the impression of reduced height, or avoid high heels. Perhaps the short boy faces similar difficulties. If he is growing up in a basketball-conscious town where status is achieved by being on the varsity team, he resents not only the "bean-poles" but also himself. He sees his height as a drawback—and it often is. One 14-year-old, for example, wrote:

> Size means a lot in the ninth grade, especially when you are small, you get pushed around by all the biger [sic] boys. To be in sports you have to be big and brawny. On the football field you always get the bad positions. When you play basketball they never pass to you. If you get the ball, they expect you to pass it immediately to them, and if you don't you're a stupid dope. You never get a chance to show how good you are. If you miss a shot they tell you that you ought to learn to shoot, but they don't let you learn to shoot because they are always hogging the ball. When you are small they never invite you to a party. [Strang, 1957, p. 237]

General body build, as well as height, influences perception of self. Biller and Liebman (1971), in a comparison of boys who were muscular with those who were fat and thin, showed the influence of build on children's views of sex-role preference and teachers' ratings of sex-role behavior. There was no relationship between boy and teacher ratings, but within the boys' preference ratings, muscular youths reported higher masculine preferences. The teachers saw the muscular boys as engaging in more masculine behavior than either of the other two groups; and thin boys

TABLE 14.3 PHYSICAL FACTORS ON THE "HOW I SEE MYSELF" SCALE

PHYSICAL APPEARANCE	*PHYSICAL ADEQUACY*
1. My hair is nice looking. 2. I am the right weight. 3. Girls like me. 4. My face is pretty. 5. I like the way I look. 6. My skin is nice. 7. My clothes are nice. 8. I like my build.	1. I have lots of energy. 2. I am good at athletics. 3. I am quite healthy. 4. I am a good dancer.

Source: I. J. Gordon, A Test Manual for the "How I See Myself" Scale, Gainesville, Fla.: Florida Educational Research Council, 1968. Adapted from P. Yeatts, Developmental Changes in the Self-Concept of Children Grades 3–12, *Florida Educational Research and Development Council Research Bulletin,* 1967, 3, 2.

were seen as behaving in a more masculine fashion than fat. What we may have here is evidence of cultural role expectation either leading to behavior or to reported behavior. In any case, body build influences not only self but also others' perceptions of a person.

On the other hand, body image is a strange phenomenon. The youth may believe his shortness to be more acute than it is. Even when he reaches his final height, which may be average for his generation, he may carry himself as though he were shorter. He may walk with rounded shoulders, slouch in his seat, look up to others who are really his own height. The impact of his stature stays with him whether he attempts to fight it or surrender to it.

Weight, too, makes its impact. The early adolescent girl is likely to put on weight, for this phenomenon is a result of the changes occurring within her body. She reads the ads in the fashion magazines and movie fan magazines and watches the TV commercials. One of the effects of these media is the dieting fad. At a time when good nutrition is so essential, she may virtually starve herself in her efforts to resemble a fashion model.

Being too fat or too thin, being different, is what creates adolescent concern. Of course, it will affect each child in its own way, but it does leave its mark.

Both physical appearance and physical adequacy are perceived as dimensions of the self by adolescents. These show up as discrete factors on the "How I See Myself" scale. Table 14.3 presents the scale items. Yeatts (1967), using this scale on over 4500 adolescents, found that on the average, these secondary school students felt a little on the positive side on both factors. The lowest scores, however, are made by seventh-through ninth-grade girls.

Rate of Maturity

Rate of maturity, as seen in the art example, poses many problems of self-acceptance. Both the extremely early and extremely late boy or girl face peer situations that put them at a disadvantage. The adolescent does not wish to be different from his peers, but his rate of growth may place him in this position.

The early-maturing boy, if he's not too far ahead, is at an advantage over the late maturer. In the American culture, height, weight, and strength all carry status. In what ways does the self-concept of the early maturing boy differ from that of the late maturer? Three approaches have been used to explore this question. Jones and Bayley (1950) used observation and ratings of the behavior of teenage boys. They found the late maturer displayed a higher activity rate and was more animated and eager in his activities. They inferred that this was compensatory behavior. If one needs to compensate, the question arises, compensate for what? The obvious answer in this case is for feelings of inadequacy due to size.

Still, although this may be a good hunch, it is an incomplete answer. An inference from behavior is one path; inference from projective materials offers another avenue. Thematic Apperception Test data was used in the California Growth Study to get a more covert expression of self-conceptions. Thirty-three boys, aged 17, upon whom there was complete physical growth data, took the TAT. In taking the TAT, a person is given, one at a time, a set of cards with somewhat ambiguous pictures on them and is asked to make up a story about each picture. The story is seen as a projection by the person of his own personality into the picture; hence the name, projective technique. There are various scoring schemes, but all are built on the above notion. The researchers conclude:

> Analysis of the data of the present study indicates that this situation [late maturity] may have adverse effects on the personalities of the physically retarded. These boys are more likely to have negative self-conceptions, feelings of inadequacy, strong feelings of being rejected and dominated, prolonged dependency needs, and rebellious attitudes toward parents. In contrast, the early-maturing boys present a much more favorable psychological picture during adolescence. Relatively few of them felt inadequate, rejected, dominated, or rebellious toward their families. More of them appeared to be self-confident, independent, and capable of playing an adult role in interpersonal relationships. [Mussen and Jones, 1957, p. 255]

A follow-up study taken when members of this sample were in their late 30s shows the lingering effects of maturity rate on personality. Skeletal age was the criterion for classification. Retrospective interviews showed that the early maturers looked back to pleasurable memories; the late maturers to peer rejection and unpleasantness. The late maturers, however, were seen as having greater insight and perceptiveness, although these may be understood as devices for coping with difficulty. There are, of course, individual differences. (Jones, 1965)

The third study used pubic hair as the index of maturity and 44 boys between 12 and 15 as subjects. Self-concept was inferred by the researchers from human figure drawings, a personality scale, and paragraph completions. Postpubescent boys, in their drawings, revealed higher images of adequacy as males than did their prepubescent peers. On the other hand, chronological age was more related to statements about emancipation from parents and heterosexual interests than was pubic age. (Smith and Lebo, 1956) We would expect that experience would play a role along with maturation in these attitudes toward others. These boys were still in early adolescence; the boys in the previous study were late adolescents who had, perhaps, already incorporated these ideas into their self-systems.

What about maturity as a problem for girls? In a parallel study to that done on the boys, the extreme cases of 17-year-old girls took the TAT. The early-maturing girls did not show negative self-conceptions. Jones and Mussen (1958) assume that the reason may have been because the critical period was already past. It may be, however, that moving into womanhood early is desired by girls in our culture. We certainly emphasize speeding up everything else!

More's intensive study of a small group of midwestern boys and girls may support this different view. He found the early-maturing girls, as measured by a battery of projective techniques, were more rational, more independent, and had better integrated systems of personal values than late maturers.

More's point of view is that our society calls upon youngsters to display competence in patterned ways of heterosexual relationships rather than in deep involvements. He concludes, therefore, "that the socially successful girl was the one who acted *as if* she were sexually mature, but who does not allow herself to feel the emotions which she appears to be acting out. Within the normal ranges of physical maturation in the sample, the girl who matures earlier has a distinct advantage in making this socially prized shift earlier. She learns it more thoroughly than her physically retarded girl friend. She is the one who is better fitted. . . ." (More, 1955, p. 117)

A third suggestion that early maturity is the desired status for girls is made by Davidson and Gottlieb (1955). According to their Rorschach data, postmenarcheal girls seem to have better self-concepts.

What conclusions can we draw? First, the rate of maturity affects the self-concept of the adolescent. Second, it seems that early maturers, regardless of sex, have, as a group, conceptions of self as more adequate, more accepted, more integrated than do their late-maturing peers. Third, the relationships are by no means simple, and the correlation between physical maturity and self-concept is far from 1.0. Many individual factors need to be considered. Of vital importance is the already developed self-concept held by the boy or girl when he reachs adolescence. Fourth, since some of these studies and others were done on late adolescents and young adults aged 33 (Jones, 1957), the effects, which last at least into young adulthood, seem to be long-range rather than situational.

Secondary Sex Characteristics

Secondary sex characteristics are evaluated by the adolescent boy or girl on the basis of their appropriateness. The male must look male; the girl must look female. Fatty deposits on hips, some breast development, lack of pubic hair, or small external genitalia all serve to make the adolescent boy a target for ridicule. The boys' shower room and locker room in the junior high school gymnasium can be a place for either exhibitionism or intense embarrassment. Although the humor is often crude, each boy becomes aware of whether or not he approaches his peers' and his own concept of the male physique.

Girls, too, must cope with the meanings assigned by both the adult and peer cultures as to what constitutes the ideal feminine form. There was a time when there was little advertising or display concerning aids to nature. Now the early adolescent girl is bombarded by manufacturers' efforts to exploit the teenage market. She is told that she doesn't have either to wait or depend upon nature. She can fill that bikini right now. But she knows her own physical self, and she may reject or be unhappy with her body because it does not measure up to cultural demands.

Further, she is confused about the shift from the tomboyish activity of prepubescence to the more feminine activities now expected of her. As one girl stated it: "There comes a time when you are baffled as to whether or not to play with boys—playing such things as football and other rough sports. If you don't, you don't get very much exercise, as an all-girl unorganized game is awful. Most of us decide to play with the boys but to take it easy." (Strang, 1957, p. 226)

Acne and body odors, both results of the changing physiological functions, are causes of great concern. Again, the world of advertising, the impact of the mass media, add to the individual's awareness. The youngster is afraid that even his best friends won't tell him. He has learned that "nervous perspiration" is worst of all and that success with the girls depends not upon your charm but your hair oil. The net effect is to make youngsters dissatisfied with something that is a natural function. They are vulnerable to the advertisements because they take them personally. At-

TABLE 14.4 PHYSICAL MANIFESTATIONS THAT DISTURBED BOYS

CHARACTERISTIC	NUMBER OF BOYS
Lack of size—particularly height	7
Fatness	7
Poor physique	4
Lack of muscular strength	4
Unusual facial features	4
Unusual development in the nipple area	4
Acne	3
Skin blemishes, scars	2
Bowed legs	2
Obvious scoliosis	2
Lack of shoulder breadth	1
Unusually small genitalia	1
Unusually large genitalia	1

Source: Reprinted from "Adolescent Problems Relating to Somatic Variations," H. Stolz and L. Stolz, *Adolescence*, 43rd Yearbook, 1944, National Society for the Study of Education. Used by permission.

tractiveness to the opposite sex holds high value, and they are crucially aware of any factor that might affect their status.

Actual body changes, such as the onset of menses, have differential meanings depending upon advance knowledge and preparation. For example, southern black girls experienced more emotions over the onset of menstruation than did their white peers. Henton (1961) assumes the difference to be due to parental guidance and sex education.

We must reiterate a word of caution. In the case of any individual youngster, his self-concepts will be the result of the totality of the transactions between his changing organism and his world. His self-system will strongly affect the new meanings he assigns to his body and his self. He is not born anew in adolescence; what modifications he makes have their origins within his self-system as it has already evolved. If he comes to adolescence with a view of himself as essentially adequate, his interpretation of any physical factors that might be negative will be tempered by his concept of self as adequate. Conversely, the youngster entering adolescence with feelings of inadequacy may view his body (which others may see as adequate) as not what he would like it to be. We cannot, therefore, apply indiscriminately to the individual our conclusions about early adolescents as a group.

Approximately one-third of the adolescents in the California Growth Study were definitely disturbed, as judged by a physician who knew them well, about their physical characteristics. Tables 14.4 and 14.5 show the

TABLE 14.5   PHYSICAL MANIFESTATIONS THAT DISTURBED GIRLS

CHARACTERISTIC	NUMBER OF GIRLS
Tallness	7
Fatness	7
Facial features	5
General physical appearance	5
Tallness and heaviness	3
Smallness and heaviness	3
Eyeglasses and strabismus	2
Thinness and small breasts	2
Late development	2
Acne	1
Hair	1
Tallness and thinness	1
Big legs	1
One short arm	1
Scar on face	1
Brace on back	1

Source: Reprinted from "Adolescent Problems Relating to Somatic Variations," H. Stolz and L. Stolz, *Adolescence,* 43rd Yearbook, 1944, National Society for the Study of Education. Used by permission.

numbers and causes. The numbers of boys and girls in these tables "who suffered known anxieties concerning physical factors represent a minimum accounting, since others undoubtedly had, at one time or another, some degree of disturbance in this area which did not come to the physician's attention." (Stolz and Stolz, 1944, p. 86)

Another indication of the extent of concern is shown by Table 14.6, compiled by Strang from compositions written by more than 1000 junior and senior high school pupils. In every IQ bracket, about one-fourth of the group expressed dissatisfaction with their own growth; a slight tendency for the brightest early adolescents to express the most was shown. Conversely, fewer of those of average IQ expressed dissatisfaction. Since the youngsters did not have to write about body growth, it is interesting that so many (over 44 percent) did.

Thus, height, weight, and sexually appropriate physique—any factor that stamps one as noticeably different—all influence the adolescent's concept of himself.

Why is this so important? "The changing body becomes a symbol not only of being different from last month or last year but of a new attitude toward self, toward others, toward life." (Stolz and Stolz, 1944, p. 82) With

TABLE 14.6 ADOLESCENTS' EXPRESSION CONCERNING BODY GROWTH

GRADE LEVEL AND IQ	NUMBER OF COMPO- SITIONS	THOSE EXPRESSING SATISFACTION WITH OWN BODY GROWTH		THOSE EXPRESSING DISSATISFACTION WITH OWN BODY GROWTH	
		NO.	PERCENT	NO.	PERCENT
7–8–9; Average IQ: 95.2	247	45	18	54	22
7–8–9; IQ: 120–129	121	39	32	29	24
7–8–9; IQ: 130 and over	35	10	29	13	37
10–11–12; Average IQ: 94.9	636	113	18	144	23
10–11–12; IQ; 120–129	65	25	38	15	23
10–11–12; IQ: 130 and over	20	6	30	5	25

Source: Reprinted by permission from *The Adolescent Views Himself,* by Ruth Strang. Copyright, 1957, McGraw-Hill Book Company.

this background, we can look at the adolescent's new attitudes toward others and then, in Chapter 16, at his new attitudes toward self.

REFERENCES AND ADDITIONAL READINGS

Bayley, N., & Tuddenham, R. Adolescent changes in body build. In NSSE, *Adolescence,* 43rd Yearbook, Part I. Chicago: The Society, 1944. Pp. 33–55.

Biller, H., & Liebman, D. Body build and sex role preference and sex role adoption in junior high school boys. *Journal of Genetic Psychology,* 1971, *118,* 81–86.

Davidson, H., & Gottlieb, L. The emotional maturity of pre- and post-menarcheal girls. *Journal of Genetic Psychology,* 1955, *86,* 261–266.

Eichorn, D. Physiological development. In P. H. Mussen (Ed.), *Carmichael's manual of child psychology.* (3rd ed.) Vol. I. New York: Wiley, 1970. Pp. 157–283.

Eichorn, D., & McKee, J. P. Physiological instability during adolescence. *Child Development,* 1958, *29,* 255–268.

Erikson, E. Eight stages of man. In C. Stendler (Ed.), *Readings in child development.* New York: Harcourt, Brace, 1954. Pp. 213–220.

Farnham, M. The adolescent. New York: Harper & Row, 1952.

Faust, M. Developmental maturity as a determinant in prestige of adolescent girls. *Child Development,* 1960, *31,* 173–184.

Frisch, R., & Revelle, R. Heights and weights at menarche and a hypothesis of critical body weights and adolescent events. *Science,* 1970, *169,* 397–399.

Gardner, G. Present-day society and the adolescent. *American Journal of Orthopsychiatry,* 1957, *27,* 508–517.

Greulich, W. Physical changes in adolescence. In NSSE, *Adolescence.* 43rd Yearbook, Part I. Chicago: The Society, 1944. Pp. 8–32.

Hart, M., & Sarnoff, C. The impact of the menarche: A study of two stages of organization. *Journal of the American Academy of Child Psychiatry,* 1971, *10,* 257–271.

Henton, C. The effect of socio-economic and emotional factors on the onset of menarche among Negro and white girls. *Journal of Genetic Psychology,* 1961, *98,* 255–264.

Holt, L., & McIntosh, R. (Eds.) *Holt pediatrics.* (12th ed.) New York: Appleton-Century-Crofts, 1953.

Jones, M. C. The later careers of boys who were early- or late-maturing. *Child Development,* 1965, *36,* 899–911.

Jones, M. C., & Bayley, N. Physical maturing among boys as related to behavior. *Journal of Educational Psychology,* 1950, *41,* 129–148.

Jones, M. C., & Mussen, P. H. Self-conceptions, motivations, and interpersonal attitudes of early- and late-maturing girls. *Child Development,* 1958, *29,* 491–501.

Lewin, K. The field theory approach to adolescence. In J. Seidman (Ed.), *Adolescence.* (Rev. ed.) New York: Holt, Rinehart & Winston, 1960. Pp. 32–42.

Lowrey, G. H. *Growth and development of children.* (6th ed.) Chicago: Year Book Publishers, 1973.

More, D. Developmental concordance and discordance during puberty and adolescence. *Child Development Monographs,* 1955, *18(56).*

Murray, C. Sociometry and athletic status of adolescents, critical review of research literature. *Perceptual & Motor Skills,* 1971, *33(3),* 1143–1150.

Mussen, P. H., & Jones, M. C. Self-conceptions, motivations and interpersonal attitudes of late- and early-maturing boys. *Child Development,* 1957, *28,* 243–256.

Powell, G., Brasel, J., & Blizzard, R. Emotional deprivation and growth retardation simulating idiopathic hypopituitarism. *New England Journal of Medicine,* 1957, *276,* 1271–1278.

Shock, N. Physiological changes in adolescence. In NSSE, *Adolescence.* 43rd Yearbook, Part I. Chicago: The Society, 1944. Pp. 56–79.

Shock, N. Some physiological aspects of adolescence. In J. Seidman (Ed.), *The adolescent.* (Rev. ed.) New York: Holt, Rinehart & Winston, 1960. Pp. 116–127.

Smith, W., & Lebo, D. Some changing aspects of the self-concept of pubescent males. *Journal of Genetic Psychology,* 1956, *88,* 61–75.

Stolz, H., & Stolz, L. Adolescent problems related to somatic variations. In NSSE, *Adolescence.* 43rd Yearbook, Part I. Chicago: The Society, 1944. Pp. 80–99.

Stolz, H., & Stolz, L. *Somatic development of adolescent boys.* New York: Macmillan, 1951.

Strang, R. *The adolescent views himself.* New York: McGraw-Hill, 1957.

Stuart, H. Normal growth and development. In J. Seidman (Ed.), *The adolescent.* (Rev. ed.) New York: Holt, Rinehart & Winston, 1960.

Tanner, J. M. *Growth at adolescence.* (2nd ed.) Oxford: Blackwell Scientific Publications, 1962.

Tanner, J. M. Physical growth. In P. H. Mussen (Ed.), *Carmichael's manual of child psychology.* (3rd ed.) Vol. I. New York: Wiley, 1970. Pp. 77–155.

Widdowson, E. Mental contentment and physical growth. *Lancet,* 1951, *1,* 1316–1318.

Yeatts, P. Developmental changes in the self-concept of children grades 3–12. *Florida Educational Research and Development Council Research Bulletin,* 1967, *3(2).*

CHAPTER 15

THE CHANGING WORLD OF THE EARLY ADOLESCENT

Although it is impossible to separate attitudes of self from attitudes toward others, we will focus here upon the ways in which self-concepts are reflected in behavior and attitudes toward others. We shall also examine the environmental field of the early adolescent—his home, culture, school, and peer group.

PARENT-CHILD RELATIONSHIPS

Parents of adolescents are often depicted as either weak, ineffectual, bemused characters who are thrown for a loss by the behavior of their offspring or as autocratic, harsh disciplinarians engaged in a running fight to keep their children in line. On the one hand, they are accused of being too lenient, on the other, of not allowing children to grow up.

This dual image of the parent probably reflects the dual struggle of the early adolescent to strengthen his identification with the parent of the same sex and emancipate himself from the home. Although this struggle is evident during the adolescent years, it is only the continuation of a trend begun at the moment of self-awareness, if not before.

Because of his changing body, the many new experiences he has, and the backlog of development, the early adolescent perceives his parents and his family in a new light. The new look at parents is not completely distinct from the old; it is fashioned upon the concepts that have been developed. Parents and their children do not suddenly exhibit behavior different from their earlier behavior, although covert thoughts may now become more overt.

The parent who is seen as weak and ambivalent in allowing the child to go with the gang, to date, and to stay out later is the same parent who cried at the loss of the child when he went off to school. The youngster who is confused and guilty about his new urges and desires has experienced this feeling before. The difference lies in the pressures from outside the family and in the increased understanding of the adolescent. Where formerly he might have surrendered to the pressure to stay tied, he may now rebel against it.

The child learned in elementary school that he was not the center of the world. He now learns what is for many parents a bitter fact: His parents are not all-good, all-wise, and all-powerful. Previously, when up against parental pressure, he may have felt that he was somehow wrong to oppose it; now he sees his parents more clearly for what they are—human beings. Perhaps he feels cheated by this discovery, and communication becomes more difficult as a result. Perhaps this discovery opens up to him chances to disagree without guilt, to apply pressure in turn, to stand up for his "rights." Whatever view he takes is related to the previous relationship between the early adolescent and his parents.

Identification

The importance of identification in normal development has been stressed in earlier chapters. It becomes heightened in early adolescence. The boy who perceives his relationships with his father to be strained may respond in unhealthy ways. He may move toward aggressive delinquent acts, hard drugs, or homosexuality. His perception of his parent depends upon the extent and type of communication that has existed throughout his life.

How closely do parent and child see alike? Helper (1958) asked parents to fill out a self-rating as they thought that their children would respond. He discovered a relationship between parental evaluation and the child's self-evaluation. A similar study by Silver (1958) indicated that the level and stability of a boy's self-concept ratings were significantly related to paternal acceptance and, to a lesser extent, to maternal acceptance.

Early adolescent boys and girls see their parents differently. In a study of working class children, for example, boys saw their parents as more controlling than did girls, and girls saw their parents as more accepting than boys. (Armentrout and Burger, 1972)

A clearer view of the importance of father-son relationships can be obtained through the careful, perceptive work of Bandura and Walters. They hypothesized that dependency relationships and patterns would be related to aggressive delinquency. Fifty-two families were studied intensively by means of interviews, self-reports, and TAT data. Twenty-six of the boys had been in trouble with the law; the other 26 were selected by school counselors as being neither especially aggressive nor withdrawn. Age, IQ, socioeconomic background, ordinal position, and neighborhood factors were all matched.

What do the data reveal? Perhaps the most significant conclusion can be conveyed by the following excerpts from interviews with the boys. In the case of the aggressive boys, a typical interview proceeded thus:

I: *How often would you say you went to your father to talk things over?*
B: *(Case 33) Never.*
I: *How about if you were worried about something or had gotten into a scrape? Do you go to him then?*
B: *No. I never go to my parents.*
I: *When your parents make a suggestion, do you usually accept it or do you prefer to work it out for yourself?*
B: *I'd rather work things out for myself. . . .*
I: *Some fellows go around with their parents quite a lot, for example on trips or to movies. Others don't like this very much. How do you feel about this?*
B: *I don't go.*

The control boys' interviews illustrate the contrast:

I: *How often would you say you went to your father to talk things over?*
B: *(Case 28) About, maybe about, do you think I should do this, or about maybe a job, or if he thinks I should take it, or if he thinks I should go someplace, or do this, or on money problems, or anything, I ask my father.*
I: *Do you do the same with your mother?*
B: *Not as much with my mother as with my father. I'm not closer to him than to my mother, but I think what I do, he's done usually and he has more insight into it. . . .*
I: *Now I'd like to ask you how often you go somewhere with your father.*
B: *I go with him, not regularly, but not just on special occasions. As much as possible, as much as I want to and, you know, not on vacations, but say there was a picnic yesterday, the office picnic. I usually go. I didn't go yesterday because I was working, but I have gone all the time. Fishing once in a while and football games, he tries to take me. He says he wants me to see everything in life and things he hasn't had the opportunity to. We try to, we do a lot things together. [Bandura and Walters, 1959, p. 72]**

The perception of father as helper, guide, and affectionate supporter seems to be a critical factor. This perception seems to have begun to develop in early childhood. There was no essential difference among these boys as to mothering in infancy. It seems the poor start and continuous disruption of opportunities for close father-son identification is the major variable.

This difficulty continues to be reinforced by the current life situation. The homes of the aggressive boys are characterized by inconsistency in

---

* Albert Bandura and Richard H. Walters, *Adolescent Aggression—A Study of the Influence of Child-Training Practices and Family Interrelationships.* Copyright © 1959, The Ronald Press Company, New York.

the handling of aggressive behavior. They seem to still face differences between parents on what types of aggression are allowed and, within each parent, on who can be a target of aggression. A study of girl delinquents also highlighted parental influence. Duncan (1971) interviewed both parents of the girls and reported that parents of normal adolescents were higher in self-esteem and expressed a more positive mother-father relationship than did the parents of the delinquent girls. She found that parents of delinquent girls are inconsistent in their feelings.

How can someone anchor to a point that shifts? How can the child make appropriate differentiations when he cannot predict? In the case of these aggressive boys, there was no feeling of home as a safe haven.

What about the boy whose father was not even physically present? Biller and Bahm (1971) reported that junior high school boys whose fathers were absent before they were 5 had less masculine self-concepts as measured by the adjective checklist. The role of the mother, however, is critical for these boys. When the mother was seen by the boys as encouraging their aggression, this enhanced masculine self-concept. Boys whose fathers became absent after age 5 did not differ in self-concept from father-present boys, nor did their perception of maternal encouragement play a role in their self-image.

Evidence of the impact of a close-knit family culture that provides a high degree of security and nurturance in the early years, that does not tolerate physical aggression, and that provides many models of approved behavior can be found in the former low delinquency rate of Chinese junior-high-age youngsters in New York's Chinatown when the population was more stable. (Sollenberger, 1968) In these studies we see again the importance of the early years, the parent-parent relationship, and the pattern of expectations and role modeling as influences on the attitudes and behavior of early adolescents.

Fortunately, for most early adolescent children, parent-child relationships are strong and essentially positive. By and large, the children accept the adult values and internalize the way of life of the family. This does not mean a lack of conflict, but it does mean that friction is kept within bounds and does not lead to the great mass of children becoming rebels without cause.

Studies of suburbia, for example, reveal that "there are few sharp conflicts between parents and children . . . the youth culture elements exist, but they are less dominant than are accepted family and authority guidance patterns." (Elkin and Westley, 1955, p. 684) This view seems to persist even in the early 1970s, in spite of the very visible (in media and print) activities of adolescent runaways, the drug scene, changes in grooming and clothing, and reported changes in sexual codes. Weiner (1971), for example, states that most adolescents are stable and closely tied to family and community. When the relative effects of kibbutz life, with its separation of children from their parents for most of the day, were compared to those of Moshav upbringing (cooperative farms, where family life is maintained), Long, Henderson, and Platt (1973) found that kibbutz adolescents identified with their parents more closely than did Moshav adolescents. Although the results may have been affected by the fact that there were youngsters from both European and North African or Middle Eastern backgrounds, the results show that adolescents, even under kibbutz conditions, have close ties to their parents. A large-scale survey of adolescents, taken from a psychoanalytic viewpoint, reinforces this view. Douvan and Adelson report:

> We think most writers have overplayed both the potency of peer norms and the amount of discrepancy between parental and peer standards. For most adolescents there is, appearances aside, no great dissonance between what parents and friends believe. We say "appearances aside" because we sometimes observe a great hue and cry of conflict between the child and his parents over "values" and "norms" which are in fact trivial. The so-called adolescent rebellion in these cases exhausts itself on issues of manners and tastes. . . . Thus a pseudorebellion helps to forestall any serious appraisal of serious value issues. Perhaps it is asking too much to expect adolescents to do more than make mock revolts, but one sometimes wonders whether the parent and child enter into a tacit understanding to disagree only over "teenage" matters. . . .
> [Douvan and Adelson, 1966, p. 812]

Kandel et al. (1970), after reviewing the literature up to about 1967, conclude that an adolescent subculture does indeed exist and has a profound effect on behavior. It is probably not an either-or situation; more likely, the youngster belongs to both the family and the peer group.

One source of conflict, perhaps even in the suburban homes mentioned above, is in the differing perceptions between the generations of what constitutes the "good" parent and the "good" child. Although the researchers fail to indicate the exact nature of the differences (on what items do people disagree?), Connor, Greene, and Walters (1958) report that there is not only difference between parents but also a greater difference between parent and child. Fathers differ most from their children in their view of the ideal role.

All these studies, viewed together, point up one significant fact: In the life of the adolescent, both parents are important. If the father has neglected his role as a conveyor of warmth and acceptance, his son stands a good chance of finding early adolescence a time of difficulty. If the mother's role in the family has been one of little importance, in which she has received little respect from her husband, the daughter's identification with and acceptance of her female role may be deficient.

As Frank points out:

> *Young girls who are involved in sex delinquencies and who have venereal infections are individuals who have never accepted, indeed have rejected, the female and feminine role . . . they have never developed any feeling of being a woman with a sense of their own dignity or worth as a woman. . . . To speak of them as the victims of passion, or weak-willed individuals who could not resist sex temptations, is to misunderstand completely their conduct and their feelings. By exercising power over men, some are getting revenge for the years of humiliation they have suffered as girls under dominant fathers and contemptuous brothers. [Frank, 1944, p. 245]*

Is such a statement still true in the 1970s? Gail Sheehy, in describing her findings on prostitution in New York, says that the girls "are generally young women of low self esteem in trouble. . . . Many of the girls have an illegitimate child. . . . Most of the time they have been thrown out of the house by their parents or expelled from school for corrupting a boy." (*Family Weekly,* 1973, p. 5)

Emancipation

The interpersonal relationships within the family serve as the field in which the youngster continues to work on emancipating himself from the home. Parents, we have seen, are ambivalent: they want him to grow, but they also expect him to remain dependent and somewhat subservient to their wishes. They hope their child will do "the right thing," but they worry that he or she will "get into trouble" without careful supervision.

The child is equally ambivalent. He or she wants to be seen as adult, yet often acts in childish, dependent ways. The timing of the shifts from dependent to independent behavior also acts to create problems. It seems that the very occasion that the parents feel calls for self-reliance and adult behavior is the one perceived by the youngster as requiring dependent behavior, and vice versa. In early adolescence, late hours, dating, and earning money are three areas in which this conflict occurs.

The sexual game is a case in point. The parents, who are worried about the behavior of their young (13–15) teenager, try to "reason" with the child with regard to why he or she (1) shouldn't date at all, (2) should play the field, (3) should avoid any sexual experimentation or intimacy. The parents' fears also reflect their own recollection of adolescence. But any adolescent pattern of behavior does not evolve from a vacuum. It grows out of the cultural milieu (see Chapter 7). We may hypothesize that this pattern might have been learned as follows: The adult world, especially in middle class neighborhoods, has promoted social dancing in the intermediate grades, formal proms in the sixth grade, and movie dates in the preteen years. Parents, before their own children reach puberty, tend to think of such activities as "cute." They encourage heterosexual relationships in preadolescence. Now, when children take the next logical step, parents throw up their hands in horror.

The horror is not completely unwarranted. The pill as a means of birth control is known to young teenagers, although, unfortunately, they may not use it. If they did, such statistics as the following probably would not occur: "The unwed mothers' division of the County Court of Philadelphia reports 2677 petitions for the support of unwanted babies were filed by unwed mothers in 1964. Junior and senior high school girls represent 40 per cent of these applicants, and 11- and 12-year-olds, still in elementary school, have become a significant group." (Sacks, 1966, p. 80) We do not yet know the effects of newer abortion laws and the dissemination of birth control information, but the problem of venereal disease is growing more serious, and statistics such as those that follow are probably still significant. "As the U.S. birthrate declined in the last decade, births to teenagers became a larger proportion of all births. In 1968, 17 percent of all births were to teenagers, compared to 14 percent in 1961. The concentration of out-of-wedlock births at young ages is even more striking. Nearly half of all out-of-wedlock births in 1968 were to teenagers, compared to 14 percent in 1961." (Menken, 1972)

Although there are many problems involved in the relationship between an adolescent and his parents, the greatest problem is the question of the degree of freedom allowed the youngster. The early adolescent, luckily, is still not old enough to drive a car legally in most states. The early adolescent, and his big brother too, tend to view freedom apart from responsibility. They tend to see freedom as the total right to do anything. In a society that theoretically emphasizes individual freedom, this is bound to be a source of tension.

As Douvan and Adelson (1966) indicate, middle class parents encourage more autonomy in boys and a greater share in decision-making for girls than do lower class parents. The payoff is shown in the self-reliance of the boys and the greater autonomy of the girls. This may be related to the fact that middle class jobs are usually more self-directive, that promotion and salary are more personal than group-oriented [although this is changing with teachers unions, collective bargaining for civil servants, etc.], and that the individuals involved are more concerned with people than with things in comparison to working class jobs. (Kohn, 1963)

Hoffman and Saltzstein (1967) indicate that power assertion is least effective in teaching the young adolescent to develop moral standards or internal controls. All it seems to do is create hostility toward the parent. Yet, we often find parents attempting to use power. When they do, they just add to their problems. They also found that mothers were more influential than fathers in effecting the development of self-control. A recent study of the effects of parental attitudes and behaviors on moral behavior of adolescent males found support for the above position.

LaVoie and Looft (1973) report that middle class boys' ability to resist temptation was positively related to maternal behavior (discussion with the child and seeking information after the son had violated a family or societal rule). Resistance to temptation was unrelated to the father, which may be due to role differentiation, that is, fathers may delegate discipline responsibility to mothers. It may be, as LaVoie and Looft suggest, that mothers are more prone to listen and seek reasons, and fathers are more prone to act. The sons respond to the willingness of their mothers to know both sides. They then feel better about being punished. Such punishment, we might infer, is not seen as power assertion. All this would fit into the idea of the utility of approaching interpersonal relationships from a decentered orientation rather than from an egocentric one.

NEW SCHOOL PATTERNS:
NEW ADJUSTMENTS

The change from the self-contained classroom, usually with one teacher in a neighborhood school, to a departmental arrangement defines part of the shift in school culture experienced by the early adolescent. Whether the youngster enters a middle school at fifth or sixth grade or the more traditional junior high in seventh grade, he faces a new set of circumstances. He must now cope with more teachers and a student body probably three times as large as at his previous school. At a time when he is still establishing his identity, when his body image is being reshaped, when he is struggling with emancipation from home, the educational system adds its share to the burden of instability. He has to establish a place for himself all over again in school. Of course, he knows many of the others from his own "feeder" school, but he may be placed in sections apart from friends. His school was populated essentially with youngsters from about the same social class; the new school brings him into contact with a wider slice of the American society.

In elementary school, even those that were grouping for ability or using the standard grading on achievement, he was generally considered by his teachers as an individual who should be helped to grow at his own rate. Now, he comes up against the multiple-track system, the accelerated and general classes, the subject-matter orientation, the assumption that each child should be judged on some absolute scale.

Historically, the junior high was created as a transitional step between the child-oriented elementary school and the college-oriented high school. In practice and in location, it often became a downward extension of the high school. That this is dangerous and unfair to the pupil has been pointed out by James Conant in his report on the junior high school: "Early adolescence is a very special period physically, emotionally and socially. It is a crucial age in the transition from childhood to adulthood and often presents many problems. He [Dr. Conant] said the junior high school program should reflect this transition. . . . He warned, too, of treating the three-year junior high as a small scale high school." (St. Petersburg *Times,* October 9, 1960)

The middle school was created in the mid-1960s to overcome these deficits. While it is too soon to tell and while such schools vary widely in staffing patterns, curriculum, and philosophy, they seem to expose the child earlier to certain pressures that he would otherwise meet in the junior high pattern. Since little research has yet been done on this school pattern, the following is still slanted to the junior high, but the student is urged to explore whether these statements are true for the middle school. What effect does team teaching, or open classrooms, or time modules have not only on the academic but also on the personal-social development of the early adolescent? What effect does the middle school have on minority cultural groups? We need to know far more than we do before accepting the middle school as a successful answer to the needs of early adolescents. Does a simple change in school organization offer any opportunities for meeting these children's needs? (Hernandez, 1973)

What does the shift in school mean to the early adolescent? Again, it will depend upon the self-concept he brings with him. If he has had success in school, if he has confidence in his ability, he may view these new circumstances as exciting and challenging. He may see the shift as evidence of growing up. He may like the idea that he'll meet and make many new friends.

However, for many youngsters the transition is difficult. They perceive the new school as a threat. Just the size of the physical plant can be a problem. Dyer's study of several midwestern cities revealed that over one-fourth of seventh-graders reported difficulties. They were troubled by the need to locate classrooms, make friends, learn the rules, become acquainted with new teachers, understand the work, and use the cafeteria. (Dyer, 1950)

They all must learn not only the formal school arrangement, but also the informal clique and status system. Belonging to the right group, going to the right place, and wearing the right clothes become intertwined with going to junior high. In the many school districts in which the junior-senior high school is actually one six-year facility, the seventh-grader is caught up in emulating the high school senior, in the welter of extraclass activities, and in the varsity athletic program. This is heady food for many and probably increases the distress of late-maturing children. It may be worthwhile for the early-maturing girl in that it gives her opportunities for boy-girl relationships that are more satisfactory than those available within her own age group.

Our knowledge of the actual impact of school upon the student is limited. Studies of the junior high as a social system are needed, as well as studies concerning the views held about self in relation to school.

We can get some indication of the way a particular child viewed school by observing classroom behavior. We might caption the following description "An Hour in the Life of Mary." (The reader is referred to R. Barker and H. Wright's *One Boy's Day* for a fuller description of the psychological ecology methodology.) It reveals attitudes toward self, toward teacher, and toward peers. It shows the way students treat one of their peers in class. It portrays the high level of energy output that often occurs in early adolescence. The behavior setting is a seventh-grade "core" class in which several periods are spent with the same teacher. The scene opens at 9:30 A.M. The observer writes:

> *Mary was wearing avocado colored bermudas, white sleeveless blouse with shirttail out, black leather flats. All the other girls in the class wore dresses. Mary had long brown hair with a white three-quarters of an inch hairband. She was wearing lipstick. The fourteen other girls were not wearing lipstick. Her figure was rounding out where the other girls were straight and flat in build.*
>
> *There was a variety of tables and chairs in the room, semicircular tables, trapezoidal tables, rectangular tables with unattached chairs, and some single chair-desk combinations. Mary was sitting in a single chair-desk. There were three boys sitting to her left. The class was finishing an English lesson when I arrived at the break. Mary was at the board diagramming a sentence. She had made a mistake and Gloria was helping her. When the class had been excused, Mary erased what had been on the board, wrote down her own sentence and diagrammed it. They all came back to the room to continue with arithmetic. The tables were in a semicircular arrangement facing the green board.*
>
> *The instructor was a young male, Mr. Smith. He sat down at a table in the middle of the semicircle with two of the youngsters. He asked them to turn to page 48 in their math books. Six children volunteered to answer the first problem. Mary did not. Mr. Smith called on one boy who had not volunteered. Boy answered wrong. Mr. Smith said, "Do you think that's the way to do it?" Silence. For the next problem Mary quickly volunteered along with four of her classmates. Mr. Smith called on her first, she answered wrong. Mr. Smith called on another, who answered correctly. Mary said, "Oh, I forgot that one-half hour."*
>
> *Mr. Smith went to the board and asked what formula to use for the next problem. He wrote on the board as they answered. As they went on to work it, it was not coming out right. Mr. Smith turned his back to the class, and Mary waved both hands violently. About six other children had their hands up. Mr. Smith turned. Mary took one hand down and held the other one still. Mr. Smith called on someone else.*

The problem was worked out. The next problem was brought up. Several of the children began to discuss it and resolve it together. Mary looked at her legs and fingers, the bermuda cuff, looked up, tossed her head.

Mr. Smith called for volunteers to work at the board. Mary and ten others volunteered. He called on Mary. He read the problem to her (fraction problem). She worked the addition of fractions and whole numbers. Mr. Smith asked her to stop, and point out to a boy where he had his trouble.

Mary went on and put wrong figures on the board. Class laughed —she said, "Oh, shut up" to her left. Had some more trouble. Boys on her right laughed, she turned to them and said, "Shut up!" Mr. Smith said, "You don't want to reduce fraction now, but break it into whole numbers and fraction." Mary said, "Oh, I forgot." Went on. Began division and made a mistake in subtraction. Boys to right began shouting and laughing. She turned to them, to board, to them, to board. She discovered her mistake and began to add this to original whole number. Forgot a digit in front of the number, more laughing, discovering mistake, and answered correctly. Mary did not laugh.

Mr. Smith announced a contest between boys and girls. Whole class began to laugh and chatter (Mary too). He called for volunteers. About twenty-four hands went up, including Mary's. Mr. Smith called on Mary and Bob (for the boys). Mary said, "Mr. Smith, you picked the dumbest girl in the class to go against the smartest boy." Class laughed. Mr. Smith read the problem. Mary and Bob wrote rapidly. Mary finished the problem first, then Bob. Both had the wrong answer. Mary flung both fists to the board, but didn't hit it. Two more pairs went up. Class got noisy until Mr. Smith said, "Control yourselves. Everybody be quiet. Work page 52 for the next ten minutes. QUIET!" Class worked until the bell rang. Mary worked quietly too.

From the above, we can visualize the impact of the total school setting: teacher, peers, and subject matter upon Mary, who happens to be an early-maturing girl. There is no assumption of "typicality" either about this classroom or about Mary. It has been selected merely to show what occurs in a classroom, so that an observer, with a sequence of such scenes, can infer both the school setting and the self-concept of the youngster.

SOCIETY AND THE EARLY ADOLESCENT

We mentioned in our discussion of the body image that the mass media tends to exploit the fears and hopes of adolescents. Sexual awareness is aroused and stimulated by movies, TV, and magazines. On the one hand, the child is told by his parents, teachers, and religious leaders to sublimate his impulses and, on the other hand, is subjected to a barrage of sexuality in the mass media and in his neighborhood. He reads the movie ads in the daily newspaper for X-rated and R-rated films and his imagination runs riot. The paperbacks and the magazine covers he sees cater to curiosity.

The early adolescent's needs to know and to understand this complex phenomenon we label sex are both magnified and denied by the adult world. This problem is not unique to the United States. A London study clearly illustrates the problem. This study is of the behavior, attitudes, and problems of youth using a facility known as Grosvenor for the Grosvenor Recreational Evening Institute, which would correspond to a combination settlement house and evening high school in a large American city. Grosvenor was used extensively by youth between the ages of 14 and 21. Jordan and Fisher report:

> *Even our limited observation of the students showed that the individual sexual needs vary within a surprisingly wide range. Our educational discipline and our social regulations may make insufficient allowance for such variation. . . . In fact a "mass-observer" from some simple society might note what would appear to him the strange form of torture prevalent in a society which decrees that the young shall postpone all expression of sex until economic maturity is attained, and at the same time by its advertising provides mass incitement to break the law. [Jordan and Fisher, 1955, p. 109]*

This inconsistency between the mores of the adult world and its expectations for the early adolescent are by no means confined to the sexual sphere. They pervade the whole structure of the society. The young adolescent is told that work is good, but there is virtually no productive work available for him to do in the city. He is told that he must accept responsibility, but in school and society he is treated as irresponsible. He is told that he must develop a moral code, that he must learn right from wrong, but a quick look at national and local news shows him that even adults are confused on these issues. How is the early adolescent to handle Watergate? How can he reconcile the cry of law and order with flagrant violations by the very people who cry for it? How can he, in social studies, bridge the gap between what he has been taught about presidential electoral processes and what he reads and sees and hears of its subversion?

Gardner's incisive 1957 statement is still applicable today:

> *Let us consider for a moment our politico-governmental climate and our communication media as societies that impinge on the adolescent endeavoring to incorporate mature values of social morality—in respect to his treatment of his fellow men. In the former, he will find the highest value placed upon the democratic process*

in juxtaposition with high value placed upon the most flagrant expressions of bigotry, prejudice and thorough circumvention of guaranteed basic rights and privileges. In the latter—in the matter of mass communication media—he is subjected to summaries of the highest achievements in social living and aesthetic productions, again in temporal sequence to an elaboration of the lowest and crassest of human motivations. We as adults seemingly must place some value on these expressions—or rather our societies in the aggregate as a society must place some value on all of them—or what is more to the point, our lack of unanimity in regard to these values evidences our own conflicts. Again, I reiterate, it is difficult for the adolescent to solve his conflicts in regard to social morality in a society that is itself conflicted.

. . .

I would emphasize again that these adolescent children of ours cannot be considered solely from the viewpoint of their internal conflicts and processes, but must on the contrary be considered biosocially, with due emphasis upon the pressures and value systems of the groups that surround them, and with emphasis upon the sometimes sharply conflicting values in the multiple roles that they must assume. [Gardner, 1957, pp. 515, 517]

In the early 1970s we often hear about a social revolution in morals and behavior. The conflict Gardner reports is even more evident. The use of drugs, the increased presence of sexual symbols, and the more open discussion of sex surround the young adolescent. Further, the conflicts between peace and war, social ills and affluence, prejudice and justice also are brought to his attention daily.

PEER RELATIONSHIPS

The way out of the dilemma of the conflict between adult cultural demands at home, in school, and in the world at large and the changing biological and developmental pressures within the early adolescent has been found for him in the peer group.

A major function of the peer group at this age is the provision of opportunities for the youngster to meet his needs for status and achievement. The real status symbols of the society are denied the early adolescent: work, cars, access to many events, mature heterosexual relationships. The peer group serves as a substitute. As Douvan and Adelson express it, ". . . it would seem that the adolescent does not choose friendship, but is driven to it." (Douvan and Adelson, 1966, p. 179)

Of course, the peer culture during adolescence mirrors the adult culture. But it is not a simple reflection. Our view is that the peer group plays a variety of vital roles for the adolescent, that it is in continuous exchange with the adult culture (it might be viewed as an open system) but that it is a separate subculture. In many respects, it does not differ from the adult world (see section on values in Chapter 18), but the adolescent may act out these values in his own particular fashion and modify them in ways to suit his particular needs.

Values

As we would expect, physical body factors play a great role in determining status in the junior high school. How a child looks to his peers is highly important. How well he can perform in physical tasks is equally important for boys.

In order to determine status, two techniques have been used. One is the social reputation test, the other is a sociometric device. Sample items from a social reputation test are:

> Which boys are restless and can't sit still, or get up and walk around a lot?
> Which are the ones everybody likes?
> Who are the good sports—the ones that always play fair, and can take it when they lose? [Hanley, 1951, p. 259]

The sociometric inventory may ask the youngster to name three people with whom he'd like to serve on a committee, or go to a dance, or see as chairman of an event. It is more situational, and the status hierarchy that emerges is partly a function of the particular question asked.

Hanley (1951) used the reputation test originally designed by Tryon (1943) to see if body build had any relationship to the way a youngster was perceived by his peers. We have seen earlier that there should be no expectation of a high relationship between any one variable, such as body build, and something as complex as peers' views of one's behavior. The relationships Hanley found were low, but they do establish that there is a link between how you look and how you are seen. The youngsters whose body build was mesomorphic (highly developed skeletal structure, thick skin, sturdy upright posture, good musculature) were seen as leaders, as daring and willing to take chances, as good at games, as grown-up, and as fighters. The transactional nature of this relationship is fairly clear. This boy looks like the typical all-American boy, and he does possess the equipment to do well in sports. His peers thus accord him prestige and provide him with a situational field in which he can lead and excel. The organism-environment transactions thus enhance his actual ability, his reputation, and his self-concept. They are mutually reinforcing.

Sociometric evidence supports the view that athletic prowess is highly related to status. Junior high school boys were asked to name the boys they liked best. Athletic ability for each boy was determined by

TABLE 15.1   CHANGES IN STATUS VALUE WITH AGE AND SEX

BOYS	GIRLS

12 YEARS

BOYS	GIRLS
1. Most related to prestige Daring, leader, active in games, friendly.	1. Most related to prestige Popular, good-looking, friendly. Enthusiastic, happy, humor about self.
2. Related to prestige Restless, talkative, attention-getting.	2. Related to prestige Restless, talkative, attention-getting. (Traits in this cluster have very different values for girls and for boys.)
3. Desirable Bossy, fights, unkempt.	3. Irrelevant Daring, leader, humor about jokes.

15 YEARS

BOYS	GIRLS
1. Very important Popular, good-looking, friendly, enthusiastic. Daring, leader, active in games, fights.	1. Important Tidy, good-looking, older friends. Popular, friendly, enthusiastic, happy, humor about jokes, daring, leader.
2. Some importance Happy, humor about jokes.	2. Related to heterosexual adjustment Active in games, humor about self (inversely related).
3. Irrelevant Restless, talkative, attention-getting.	3. Irrelevant Restless, talkative, attention-getting, bossy, fights.

Source: Reprinted from I. J. Gordon, *The Teacher as a Guidance Worker*, Harper & Row, 1956.

physical tests, by peer judgment, and by experience in intramural and interscholastic athletics. There was a moderately high relationship between sociometric status and athletic ability, and it was "possible that the boys achieved their popularity through participation in interschool athletics more than any other factor included in this investigation." (McCraw and Tolbert, 1953, p. 79)

A girl's appearance also affects her status. She's not expected to be athletic, but she is expected to be good-looking. Although standards of good looks change to some degree with each generation, being considered good-looking by peers is highly important. Table 15.1, compiled from data gathered through social reputation tests by Tryon (1943), shows the place of appearance.

Personality factors are also related to status in early adolescence and thus reveal the value system. Table 15.1 shows the traits that peers associated with success in peer relations. It reveals the change from pre- to postpubescence in boys. Good looks, enthusiasm, and an already-established reputation as popular become functional as status symbols in the 15-year-old's group.

The popularity of the 15-year-old girl depends heavily upon what might be called the social skills. She must exude happiness and enthusiasm and be able to lead. She should be unself-conscious or, in Riesman's terms, "other-directed." The outgoing youngster, in Tryon's study, is the one accorded prestige. Gronlund and Anderson found similar results (1957).

Girls in their middle-teens are concerned about the ability to confide in another. This is the period of emerging sexuality, and a girl needs to feel secure in her friends. She seems more concerned about her reputation with girls than with boys. The boy uses his group for autonomy from adults and in the process, ironically, accords it more power over him.

These trait names, such as "leader" or "enthusiastic," conceal as much as they reveal. What does an early adolescent do that makes him a leader? What roles must he play and how broad must be his repertoire? Elkins' (1958) research provides some clues. Sociometric tests, interviews with pupils and parents, diaries of out-of-school activities, and open-ended questions (my worries, etc.) were secured. In addition, social class and physical and intelligence test data were obtained on the 90 junior high pupils in the study.

If we view the ability to participate in a variety of activities as equivalent to playing many roles, then we can accept Elkins' conclusions that "children who were flexible in role performance, who had the ability to meet the needs of others, who could further the goals of the group, who displayed certain acceptable behavior patterns, were among the highly chosen. . . . Children who displayed rigidity of role performance, who were unable to meet the needs of peers, who blocked the goals of the group, who displayed certain objectionable behavior patterns, were among the least chosen." (Elkins, 1958, p. 267) In effect, those who were group-oriented were rewarded; those who lacked skills or were not "groupy" were excluded.

Costanzo and Shaw (1966) placed youngsters between the ages of 7 and 21 in a conformity situation; those between 11 and 13 conformed the most. Of special interest is the finding that they didn't see their behavior as being governed by the group. Collins and Thomas (1972) found that Australian youngsters between 13 and 16 conformed more to peer pressure in a judgment task than both younger and older age groups.

There was a relationship between the number of activities (seen by

Elkins as roles) and status. The high-status boys and girls participated in more activities, were visitors in others' homes, were sought out by others more often, and both gave and received more thoughtful gestures than the lower-status children. This raises the question of what leads a child into this activity pattern.

To some degree, family background in both its emotional climate and socioeconomic aspects plays a role. Generally, children of the middle class have more opportunities for learning social skills than do lower class children. But mobile youngsters going upward socially make it their business to find out how to behave and gain acceptance.

Generally, the early adolescent peer group values physical adequacy for boys, group-oriented behavior, high energy rate, good looks, and social skills. The youngster who, for physical, familial, or personal reasons, cannot function effectively is ignored and lost in the shuffle. It is a rough league, with little compassion or mercy.

The Peers and Self-Concept

A poignant picture of the effect of rejection is portrayed by Kit, a Grosvenor student:

> My little brother is delicate and has a speech defect. He has a gang of school and street friends. Sometimes the leader of the gang expels him. Nothing upsets him so much as this. Once he was expelled for three days. He sat at home and moped and wouldn't eat or drink. He won't eat much at the best of times but my mother got really worried during these three days. Then the gang had him back and he picked up again in health. [Jordan and Fisher, 1955, p. 150]

That peer acceptance affects the self-concept cannot be doubted, although the relationship is not simple. We could easily guess how the successful and unsuccessful view themselves. In addition to our guesses, we have some empirical data, although certainly far from enough. Feinberg reports that "accepted boys considered themselves most successful in getting along with their classmates, and they also felt that they make friends quickly and have many more close friends than most of the boys in their class. . . ." (Feinberg, 1953, p. 211) Hartup, in his review of peer research, concludes that "there is clear consensus that a child's general adjustment is related to his popularity with peers." (Hartup, 1971, p. 391)

Prestige position influences self-concept and behavior, and behavior, in turn, plays back into the group system for granting prestige. Once a youngster has a "reputation," his behavior tends to reinforce this image. The psychologist, parent, teacher, or group worker who understands both this phenomenon and the value system of a particular group can begin to be effective in helping individuals. He may not be able to change a child's reputation, but he can help him learn new behaviors that will have this effect. Once a new prestige position is attained, further new behaviors and concepts of self become possible.

Activities

When peer group members get together, what do they do? First, the boys spend considerable time in team games and contact horseplay. Even in class or in the halls, they push, shove, and wrestle. The girls spend hours on the telephone or in hen parties, slumber parties, and gossip sessions. There is a trend, however, away from the all-boy or all-girl group that was typical of preadolescence. Heterosexual groups now complement the continuing one-sex group.

With this change, dating enters the picture. It is primarily a group activity in early adolescence. It begins for many youngsters sometime between the ages of 14 and 15, but it may occur earlier. There are some movie dates, coke dates, parties-in-the-home dates, walking dates, and sports dates. They usually involve several couples and may involve some sex play as couples pair off.

There seem to be changes in this pattern that are related to the drug scene and to adolescents' general reactions to school and society, but no clear picture is presently in the literature. The reader might want to try to study this with interviews, rap sessions, and observation in public places in order to find out for himself what is going on. Unfortunately, research is often behind the times and may even be invalid because of the ability of adolescents to misinform the adult about the peer group's business.

The original push to date is more cultural than biological, however. It is the expected thing to do. In the next chapter we shall see some of the youngsters' concerns about dating.

A phenomenon of the middle and late 1960s and early 1970s is the development of electronic band groups based on the guitar. It may reflect the affluent culture, because the equipment is expensive, but it seems to have great meaning to youth. The main emphasis is on the beat, with noise level geared to allow one not just to hear the music but to feel it and be immersed and absorbed in it. The effect is heightened with strobe lights and colored lights that enable one to "blow his mind" without drugs.

Peer group activities during this age serve the value arrangements and status efforts of individual members. They are important in providing youngsters with opportunities to socialize, to demonstrate skills, to gain skills, and to evaluate self and others.

SUMMARY

In this chapter we have examined the interpersonal world of the adolescent and some of the effects this changing world has upon him. We have seen that self-definition is a vital task for this age group and that both biological and cultural forces combine to make this so. In Chapter 16 we shall examine more thoroughly the impact this has upon him and how he works at the problem of self-definition and development.

REFERENCES AND ADDITIONAL READINGS

Adams, J. (Ed.) *Understanding adolescence.* Boston: Allyn & Bacon, 1968.

Armentrout, James A., & Burger, Gary K. Children's reports of parental child-rearing behavior at five grade levels. *Developmental Psychology,* 1972, *7,* 44–48.

Bandura, A., & Walters, R. *Adolescent aggression.* New York: Ronald Press, 1959.

Barker, R., & Wright, H. *One boy's day.* New York: Harper & Row, 1951.

Biller, H., & Bahm, R. Father absence, perceived maternal behavior, and masculinity of self-concept among junior high school boys. *Developmental Psychology,* 1971, *4,* 171–181.

Bowerman, C. E., & Elder, G. H. Variations in adolescent perception of family power structure. *American Sociological Review,* 1964, *29,* 551–567.

Campbell, J. D. Peer relations in childhood. In M. Hoffman & L. Hoffman (Eds.), *Review of child development research.* Vol. 1. New York: Russell Sage Foundation, 1964. Pp. 289–322.

Collins, J., & Thomas, N. Age and susceptibility to same sex peer pressure. *British Journal of Educational Psychology,* 1972, *42,* 83–85.

Connor, R., Greene, H., & Walters, J. Agreement of family member conceptions of "good" parent and child roles. *Social Forces,* 1958, *36,* 353–358.

Costanzo, P., & Shaw, M. Conformity as a function of age level. *Child Development,* 1966, *37,* 967–975.

Douvan, E., & Adelson, J. *The adolescent experience.* New York: Wiley, 1966.

Duncan, P. Parental attitudes and interactions in delinquency. *Child Development,* 1971, *42,* 1751–1765.

Dyer, C. Problems of transition between the elementary school and the junior high school. Unpublished doctoral dissertation, University of Oklahoma, 1950.

Elder, G. *Adolescent socialization and personality development.* Chicago: Rand McNally, 1968.

Elkin, F., & Westley, W. The myth of adolescent culture. *American Sociological Review,* 1955, *20,* 680–684.

Elkins, D. Some factors related to the choice-status of ninety eighth-grade children in a school society. *Genetic Psychology Monographs,* 1958, *58,* 207–272.

Feinberg, M. Relation of background experience to social acceptance. *Journal of Abnormal and Social Psychology,* 1953, *48,* 206–214.

Frank, L. K. The adolescent and the family. In NSSE, *Adolescence.* 43rd Yearbook, Part I. Chicago: The Society, 1944. Pp. 240–254.

Gardner, G. Present day society and the adolescent. *American Journal of Orthopsychiatry,* 1957, *27,* 508–517. Copyright 1957, the American Orthopsychiatric Association, Inc. Reproduced by permission.

Gordon, I. J. *The teacher as a guidance worker.* New York: Harper & Row, 1956.

Gronlund, N., & Anderson, L. Personality characteristics of socially accepted, socially neglected, and socially rejected junior high school pupils. *Educational Administration and Supervision,* 1957, *43,* 329–338.

Hanley, C. Physique and reputation of junior high school boys. *Child Development*, 1951, *22*, 247–260.

Hartup, W. Peer interaction and social organization. In P. Mussen (Ed.), *Carmichael's handbook of child psychology.* (3rd ed.) Vol. 2. New York: Wiley, 1971. Pp. 361–456.

Helper, M. Parental evaluational of children and children's self evaluations. *Journal of Abnormal and Social Psychology*, 1958, *56*, 190–194.

Hernandez, N. Variables affecting achievement of middle school Mexican-American students. *Review of Educational Research,* 1973, *43*, 1–40.

Hicks, J. (Ed.) The RAP, Reports on adolescent pregnancy. Vol. 2. Number 1. Atlanta, Ga.: ICC-MIC Projects, Grady Memorial Hospital, March 1973.

Hoffman, M., & Saltzstein, H. Parent discipline and the child's moral development. *Journal of Personality and Social Psychology*, 1967, *5*, 45–57.

Jordon, G., & Fisher, E. *Self-portrait of youth.* London: Heinemann, 1955.

Kagan, J., & Coles, R. (Eds.) *Twelve to sixteen: Early adolescence.* New York: Norton, 1972.

Kandel, D., Lesser, G., Roberts, G., & Weiss, R. The concept of adolescent subculture. In R. Purnell (Ed.), *Adolescents and the American high school.* New York: Holt, Rinehart & Winston, 1970. Pp. 194–205.

Kohn, M. Social class and parent-child relationships: An interpretation. *American Journal of Sociology,* 1963, *68*, 471–480.

LaVoie, J., & Looft, W. Parental antecedents of resistance-to-temptation behavior in adolescent males. *Merrill-Palmer Quarterly,* 1973, *19*, 107–116.

Levitt, E. E., & Edwards, J. A. A multivariate study of correlative factors in youthful cigarette smoking. *Developmental Psychology*, 1969, *2(1)*, 5–11.

Long, B., Henderson, E., & Platt, D. Self-other orientations of Israeli adolescents reared in Kibbutzim and Moshavim. *Developmental Psychology,* 1973, *8*, 300–308.

Lowrie, S. Sex differences and age of initial dating. *Social Forces,* 1952, *30*, 456–461.

McCraw, L., & Tolbert, J. Sociometric status and athletic ability of junior high school boys. *Research Quarterly, American Association for Health, Physical Education and Recreation,* 1953, *24*, 72–80.

Menken, J. The health and social consequences of teenage childbearing. *Family Planning Perspectives,* 1972, *4(3)*.

Muma, J. Peer evaluation and academic performance. *Personnel and Guidance Journal,* 1965, *44*, 405–409.

National Education Association. Contemporary youth culture. *NEA Journal,* 1967, *56*, 8–20.

Reese, H. Relationships between self-acceptance and sociometric choices. *Journal of Abnormal and Social Psychology,* 1961, *62*, 472–474. Reprinted in I. J. Gordon (Ed.), *Human development: Readings in research.* Glenview, Ill.: Scott, Foresman, 1965.

Reevy, W. Adolescent sexuality. In A. Ellis & A. Abarbanel (Eds.), *The encyclopedia of sexual behavior.* New York: Hawthorn Books, 1961. Pp. 52–67.

Rosen, S., Levinger, G., & Lippitt, R. Desired change in self and others as a function of resource ownership. *Human Relations,* 1960, *13*, 187–192.

Rosenfeld, H., & Zander, A. The influence of teachers on aspirations of students. *Journal of Educational Psychology,* 1961, *52*, 1–11.

Sacks, S. Widening the perspectives on adolescent sex problems. *Adolescence,* 1966, *1*, 80.

Sheehy, G. Beware the white slaver. *Family Weekly,* May 20, 1973, p. 5.

Silver, A. W. The self-concept: Its relationship to parental and peer acceptance. Doctoral dissertation, Michigan State University, 1958.

Smith, G. M. Relations between personality and smoking behavior in preadult subjects. *Journal of Consulting and Clinical Psychology,* 1969, *33(6),* 710–715.

Sollenberger, R. Chinese-American child-rearing practices and juvenile delinquency. *Journal of Social Psychology,* 1968, *74,* 13–23.

Strang, R. The transition from childhood to adolescence. In J. Adams (Ed.), *Understanding adolescence.* Boston: Allyn & Bacon, 1968. Pp. 13–42.

Tec, N. Drugs among suburban teenagers: Basic findings. *Social Science and Medicine,* 1971, *5,* 77–84.

Tryon, C. Evaluations of adolescent personality by adolescents. In R. Barker, J. Kounin, & H. Wright (Eds.), *Child behavior and development.* New York: McGraw-Hill, 1943. Pp. 545–566.

Tuma, E., & Livson, N. Family socioeconomic status and adolescent attitudes to authority. *Child Development,* 1960, *31,* 387–399. Reprinted in I. J. Gordon (Ed.), *Human development: Readings in research.* Glenview, Ill.: Scott, Foresman, 1965.

Weiner, I. B. The generation gap: Fact and fancy. *Adolescence,* 1971, *6(22),* 156–166.

CHAPTER 16
THE CHANGING SELF

CONCEPTUAL DEVELOPMENT
Intellectual Development: Test Scores

The period of early adolescence is characterized by the widening of intellectual pursuits. The child's horizons expand considerably throughout the junior high school years. To list what a "typical" youngster might know is meaningless, because if there is anything typical about his intellectual development, it is that his pattern is unique. The gap between those who do relatively well on intelligence tests and those who do poorly widens during these years, but virtually all youngsters make progress.

Individual growth rates are subject to fluctuations because of the many factors that influence an individual's performance at any given time. Early adolescence seems to be a period in which such fluctuation occurs. Figures 16.1 and 16.2 indicate individual curves for some boys and girls in the California Growth Study. In this major longitudinal study, a group of children were followed from birth and are still being followed in their adult years. A wide variety of measurements were made, including IQ scores on different tests at different ages. In order to assess patterns of individual growth as well as general (or normative) data about this population, techniques were developed for translating scores on these different measures into uniform scores. A 16D score was calculated on the basis of the person's position at age 16 relative to his peers.

Scores on intelligence tests were converted on the basis of means (averages) and standard deviations (dispersion around the means), which allowed the researcher to use data from several different tests. In this fashion, a curve of the youngster's own growth, as measured by intelligence tests, could be developed. This curve gives a picture of both his growth as an individual and his relative position. Analysis of Figures 16.1 and 16.2 for the ages 12 to 16 shows that the boys maintained their relative positions, but 7M and 22M both dipped markedly and recovered. Girls 13F and 5F temporarily changed position while 21F's curve shows great fluctuation

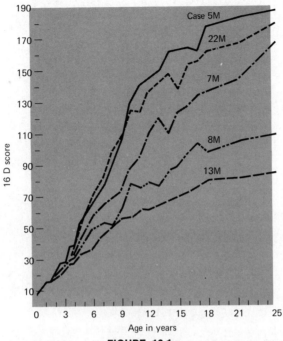

FIGURE 16.1

Individual curves of intelligence of five boys, from 1 month to 25 years. Reprinted from N. Bayley, On the growth of intelligence. *American Psychologist,* 1955, **10,** 805–818. Copyright 1955 by the American Psychological Association. Reprinted by permission.

from year to year. The long-range trend is upward, though this period is unstable.

Why might this be so? Bayley postulates two main reasons: (1) differences in rate of maturity and (2) differences in inherent capacity. (Bayley, 1956, p. 66) Concerning rates of maturity, we do not find the correlation between physical and mental growth in the expected direction. In fact, "within the individual child his own mental and physical rates of growth are not concomitant. If anything, there is a suggestion that those who are slower in physical maturing approach their 21-year intelligence sooner." (Bayley, 1956, p. 71)

We are dealing here with *rate* of growth, not *amount* of intelligence. The child who grows slower physically seems to reach his adult level of intelligence sooner, although his adult level may be less than that of his rapidly developing peer. It may be that the relationship exists because of a third factor, socioeconomic class. Lower class youngsters suffer from experiential, dietary, and prenatal deprivations, all of which influence both physical and intellectual development.

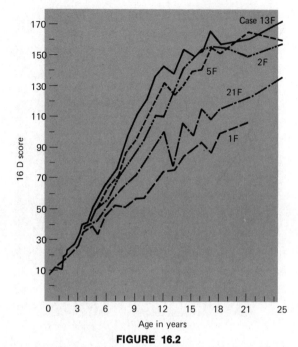

FIGURE 16.2

Individual curves of intelligence of five girls, from 1 month to 25 years. Reprinted from N. Bayley, On the growth of intelligence. *American Psychologist,* 1955, **10,** 805–818. Copyright 1955 by the American Psychological Association. Reprinted by permission.

The relationships are extremely complex because so many variables contribute to the intelligence test score. We know that range in physical and physiological development is wide during these years; therefore, we would expect, if there is a rate at which intelligence grows, that the range would also be wide. Overlaid upon this biological base are the myriad factors that become organized into the self of the individual child:

> They will include the emotional climate in which he grows; whether he is encouraged or discouraged, whether his drive (or ego-involvement) is strong in intellectual thought processes, or is directed toward other aspects of his life-field. And they will include the material environment in which he grows: the opportunities for experience and for learning, and the extent to which these opportunities are continuously geared to his capacity to respond and make use of them. [Bayley, 1955, pp. 813–814]

It has become increasingly clear that extreme environments, at home or in schools, influence the development of intelligence, whether it is conceived as a unitary trait or as a combination of discrete abilities. Bloom (1964) reviewed the longitudinal research and concluded that a spread of as much as 20 IQ points may be accounted for by environmental factors. The impact of environment does not begin, obviously, in adolescence; we simply see a part of its results at that time.

Two major conclusions emerge: (1) The interindividual range of intellectual ability becomes increasingly wider during the early adolescent period. (2) Each child's rate of intellectual growth, based upon his own particular unique organization (his self-system), may be irregular for short periods of time but follows an upward trend reaching beyond this age period. Any notion that the 15-year-old has reached his final point in intellectual development is not supported by the data. He has perhaps reached about 80 percent of his adult status. This "room for growth" does not reflect any notion of ceiling, or mere unfolding. The figure is a statistic, based on longitudinal studies. As we have said before about such numbers, it reflects what is, not what might be if the school and the society provided different experiences.

We should therefore avoid diagnosing or predicting from any single score on tests taken during this age or any period. We must be especially wary because of the many cultural pressures to identify the "special" child and accord him special treatment in the secondary school. The "slow learner" also is a dangerous label that leads to deceptive forms of discrimination in "track" programs. Since rate of growth seems to be a factor, we might very well expect some youngsters temporarily to lose ground in relation to their peers and then gain substantially later on. The major factor of motivation, too, is often overlooked when judgments are made upon such slim evidence as a single IQ score. Especially in early adolescence, with so much happening to the total self of the child, selection or stigmatization on the basis of IQ scores seems unwarranted.

Intellectual Development:
Cognitive Organization

Standardized IQ scores reveal only a portion of our current view about intellectual development in adolescence. As we saw in previous chapters, it is possible to describe the mode of thought, the style of thought, and the type of operations or problem-solving techniques used by children at different age levels.

As Piaget sees the transition, the adolescent is capable of performing formal operations as distinct from the concrete operations of the preadolescent. This represents a major shift in that now the adolescent's thought pattern resembles the adult. The adolescent can deal with abstract symbol systems in the absence of concrete materials; he can hypothesize and reverse his thinking by the manipulation of words—certainly a high-powered tool. If we turn to Figure 12.1 in Chapter 12 (page 240), we can now contrast how the preadolescent and the adolescent deal with the same problem. The 15-year-old approaches the same task, but responds:

> *VUL (15;6) determines 4W for M when the rail is vertical; then:* "At 33° I find 2; at 15° I find 1: at 60° it should be 4 but it isn't. If it isn't proportional to the angle, then. . . ."—*"Is there something else you might consider?"*—"The height corresponds to the angle. If I take twice the height: height 2 corresponds to 2 weights. Let's see: elevation 3 gives 3 in weight. Good, it's in proportion to the height. Each time you increase the height by a certain amount, you have to add a proportionate amount of weight." *Summary:* "The height is proportional to the weight." [*Inhelder and Piaget, 1958, p. 195*]

As Elkind reports on the basis of some comparative studies of children ages 8 and 9 with adolescents ages 13 and 14, adolescents raised hypotheses and checked against them when they attempted to solve a problem, whereas the children seemed to be bound to the perceptual stimulus. (Elkind, 1966) The essential difference, supported by Weir (1964) is the hypothesis-making strategy of the adolescent. He uses an "if . . . then" approach to tasks rather than a more simple plugging ahead.

This doesn't mean that hypothesis-making is always the best strategy; indeed, Bruner's (1958) study of thinking shows that conservative focusing (that is, eliminating one variable at a time) may be a more effective approach in certain situations. Some data on junior high school students (Doyle, 1966) indicate that, although they use several strategies, they seem to function best when they use the approach of a single variable at a time. Even here, however, Piaget's notion of the 16 binary operations, with all the various logical arrangements for testing the validity of the response, are present in the strategy. The adolescent can deal with the empty set, that is, the chance that nothing fits.

This is a particularly difficult concept for the younger child. For example, if children and adolescents were faced with the problem that a rocket going to Mars could bring back information about four possible things on the planet—the presence of rocks, green cheese, water, and iron —and they were asked to list all possible things they could learn from the rocket, two types of differences would become manifest. First, the children would probably get into a discussion about the silliness of green cheese, whereas the adolescents would recognize it as simply a symbol or an abstraction for which anything else might be substituted. They would not be as "reality" based. The second difference, however, is that the children most likely would say we could know whether or not there was green cheese, or rocks, or water, or iron, but they would probably not go beyond this. The adolescent might see all the sixteen different pieces of information that could possibly be learned from the four message circuits, ranging

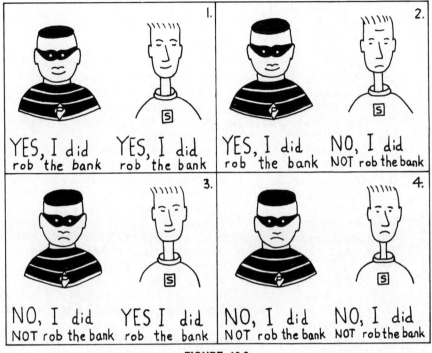

FIGURE 16.3
From J. Ward, The saga of Butch and Slim. *British Journal of Educational Psychology,* 1972, **42,** 269. Used with permission of the British Psychological Society.

from the message in which none of the four items is present to the existence of all four of them (see the list of 16 combinations shown below). This is what Piaget means by the 16 binary operations. It is interesting to see the computer analogues, in that each separate message is a yes-no, very much like the way the computer processes data.

1. None of them
2. Only rocks
3. Only green cheese
4. Only water
5. Only iron
6. Rocks and green cheese
7. Rocks and water
8. Rocks and iron
9. Green cheese and water
10. Green cheese and iron
11. Water and iron
12. Rocks, green cheese and water
13. Rocks, green cheese and iron
14. Rocks, water and iron
15. Green cheese, water and iron
16. All of them

The British are developing a new British Intelligence Scale (BIS) that includes an operational thinking subscale based on these 16 binary operations. Figure 16.3 presents Butch and Slim, who are their cast of characters. Children from age 10 and adults can play the game. The directions are:

> *Spread out four cards before the subject and say, "This is a game about a bank robbery. There has been a bank robbery and two well-known criminals, 'Butch' and 'Slim' are suspected. Here is Butch—(point), and here is Slim—(point). Now, supposing these two were taken in and questioned together, in the same room, as to whether they committed the crime, they could only really answer four different ways: both of them could say, 'yes,' they did it, like this—(point to Card 1) or Butch might say that he did it and Slim deny it, like this—(point to Card 2). Or Butch might deny he did it but Slim admit it like this—(point to Card 3). Then, of course, both might say 'No' like this—(point to Card 4). So when they were asked if they committed the crime, they could answer in the four ways shown on these cards. Now I am going to tell you some statements Butch might have made to the police, and each time I want you to look at each of these cards in turn and tell me whether Butch and Slim's answers on the cards could be true or not. You are looking for cards which could agree with what Butch said." [Ward, 1972, p. 269]*

Answers fit into the 16 propositions. Try it and see. One of the problems that Ward points out is that the answer format only tests whether the person sees that such a statement could be true; and he is not asked to hypothesize. He indicates that analysis of the types of errors is a useful device for seeing how people think (for another example, see Sigel, 1963). When this was done, it showed that many youngsters could not handle negation, nor did they recognize the possibility that different combinations could be true. The research is still underway, but the preliminary findings are useful.

When we look at the development of religious concepts, the same type of shift occurs. Goldman (1964) analyzed children's responses to Bible information. He attempted to explore children's concepts of divine justice by seeking their answers to a question such as "Was it fair that all the men in the Egyptian army should be drowned?" in reference to the Exodus. He found that the emergence of what he called moral consistency begins to dominate thinking from about the age of 12. That is, from this point on, for God to be unfair would be a contradiction in terms. This resembles the stage of moral judgment which Piaget called distributive justice—that all must be treated alike. Later in this chapter, when we look at the developing value system, we shall see the interplay between arriving at formal logical thought and arriving at mature levels of moral judgments.

What does this transition from concrete to formal mean in practice? According to Ausubel (1962) it means that gearing instruction to discovery and concrete problem solving is inefficient, because the adolescent is now able to learn by dealing directly with words and the relationships between words. It is only when they are faced with very new subject matter that it seems worthwhile, according to Ausubel, to revert to concrete empirical experience in the curriculum. Many of the new science curricula designed for high schools, however, use the discovery approach based upon the development of strategies more closely related to Bruner. The issue is unresolved as are many when we try to take ideas from human development and translate them or engineer them for education. The questions are pretty clear, however, and research in time should give us some reasonable answers as to the best way to capitalize on the present level of functioning of the child and help him move to higher levels of thought. All we can do in this book at this time is make the reader aware of the issue.

The Developing Value System

The early adolescent is concerned with value judgments and with the question: How should one behave? He writes to the advice-giving newspaper columnists; he sees the discrepancies in the adult world; and he seeks solutions to moral questions.

The developing value system is a function of both the developing cognitive power of the youngster and the developing views of self. The concept of decentering is one useful way to see this integration. Elkind (1967) conjectures that adolescent egocentrism is manifested by the belief of the adolescent that everyone is interested in his appearance and behavior. He can only hold such a belief, according to Elkind, because he can now engage in formal operations and thus is able to conceptualize the thought of others. It might be, if Elkind is right, that because he can do this, he can also be more concerned about the meaning, especially the moral meaning, of his behavior. The switch might be that egocentrism (or centering upon the self) in infancy and early childhood meant the child thought everybody thought like him; now he is concerned because he realizes that everybody does not, and he would like their approval. This requires that he produce values and behavior that he believes others value.

Kohlberg and Gilligan (1972) have also explored the connections between Kohlberg's stages of moral development and Piaget's stages. Table 16.1 presents their scheme. Note that moral stage 0 is the height of infantile egocentrism, as we would expect. The early adolescent is somewhere within moral stages 2 and 4 and the logical substages of formal operations 1 and 2. Kohlberg and Gilligan state that it takes arrival at formal operations in order to move "from conventional to principled moral reasoning. . . . The rejection of conventional moral reasoning begins with the perception of relativism, the awareness that any given society's definition of right and wrong, however legitimate, is only one among many,

---

TABLE 16.1 RELATIONS BETWEEN PIAGET LOGICAL STAGES AND
KOHLBERG MORAL STAGES*

LOGICAL STAGE	MORAL STAGE
Symbolic, intuitive thought	*Stage 0:* The good is what I want and like.
Concrete operations, Substage 1 Categorical classification	*Stage 1:* Punishment-obedience orientation.
Concrete operations, Substage 2 Reversible concrete thought	*Stage 2:* Instrumental hedonism and concrete reciprocity.
Formal operations, Substage 1 Relations involving the inverse of the reciprocal	*Stage 3:* Orientation to interpersonal relations of mutuality.
Formal operations, Substage 2	*Stage 4:* Maintenance of social order, fixed rules, and authority.
Formal operations, Substage 3	*Stage 5A:* Social contract, utilitarian law-making perspective.
	Stage 5B: Higher law and conscience orientation.
	Stage 6: Universal ethical principle orientation.

* All relations are that attainment of the logical stages is necessary, but not sufficient, for attainment of the moral stage.
Source: Reprinted from The adolescent as a philosopher: The discovery of the self in a post-conventional world by L. Kohlberg and C. Gilligan, in *Twelve to sixteen: Early adolescence,* edited by Jerome Kagan and Robert Coles. Copyright © 1972, 1971 by The American Academy of Arts and Sciences.

---

both in fact and theory.'' (Kohlberg and Gilligan, 1972, p. 165) From our view, this is the ultimate in decentering. It is not arrived at in early adolescence, and many people never make it at all.

Moral development in early adolescence, then, can be seen as in a transition zone between (1) the simpler approach represented by concrete thought and stages 1 and 2 of Kohlberg's scheme and its equivalent in Piaget of punishment through retribution and rendering judgment on the basis of the consequences of behavior, and (2) the more complex approach of relativism, decentering, and individual responsibility represented by Kohlberg's higher stages and Piaget's punishment by restitution, individual rather than collective responsibility, and judgment based on intent.

However, the early adolescent is living in a real world of conflicting values, in which logic does not necessarily apply, and truth does not out, and one man's logical intention is another man's treason or fascism. There is a discrepancy between should and would. Youngsters seem to know what is right. There has been continued development of recognition of the social norm, the origins of which began during preadolescence. These origins include the internalization of parental values through the identification process. Hoffman (1971), for example, found that the judgments of seventh-graders involving conforming to rules were related to identification with both parents, especially with fathers for middle class boys and girls. In his view, the moral development of children is a function of the way parents handle discipline situations. The use of reasoning, the amount of parent self-evaluation, and the feeling involved are all positively related to development of conscience. However, when it comes to behavior, knowledge of the norm is an insufficient predictor of an individual's response. (Berkowitz, 1962) There is also increasing individuality of judgment. Not only does the individual become more consistent with age; his interindividual differences also increase.

In addition, moral judgment depends not only upon the situation but also upon the cultural patterns of a society. Morris concludes, on the basis of his survey of the literature and his research in London and Manchester, England, schools, that there are "social-class differences in 'moral realism' and differences in 'moral realism' between some primitive societies and modern industrial societies." (Morris, 1958, p. 1) Kohlberg, however, reports that, as with Piaget's stages, there seems to be a universal pattern of development. (Kohlberg and Turiel, 1971; Kohlberg and Gilligan, 1972; Turiel, 1973) When middle class, urban boys in the United States, Taiwan, and Mexico were compared, stage 3 was used most by 13-year-olds, and the developmental patterns were similar.

Early adolescence has often been cited as a time in which youngsters begin to doubt their religious heritage and become cynical. It has been seen as a time of conflict between parent and child over attendance at religious services as well as belief. The combination of emerging sexual strivings versus the "thou shalt nots" or parents and preachers and the ongoing struggle for independence leads to conflict within the child. We saw in Chapter 15 that the child now can view his parent more distinctly; he looks at religion in the same way. This is not to imply that he becomes irreligious, but it does mean that he moves from an unquestioning belief to a search for personal belief based upon his own experiences and interpretations. This again can be understood from our earlier discussion of decentering.

Generally, the early adolescent examines values more carefully and thoughtfully than the preadolescent. His value system is based upon his own organization of parental, community, and peer values and resembles, at least verbally, the adult world. If there is a difference, it lies in the particular interpretations he makes in the meaning of an adult value. Courage, honesty, and religion are merely cases in point, not the totality of his values. His perceptions of other groups and his perceptions of the world as idealistic or materialistic are screened through his own unique experience.

As we noted in relation to physical and intellectual development, the time of early adolescence is marked by increasing differences in the development of an integrated, individual value system. The early adolescent makes increasing differentiations in his field and looks at events in a fashion that is more relativistic than conventional. Thus his behavior, which reflects his value system, depends upon his assessment of the immediate situation, the presence or absence of peer-group members, and his general level of cognitive and moral development.

Except in certain delinquent groups, the early adolescent views acts that hurt individuals as repugnant. He has developed to the point where he sees others as having needs, rights, and privileges of their own, which he will not purposely violate. However, he may not yet have extended his horizons beyond his own group-class, neighborhood, race—so that he can be inconsistent. He can treat his "own" as individuals, but regards those who are different as not entitled to equal treatment. Of course, he comes by this naturally; his parents often engage in the same behavior. The struggles for civil rights clearly indicate the problem. In turn, he will vigorously defend himself against what he perceives to be violations of his individual integrity. This value placed on the individual probably reflects his growing sense of self-awareness.

Developing Interests

Reading.   The development of reading-interest patterns in junior high school continues, though, interestingly enough, these patterns seem to emerge earlier now. Formerly, early adolescents read science fiction and career books; now these are read by the preadolescent. The young teenager seeks books that used to be read in high school. Girls look for books about developing "personality," poise, and all the other manifestations of the social graces. This seems to be another indication of the movement toward behaving in "other-directed," externally appropriate patterns; this may be evidence of the trend toward conformity.

Boys read biography (but not about women!), history, and books of high adventure and athletic prowess. Girls' interests are in the direction of books about home and family life, biographies, mostly of women, and milder adventure stories. We can see in these choices the role played by sex identification as well as the use of reading to enhance a youngster's sense of self.

Wickens' (1960) survey of reading research reveals that the junior high school years are a turning point. Although it is the age of maximum reading, it is also the age when reading begins to decrease in quantity. That is, the curve of reading reaches its peak and begins to decline. The avid reader continues to read many books, but on the average, the number decreases in the ninth grade. The pressures of social life, increased homework, great needs for bodily activity, and diversification of interests are all possible reasons for this pattern. The youngster just gets involved in so many things that he cannot sustain them all at an increasing pace.

There may be another explanation. It may be that many of the books the early teenager would prefer to read are categorized in libraries as "adult" or are not purchased by school libraries. There were several incidents in the 1960s in which books were removed from high school libraries because of adult pressure. Could it be that we underestimate many of these youngsters and try to force-feed them "children's books" when they are both intellectually and developmentally ready to read adult works? They have been exposed to information through the mass media that other generations did not possess. This may serve not only to stimulate many to read but also to read different books. Perhaps a survey of paperback books would reveal data we could not know from library studies. It may be that the amount of reading has not decreased but that the use of the library as the main source for reading materials has been supplemented by the drugstore paperback rack.

Vocational Interests.   There continues to be, at both federal and local levels, discussion about career education, although no one has carefully defined the term. The concern stems partly from drop-out rates and student dissatisfaction with school, coupled with high rates of unemployment and unemployability at semiskilled or skilled jobs on the part of urban youth. Some people have advocated that youngsters in junior high be separated on the basis of ability and interest into different programs, or "tracks," that would lead to specific kinds of work in high school. Some have felt that youngsters should make decisions early with regard to their future careers, so that they could save time and get started early. How realistic are these expectations in the light of the evidence about the development of vocational interests and the reality of the work world, with its prejudices against women and minority groups?

We can examine (1) the level and type of vocational interests, (2) the accuracy of self-estimate, and (3) the attitudes that reflect cultural bias. First, we again find the phenomenon of individuality. Thompson, in a symposium on occupational information for junior high school youth, stated:

> Junior high students exhibit a fairly wide range of vocational development: Some are ready for work, having already sampled work activities through after-school jobs; some are thinking about long-term plans; most are thinking more about educational than vocational problems; some are uninterested or unable to concern themselves with career planning. The modal stage is probably characterized by "thinking about the planning for high school careers" so far as future planning is concerned. [Thompson, 1960, pp. 116–117]

This would suggest that any expectation of readiness on the part of all but a few junior high students to make realistic decisions is unwarranted. Super's research bolsters this position. On the basis of research utilizing school records, testing, and interviews, he reports: "Our typical ninth grade boys, in a typical small city high school, with a typical guidance program, were at a stage of vocational development which is characterized by readiness to consider problems of prevocational choice but also by a general lack of readiness to make vocational choices." (Super, 1960, p. 108) Further, Super (1961) indicates that choice at this time is unwise.

Second, how well does the early adolescent know himself in terms of vocational interest? The characteristic pattern for early adolescents seems to be highly governed by what they view as self-enhancing. Their needs for prestige and achievement affect their views of their interests, as judged by others and by tests. Further, lower class youngsters, with fewer models of professional and middle class occupations to emulate, with school situations that have often denigrated them, seem to have particular difficulty. In addition, schools often "counsel" such youngsters into low-level jobs. (Kohrs, 1968) Further, Hollander and Parker (1972) found that occupational choice was related both to self-description and stereotypic views of occupations. Since these views and self-descriptions also reflect the youngster's culture, we should be wary of any efforts to "track" or "guide" on the basis of his stated preference at this age.

Junior high school students are not aware of the interest patterns of adults in various professions. Their own estimates of their interests do not correspond with the interest patterns of people in their chosen fields, as measured by the Kuder. This "inaccuracy" can be seen as a function of their development, their experiences, and perhaps most significantly, of their needs for self-enhancement. We should not assume that this "vocational unreality," to borrow Ausubel, Schiff, and Zeleny's (1953) term, is necessarily an indication of poor adjustment. It might be better understood as an indicator of the lack of significance the 15-year-old still attaches to adult concepts of the world of work. He is still more interested in other things. He does not view the future in terms of actuality, but through the perceptual distortion of wish fulfillment.

In one way, however, early adolescents' views of work match that of the adult occupational world. Ninth-grade boys and girls were asked three questions: "What do you think women should be like?" "How do you think women see the world?" and "What do you think women should do?" Both boys and girls felt women should do different work than men do, and both sexes saw women as curious and exploring. But girls were more positive about women working; boys were more likely to see them as homebodies. Generally, the boys' responses were the more traditional. Entwisle and Greenberger (1972) conclude that such attitudes lower girls' level of aspiration and achievement because of peer-group pressure and that there is a conflict between school expectations and the peer view of women's role.

Adults should not expect youngsters to make vocational decisions by the ninth grade. Such decisions, for many youngsters, would bind them to choices that are unrealistic or prevent the exploration that is so necessary to a wise personal judgment. Rather, research on interest patterns should be used to see how the early adolescent views his world and to then provide opportunities for explorations leading to realistic vocational choice.

THE SELF-CONCEPT

One view of the importance of this period is presented by Douvan and Adelson:

> For many of us, the self—what we are now—begins at puberty. . . . The autobiographical fiction, the myth of the self in time, the narrative of what we were and then became are all, in some distinctive sense, dated from adolescence. We view childhood as a preparation. The true life, the true self, began when childhood was over, at 11, 12, 13. Nowadays, people (especially when they are patients) have that half or quarter knowledge of psychoanalysis which leads them, dutifully, to tell their stories from early childhood—the earlier the better. But if they are naive enough, or if we can get them to be naive enough, they will date the self (the present self) from puberty. [Douvan and Adelson, 1966, p. 3]

They see adolescence as a period of transition and assume that successful adaptation "directly depends on the ability to integrate the future to their present life and current self-concept." (p. 229) Our position is that the self-concept in adolescence reflects pubertal changes but is a natural extension and further development of the self that began in very early childhood. Both positions recognize the role of self in adolescence.

Basic, then, to the adolescent is the problem of his identity. Earlier in this chapter, we stressed the synthesis of cognitive and value development and the utility of the concept of egocentrism-decentering. We have seen that vocational interests are a function of self-perception. According to Erikson (1970), the inability to attain an occupational identity makes it hard on the adolescent to have a self-made identity. Taborn (1972) points out the double problem of black youths because "the 'individuation process' for Blacks not only means defining 'self' versus society, it also means achieving a constructive sense of Black identity with reference to society which historically has defined Blackness as negative." (Taborn, 1972, p. 6) But this is equally true of other groups—women, Chicanos, and Indians in the present United States culture; Jews for a long period in

Europe (not ending with the Hitler holocaust but continuing in the Soviet Union at least); and eastern and southern European immigrants, who came in waves into the United States. Anyone in either a self-defined or society-defined negative minority position faces the double problem. Perhaps all teenagers, by virtue of the label, belong in such a category.

How then, does the early adolescent define himself? Three questions form the basis of our analysis: (1) How does he conceive of himself? And, as a corollary, how accurate is this view? (2) In light of the variability both within and between individuals that is characteristic of this period of development, how stable is his image? (3) What is the effect of his self-concept on behavior?

How Does He Conceive of Himself?

Just what ideas do early adolescents hold of themselves? Attempts to answer this question have been made through the obvious means of asking them (questionnaires, interviews, essays, problem check lists) and through projective techniques. The one great weakness of these approaches is that they are all verbal and perhaps overlook the many nonverbal means by which the adolescent makes himself known to peers and adults. Nevertheless, these techniques provide us with a view of how the youngster looks at himself.

Boys.   Over half the boys in a sample of Canadian ninth graders (N = 190 boys, 194 girls) rated the following items as true of themselves: being honest, truthful, loyal to friends, kind, getting along with others, capable of looking after self, liking parents, being happy, and having many friends. About 40 percent of the boys indicated restlessness and envy of others, but only a small group (16) expressed conflict with teachers. If there was any area of concern, it was not over controlling feelings and interpersonal relations; it was concern over the physical body—being attractive, being able to dance, and being the right height and weight. (Taschuk, 1957)

Meissner (1961) used a survey questionnaire with more than 1000 high school boys in Catholic schools in the middle Atlantic states. He found that 14- and 15-year-olds report themselves as feeling pretty well satisfied with their lives, although they did indicate worrying over their studies. He also found that they felt misunderstood and had feelings of being sad and depressed. About the same percentage felt pretty well satisfied with life as those who responded "yes" to the question of ever feeling sad and depressed. This may reflect the mixture of levels of questioning that often causes trouble in interpreting self-reports. It is perfectly possible for one to feel pretty well satisfied and occasionally sad and depressed.

The Gordon How I See Myself data (Yeatts, 1967; Gordon, 1968) yield some interesting sex differences. Junior high school boys have a peer factor on which they scored, on the average, on the positive side. It consists of these items: "I play games well, the girls like me, I want the girls to admire me, I'm a good dancer, I'm smarter than most others, the boys admire me." There were no comparable factors for girls; that is, the items did not correlate with each other when girls completed the HISM scale. On factors shared by both sexes, the boys were more positive about themselves than the girls on physical appearance and autonomy, with no differences in physical adequacy. The girls were more positive than the boys on teacher-school and interpersonal adequacy factors. This last factor consists of 18 of the 42 items of the scale and includes handling feelings, attitudes toward one's body, school, teachers, peers.

It must be recalled, however, that factors derived from self-report data, on any scale, have serious limitations, not the least of which is that what comes out as a factor, or cluster of interrelated items, depends upon what items are on the scale. The HISM, for example, does not include family items.

It seems to be easier for boys to express concern over their bodies than over their more intimate feelings. The Purdue Opinion Poll, using a combination checklist and blank page for problems, found that over 50 percent of ninth-grade boys and girls indicated problems in connection with their bodies. The only other percentages approaching this (and other data indicate that girls contributed more to these percentages than boys) related to temper, worry about little things, feelings about not being as smart as others, and heterosexual relationships. Of course, a problem checklist needs interpretation, because our concern is with the more central self-concept. The mere fact that about 30 percent indicate problems of temper and worry does not tell us much about the other 70 percent. Do they feel secure and adequate in self-control? Or do they see this as insignificant to their self-view? We get no indication of the relative importance of these problems to the individual boy or girl.

Perhaps the best we can say is that most boys report favorably on themselves. The impact of the culture may contribute to this. Male sex-role identification seems to be a potent source of self-esteem. (Connell and Johnson, 1970) Singer and Singer go so far as to state: "For the early adolescent, it would appear that the male role has value as a basis for self-esteem beyond that of the female role, regardless of whether the role is accepted by male or female." (Singer and Singer, 1972, p. 399) Whether this view will be maintained as women's liberation gains ground remains to be seen.

Boys indicate concerns about their bodies, suggesting that they have not yet resolved their body image. Their other statements indicate that they have differentiated their perceptual world into two major environmental anchorage points: the family and the peer culture. Of these two, they are still clarifying their view of themselves in relation to peers, especially opposite-sex peers. On the whole, they see themselves as adequate, but a substantial number recognize their needs to control feelings and meet cultural demands.

Girls. Girls seem to experience more tension in establishing their self-identity. The lack of self-acceptance depicted by Milner (1949) is supported by Roff. She used the Q-sort technique with girls of 11, 14, 17, and 20. The girls sorted statements for self, ideal self, and mother. Roff reports that not only does self-satisfaction decline throughout adolescence but also that self-mother identification declines, reaching a low at age 17. (Roff, 1959)

Again the Canadians studied by Taschuk (1957) present a more optimistic picture. Self-reports showed that about half the girls perceived the following items as being true about themselves: being honest, kind, friendly, self-reliant, truthful, loyal to friends, being able to get along with both sexes, being a good sport, and being dependable. Only about one-third of the girls expressed feelings of being stubborn or daydreaming too much. We can see that they present themselves as the very model of good behavior. The How I See Myself data resemble the Taschuk material much more than they do Milner (1949) or Roff (1959). Three factors appear in junior high school girls that are absent from junior high school boys: emotional control, on which the girls' average is positive; body build, on which the average is negative; and academic achievement, positive. There is a clear recognition here by the girls of their emotions, but what is most significant is their perceptions of self as inadequate in physical appearance. We noted earlier in discussing the boys that the boys' scores were higher than the girls' on physical appearance, and now we have the body-build factor to complement this view.

What can we say, then, about the self-concept of early adolescent girls? They present a perception of selves as more inadequate generally than do the boys. Their major area of concern seems to lie in acceptance of their bodies and in seeing their own autonomy or individuality. The girls' concerns about peers are mixed in with their general views of interpersonal adequacy rather than being discrete, as it is for boys.

A further difference between the self-concept of boys and girls during early adolescence seems to be the way they organize their feelings and meanings about aggression. (Lansky et al., 1961) As a part of the longitudinal study of middle class youngsters at the Fels Research Institute, they found that boys reported more aggressive tendencies than girls but also had a different constellation of patterns of aggression than did the girls.

In general, from the mixture of projective techniques and self-reports described above, we might speculate that boys conceive of themselves as more independent, more accepting of their bodies, and more concerned with peers as a separate group than girls do. The girls tend to view school and teachers in a more positive light, to acknowledge feelings as a separate area of concern, and to view academic achievement as a distinct dimension of themselves. Generally, the boys seem to be more secure in that they express fewer problems.

But the standard approaches of the researcher seem to miss some of the essence of what it means to be an early adolescent. Cottle's (1971) descriptions of his long-term conversations with early adolescents, Goethals' and Klos' (1970) case studies, or Robert Coles' (1972) individual portraits may take us closer to the "real" youngster. Cottle, for example, describes a 15-year-old girl and gives her reactions to school, sex, drugs, herself. She says, for example, about a D— in a French test, " 'I felt this high.' Marty lay her hand perfectly still, flat out, palm down, parallel to the ground an inch above the top of her shiny loafers. . . . 'I could have crawled into my socks except they were too high. Poor grades do something to your ego. They make you feel so small and unimportant.' " (Cottle, 1971, p. 23)*

Her reactions to a party also reflect tension. "What comes out of these moments of talks and reminiscences is precisely that question: how does one know if he or she is a prude? How does one learn what practically amounts to hard sociological data, about sex, about making out, about potency and impotency, about beauty and ugliness? . . . What comes out of these moments is how one learns that he or she is doing all right, what in fact is 'all right'; and how what is 'supposed' to be happening at fifteen hasn't already happened at twelve and should have, or won't happen until seventeen and should have way before then. But how is one supposed to know when she cannot confess to the fright and nausea and physical illness. . . ." (Cottle, 1971, p. 38)

Cottle summarizes, "Most of the conversations of those three cherished summer months came around to the same themes: boys and sex, popularity, clothes and appearance. But it is almost as if the language itself contained pockets of feelings often having nothing whatever to do with what was being spoken about, or for that matter, with the feelings that popped up here and there: the anxiety with the willingness, the fear with the daring, the reservations with the plotting." (Cottle, 1971, p. 41)

The "Ideal" Self. Both boys and girls are still dealing with the as-yet-unfinished task of defining self. They are still finding out about areas of themselves and about interpersonal relationships. We know how important identification is to them and how their needs for prestige, acceptance, and achievement color their views of their world. Perhaps of primary importance in these years is the resolution of what C. Gordon (1972) called "the

---

* Quotes on pages 339, 360, and 368 from Thomas J. Cottle, *Time's Children: Impressions of Youth,* pp. 23, 38, 41, 84, 327, and 331. Copyright © 1967, 1969, 1970, 1971 by Thomas J. Cottle. Reprinted by permission.

acceptance/achievement dilemma'' (1972, p. 37), in which the youngster is expected to do well in school and at the same time relate to the peer culture. As we have stated above, this seems to pose particular problems for girls in the present American culture.

Another way in which they use identification in developing their self-concepts is through the creation of an ideal. They select people, either real or fictional, and engage in both hero-worship and emulation. Bray (1964) asked English adolescents, both middle and lower class, ''Of all the persons you have yourself known or that you've got to know about in any way as in reading, or watching, or listening, who would you most wish to be like?'' Boys tended to choose from people they did not know (remote environment), whereas girls chose to select their models from people they did know. Both tended to choose same sex figures, with the boys' choices centering around athletes and the girls' choices around entertainers.

His study bears out previous studies conducted in the United States. In early adolescence, the hero is often a glamorous, romantic adult or one who is invested with glamor. Each generation seems to have its version of the Pied Piper of Hamlin, the musician who attracts a following. It may be that the same parents who jitterbugged to the name bands of immediate pre–World War II years were the loudest objectors to the rock and psyche-delic groups of the late 1960s. The media in the early 1970s, following a trend begun in the late 1960s, developed an ''antihero'' type and seemed to move away from the handsome or beautiful star doing fine things. Instead we had *The Graduate, Midnight Cowboy, MASH, Catch 22,* and *Slaughterhouse Five.* It became cool to be cool. How much this has influenced the early adolescent is speculative, but if he is searching for idols, the models are different from those presented to his parents.

How Accurate Is the Self-concept?

A basic problem in answering such a question is the definition of accuracy. If self-concept is the way one views himself, then there can be no external standard of accuracy. The self is the only judge. Such a definition not only makes self-concept unscientific (because it becomes completely internal and private); it also makes it useless (because there is no common standard). Another way to define accuracy, the way used here, is the degree of similarity between the way one reports on himself and the way he is seen by others or performs on standard measures. Accuracy, then, is ''to see ourselves as others see us.'' Admittedly, this does some violence to the notion of one's own internal assessment, but it is all we can deal with scientifically.

Self-estimates of scholastic ability and school achievement (Ausubel, Schiff, and Zeleny, 1953; and O'Hara and Tiedeman, 1959) were far from accurate when 14- and 15-year-olds were asked to look at their overall ability. The Illinois study illustrates the pattern: Girls showed much more variability than boys. "Individuals who tended to overestimate past performance also tended to have relatively high academic aspirations for the future in terms of past performance." (Ausubel et al., 1953, p. 159) Teachers and pupils disagreed on their estimates of pupil ability. It is not only that early adolescents are inaccurate; some individual adolescents are systematically so. When the Coopersmith Self-esteem Inventory was used with a group of ninth-graders, only moderate relationships were found between it and academic achievement. (Kunce, Getsinger, and Miller, 1972)

Many children are accurate in assessing their academic achievement. For example, Brookover's study of junior high school youngsters indicated that there was a high relationship for both boys and girls between self-concept of ability and school achievement. There were more than 500 boys and 500 girls in the study. He also found, however, that children were specific in their concepts of school subjects and realized that they did not hold a single view about their ability. The data on the Gordon How I See Myself Scale also indicated a reliable relationship between the academic achievement factor and actual school achievement.

Brandt's (1958) study (described in Chapter 13) showed superiority of boys over girls in accuracy of self-estimate of academic achievement. However, there was no sex difference on estimates of physical ability and social reputations. We might infer, from all we've said about the varying impacts of schooling and cultural demands upon boys and girls, that the difference in their responses is partially due to threat. Girls are supposed to be good, to follow directions, and to do their work. We have seen that early adolescent girls are torn between meeting this cultural demand and the internal pressures to do what they'd like to do. They tend to devaluate themselves, and this may show up in their greater inaccuracy of estimate of scholastic achievement.

On the other hand, both sexes are caught in the redefinition of physical and social aspects of self. We would, therefore, expect them not to differ, and they do not. Another indication of discrepancy between what might be expected (externally) and self-report can be found in the results of the Trowbridges' (Trowbridge, Trowbridge, and Trowbridge, 1972) study, using Coopersmith's scale. They found that black, lower social class, and/or rural children reported more positive views of self than did white, middle class, and/or urban eighth-graders. Further, the latter tended to express more positive views toward self in relation to home and parents; the former, toward general self-esteem and self in relation to peers and school.

Taschuk (1957) and Brandt (1958) both found that the various aspects of self-estimate were related to each other. This seems to indicate that in back of the discrete self-concepts there is an organizing or integrating factor. These interrelationships were not high, but they were positive and reliable beyond chance. Self-estimates in early adolescence (and all through life) are functions of this self-concept and the total organization of the self. We should not expect anything resembling perfect agreement between an internal and external view; the best we can hope for is that there is a sufficient relationship to enable us to understand another's view of self, and thus his perspective, from observing his behavior or from what he chooses to tell us about himself.

How Stable Is the Self-concept?

Is the early adolescent's view of himself reliable as a predictor, or how he will see himself a few years later? Is there any consistency at this time?

The extent of stability seems to be related to the amount of positive view already held by the individual boy or girl. We may hypothesize that if, as a youngster entering adolescence, I feel good about myself, the chances are I will become more positive in my view and more consistent too. If I enter adolescence with a negative view of myself, then my opinion of myself becomes unstable. I'm not sure of myself, and so I "latch on" to cues from my gang and other people that tell me how they see me. I shift my view to take into account their ideas, and so I do not stay the same. I may end up thinking I'm better or worse, but at least I change.

We have little current data to go on. One study done by Tyler (1957) compared the self-reports that 30 boys in the California Growth Study (born in the late 1920s) gave on themselves when they were 11, 13, and 17. He concluded that there was no support for the idea of stability in adolescents' self-reports. However, another longitudinal study (Faterson and Witkin, 1970) examined the figure drawings of the children when they were 8 and again at 13 for one group and at ages 10, 14, 17, and 24 for another group. They report a high degree of individual stability was established by age 14 in the way these people drew their bodies.

The only real way to deal with individual stability is through longitudinal studies. But cross-sectional studies in which people at different ages complete the same questionnaire or instrument can help us see trends. Beemer (1972) used a Q-sort with over 4000 children in grades 1 through 12. Her measures for preadolescents and adolescents were verbal (see Perkins in Chapter 11). She found a movement with age toward more positive views of self. We noted earlier that both Brandt (1958) and Taschuk (1957) found interrelationships among the various aspects of self-estimate they measured. Mullener and Laird (1971) used a questionnaire with seventh- and twelfth-graders. These adolescents evaluated themselves in five skill areas: achievement, interpersonal, intellectual, physical, and social. There was a definite trend for the older teenagers to differentiate their views across areas; that is, the older adolescents did not have a single view of self.

This fits in with our concept that "as the child grows he goes through periods of being more unified and more global and through periods of being more differentiated." (Gordon, 1968, p. 4) Early adolescence may be a time of more global view than late adolescence, because it is a time of rapid change that might require the youngster to mobilize himself. Such mobilization might be analogous to the circle of wagons—a tight defensive ring requiring uniformity of effort. This is speculative; we need far more data of the longitudinal type to really understand both individual stability and developmental trends.

Self-concept and Behavior

The empirical evidence demonstrating direct connections between self-concept (as measured by self-report or other testing techniques) and behavior (as judged by outsiders) is extremely limited and somewhat conflicting.

We find, for instance, evidence of relationships between anxiety and fantasy as measured by TAT, personality scales, and the self-reports of boys and girls. The youngsters who expressed dissatisfaction with self and others also showed anxiety (Phillips et al., 1960), and those whose fantasy productions on the TAT were inferred as indicating certain attitudes toward self in the family also tended to report these same attitudes. (Calogeras, 1958) We have also indicated above the relationship between academic self-concept and academic achievement. Because correlations cannot be used to indicate cause and effect, we cannot, of course, postulate the direction.

Suggestions of relationships between self-concept and behavior can also be found in a Columbus, Ohio, study of delinquency. The question often asked by laymen and students alike is: Why do some youngsters who grow up in high delinquency areas become law-abiding, whereas others become delinquent? Reckless and his colleagues (1956) report the difference lies in self-concept. They found that the nondelinquent boy saw himself as obedient to adults, was stricter about right and wrong than the delinquent, and was concerned about the reaction of others. In general, he had insulated himself against delinquency by taking over as a part of his self the values of significant nondelinquent others. A type of replication of the Reckless study was conducted by Schwartz and Tangri (1965), who used a semantic differential scale in which children responded in terms of "I am," "My friends think I am," "My mother thinks I am," "My teacher thinks I am." They attempted to examine the discrepancy among these for sixth grade boys in the inner city of Detroit. They found no positive relationship between the way a boy thought he was and the way he thought his friends thought he was for either "good" (delinquency-immune) or "bad" (delinquency-prone) boys. The "bad" boys seemed to have a higher correlation between their self-concepts and perceived mothers' concepts of them, whereas the "good" boys had their highest relationships between self-views and teachers' views of them. Schwartz and Tangri indicate that, although Reckless' conclusion is probably correct, the self-concept is not a single dimension but a complex organization.

In their study of delinquents, Fitts and Hamner (1969) used the Tennessee Self-Concept Scale (TSSC), a self-report that produces scores on physical, moral-ethical, personal, family, and social self as well as ratios of conflict, self-criticism, and psychological harmony. On the basis of use over a wide range of populations, empirical scales were developed that seem to use the patterns of neurotics, psychotics, and normals to differentiate them by psychiatric category. They found, not only on their sample in Tennessee but also when others in a wide range of states and in Mexico used the scale, that there was a characteristic test pattern for delinquents. The pattern was one of negative self-concept—especially in respect to behavior, moral-ethical concepts, and family self-report. The pattern also reveals conflict, and confusion, and little personality strength.

The Tennessee Scale has also been used to examine the relationship between self-concept (as measured by this self-report device) and school performance in junior high. Fitts (1972) reports that 90 studies are underway or have been concluded. There have been mixed results, but few direct, reliable relationships have been found between scores on the TSSC and achievement-test or grade-point average. TSSC scores were related to other nonacademic measures, such as attitude toward school, morale, and motivation. On the basis of these studies, self-concept as measured by the TSSC seems to have little influence or to be little influenced by academic performance.

But self-concept includes more than the type of self-esteem items or judgments on such scales as the TSSC, Coopersmith, or How I See Myself. One aspect of self, which we have mentioned in several chapters, is sex-role identification. Stein (1971) assessed sex-role standards of sixth- and ninth-grade students. The students indicated for each of 42 items in 6 achievement areas whether they considered the item as more boyish or girlish. There were significant differences at the ninth-grade level on 5 of the 6 areas (mechanical and athletic were male; reading, artistic, and social were female, and there was no difference on math) in motivation. Boys thought it more important to achieve in their areas; girls, in their self-chosen, sex-related areas. Stein concludes that sex-role standards influence achievement. Her approach is especially useful because it sheds light on one of the complications that has been inadequately dealt with in the usual correlational study of self-concept (self-reported esteem) and performance. What is the person's own hierarchy of values? The fact that I, as a ninth-grade boy, may not value reading as much as I value athletics may mean that my self-esteem is therefore more a function of athletic skill than of reading. On an overall, self-concept measure, I may rate myself high on self-esteem, even though, objectively, I am not doing well in reading. This will lead to a low correlation between self-esteem and academic performance. But it fails to take into account the true sources of my self-esteem, and thus it leads to false conclusions about the real relationship between self-concept (broadly conceived and including sex-role identification) and performance.

Another aspect of self-concept often neglected in the usual self-report research is the degree to which one feels control over reinforcement; that is, whether one feels he is a victim of circumstances or can influence what happens to him. Buck and Harvey (1971) compared the beliefs in internal-external control of 50 black adequate achievers with 50 black underachievers who were matched for IQ, sex, age, and family background. These youngsters were also rated by teachers. They used the Intellectual Achievement Responsibility (IAR) (Crandall, 1965) as the measure of belief in control over intellectual-academic activities. Adequate achievers, within each sex and across the total group, scored higher on internal control. Further, those who had a belief in their own ability to influence the academic situation (internals) were seen by teachers as more active, striving, and involved.

What these studies suggest is that there are relationships between aspects of self-concept, and behavior and performance. They tend to support our view that self-concept is not a unitary trait but that there is a hierarchical organization of concepts of self, including self-definition, esteem, potency, and values, that are in complex interplay both within the self and between the self and the world. This view rules out simplified expectations concerning the relationship between self-concept and behavior.

SUMMARY

In this chapter we have examined the development of intelligence, interests, values, and self-concept in early adolescence. We have seen that these are not independent developments but are all related to each other and to the physical development and body image discussed in Chapter 14. These various developments are all organized as a result of the functioning of the previously developed self-system. Since the self is an open system in constant transaction with its environment, it is subject to modification. The early adolescent period is a major period for such modification. Because the early adolescent experiences changes both within and without his skin, his self goes through a reorganization stage. Preadolescence was characterized by movement toward integration; early adolescence might be seen as a period of increased differentiation, instability, and reintegration. The general view the youngster holds of self and world has not necessarily changed fundamentally, but many bits of information formerly not perceived or integrated now become part of the self.

A most important generalization emerging from the data is the systematic way in which the individual boy or girl selects both internal and external events from the welter of stimuli to include into his self-system. This seems to be more than a chance operation and suggests the presence of organizing processes by which the person is able to maintain and enhance his ongoing self-system. His uniqueness in all aspects of his existence is unquestionable; his organization and his self belong to him alone.

By the end of early adolescence, the period of readjustment enters a new phase: reintegration. The metamorphosis, physiologically and in many other ways, is essentially complete. Youth now turns to the job of building upon the newly broadened self. He begins to work on becoming adult.

We also saw, in this chapter, that our theory is ahead of our data. The need for careful, rigorous research must be emphasized. We have made a number of hypotheses in the above chapter and have used others' hypotheses. These should open up numerous ideas for research.

REFERENCES AND ADDITIONAL READINGS

Anderson, W., & Bosworth, D. A note on occupational values of ninth grade students of 1958 as compared to 1970. *Journal of Vocational Behavior,* 1971, *1,* 301–303.

Ausubel, D. Implications of preadolescent and early adolescent cognitive development for secondary school teaching. Paper presented at Symposium of the American Educational Research Association, Atlantic City, N.J., February 20, 1962.

Ausubel, D., Schiff, H., & Zeleny, M. Real-life measures of level of academic and vocational aspiration in adolescents: Relation to laboratory measures and to adjustment. *Child Development,* 1953, *24,* 155–168.

Bayley, N. On the growth of intelligence. *American Psychologist,* 1955, *10,* 805–818.

Bayley, N. Individual patterns of development. *Child Development,* 1956, *27,* 45–74. Reprinted in I. J. Gordon (Ed.), *Human development: Readings in research,* Glenview, Ill.: Scott, Foresman, 1965.

Beemer, L. C. Developmental changes in the self-concepts of children and adolescents. *Dissertation Abstracts International,* 1972, *32,* 5031–5032.

Berkowitz, L. *The development of motives and values in the child.* New York: Basic Books, 1962.

Bloom, B. *Stability and change in human characteristics.* New York: Wiley, 1964.

Brandt, R. The accuracy of self-estimate: A measure of self-concept reality. *Genetic Psychology Monographs,* 1958, *58,* 55–99.

Bray, D. H. Attributes of ideal persons and of the self as conceived by some English secondary school children. *Journal of Experimental Education,* 1964, *33,* 93–97.

Brookover, W., Paterson, A., & Thomas, S. *Self-concept of ability and school achievement.* East Lansing, Mich.: Michigan State University, Final Report, Cooperative Research Project No. 845, 1962.

Bruner, J. et al. *Studies of thinking.* New York: Wiley, 1958.

Buck, M. R., & Austrin, H. R. Factors related to school achievement in an economically disadvantaged group. *Child Development,* 1971, *42,* 1813–1826.

Calogeras, R. Some relationships between fantasy and self-report. *Genetic Psychology Monographs,* 1958, *58,* 273–325.

Coles, R. The weather of the years. In J. Kagan & R. Coles (Eds.), *Twelve to sixteen: Early adolescence.* New York: Norton, 1972. Pp. 258–276.

Connell, D., & Johnson, J. Relationship between sex-role identification and self-esteem in early adolescents. *Developmental Psychology,* 1970, *3,* 268.

Cottle, T. *Time's children, impressions of youth.* Boston: Little, Brown, 1971.

Crandall, V. C., Katkovsky, W., & Crandall, V. J. Children's beliefs in their own control of reinforcements in intellectual-academic achievement situations. *Child Development,* 1965, *36,* 91–109.

Deitz, G. The influence of social class, sex and delinquency-nondelinquency on adolescent values. *Journal of Genetic Psychology,* 1972, *121,* 119–126.

Douvan, E., & Adelson, J. *The adolescent experience.* New York: Wiley, 1966.

Doyle, J. The effect of cognitive style on the ability to attain concepts and to perceive embedded figures. Unpublished doctoral dissertation, University of Florida, 1966.

Elkind, D. Conceptual orientation shifts in children and adolescents. *Child Development,* 1966, *37,* 493–498.

Elkind, D. Egocentrism in adolescence. *Child Development,* 1967, *38,* 1025–1034. Reprinted in I. J. Gordon (Ed.), *Readings in research in developmental psychology.* Glenview, Ill.: Scott, Foresman, 1971. Pp. 306–311.

Engel, M. The stability of the self-concept in adolescence. *Journal of Abnormal and Social Psychology,* 1959, *58,* 211–215.

Entwisle, D., & Greenberger, E. Adolescents' views of women's work role. *American Journal of Orthopsychiatry,* 1972, *42,* 648–656.

Erikson, E. Identity versus identity diffusion. In J. Duffy & G. Giuliani (Eds.), *Selected readings in adolescent psychology.* Berkeley, Calif.: McCutchan, 1970. Pp. 43–48.

Faterson, H., & Witkin, H. Longitudinal study of development of the body concept. *Developmental Psychology,* 1970, *2,* 429–438.

Fitts, W. *The self concept and performance.* Research Monograph *V,* Dede Wallace Center. Nashville, Tenn.: Fitts, April 1972.

Fitts, W. *The self concept and behavior: Overview and supplement.* Research Monograph *VII,* Dede Wallace Center. Nashville, Tenn.: Fitts, June 1972.

Fitts, W., & Hamner, W. *The self concept and delinquency.* Research Monograph *I.* Nashville, Tenn.: Nashville Mental Health Center, July 1969.

Gecas, V. Parental behavior and dimensions of adolescent self-evaluation. *Sociometry,* 1971, *34,* 466–482.

Goertzen, S. Factors relating to opinions of seventh grade children regarding the acceptability of certain behaviors in the peer group. *Journal of Genetic Psychology,* 1959, *94,* 29–34.

Goethals, G., & Klos, D. *Experiencing youth, first person accounts.* Boston: Little, Brown, 1970.

Goldman, R. *Religious thinking from childhood to adolescence.* London: Routledge & Kegan Paul, 1964.

Gordon, C. Social characteristics of early adolescence. In J. Kagan & R. Coles (Eds.), *Twelve to sixteen: Early adolescence.* New York: Norton, 1972. Pp. 25–54.

Gordon, I. J. *Studying the child in school.* New York: Wiley, 1966.

Gordon, I. J. *The How I See Myself Scale: A manual.* Gainesville, Fla.: Florida Educational Research and Development Council, 1968.

Havighurst, R., & MacDonald, D. Development of the ideal self in New Zealand and American children. *Journal of Educational Research,* 1955, *49,* 263–273.

Hoffman, M. Identification and conscience development. *Child Development,* 1971, *42,* 1071–1082.

Hollander, M., & Parker, H. Occupational stereotypes and self-descriptions: Their relationship to vocational choice. *Journal of Vocational Behavior,* 1972, *2,* 57–65.

Inhelder, B., & Piaget, J. *Growth in logical thinking from childhood through adolescence.* New York: Basic Books, 1958.

Johnson, R. C. A study of children's moral judgments. *Child Development,* 1962, *33,* 327–354. Reprinted in I. J. Gordon (Ed.), *Human development: Readings in research.* Glenview, Ill.: Scott, Foresman, 1965.

Kagan, J., & Coles, R. (Eds.) *Twelve to sixteen: Early adolescence.* New York: Norton, 1972.

Ken-Ichiro, I. On conscience of Japanese junior high school students—their moral awakening. *Japanese Journal of Educational Psychology,* 1959, *7,* 79–83.

Kohlberg, L., & Gilligan, C. The adolescent as a philosopher: The discovery of the self in a postconventional world. In J. Kagan & R. Coles (Eds.), *Twelve to sixteen: Early adolescence.* New York: Norton, 1972. Pp. 144–179.

Kohlberg, L. & Turiel, E. Moral development and moral education. In G. Lesser (Ed.), *Psychological and educational practice.* Glenview, Ill.: Scott, Foresman, 1971. Pp. 410–465.

Kohrs, E. V. The disadvantaged and lower class adolescent. In J. Adams (Ed.), *Understanding adolescence.* Boston: Allyn & Bacon, 1968.

Kunce, J., Getsinger, S., & Miller, D. Educational implications of self-esteem. *Psychology in the Schools,* 1972, *9,* 314–316.

Lansky, L. M. et al. Sex differences in aggression and its correlates in middle-class adolescents. *Child Development,* 1961, *32,* 45–58.

Mead, M. Early adolescence in the United States. *Bulletin of the National Association of Secondary School Principals,* 1965, *49,* 5–10.

Meissner, W. W. Some anxiety indications in the adolescent boy. *Journal of General Psychology,* 1961, *64,* 251–257.

Milner, E. Effects of sex role and social status on the early adolescent personality. *Genetic Psychology Monographs,* 1949, *40,* 233–325.

Morris, J. The development of adolescent value-judgments. *British Journal of Educational Psychology,* 1958, *28,* 1–14.

Mullener, N., & Laird, J. Some developmental changes in the organization of self-evaluations. *Developmental Psychology,* 1971, *5,* 233–236.

Muuss, R. E. (Ed.) *Adolescent behavior and society: A book of readings.* New York: Random House, 1971.

O'Hara, R., & Tiedeman, D. The vocational self concept in adolescence. *Journal of Counseling Psychology,* 1959, *6,* 292–301.

Phillips, B., Hindsman, E., & Jennings, E. Influence of intelligence on anxiety and perception of self. *Child Development,* 1960, *31,* 41–46.

Piaget, J. Intellectual evolution from adolescence to adulthood. *Human Development,* 1972, *15,* 1–12.

Powell, M., & Frerichs, A. H. (Eds.) *Readings in adolescent psychology.* Minneapolis, Minn.: Burgess, 1971.

Reckless, W., Dinitz, S., & Murray, E. Self-concept as an insulator against delinquency. *American Sociological Review,* 1956, *21,* 744–746.

Roff, C. The self-concept in adolescent girls. Doctoral dissertation, Boston University, 1959.

Schwartz, M., & Tangri, S. A note on self-concept as an insulator against delinquency. *American Sociological Review,* 1965, *30,* 922–926.

Sigel, I. How intelligence tests limit understanding of intelligence. *Merrill-Palmer Quarterly,* 1963, *9,* 39–56. Reprinted in I. J. Gordon (Ed.), *Readings in research in developmental psychology.* Glenview, Ill.: Scott, Foresman, 1971. Pp. 279–289.

Singer, J., & Singer, D. Personality. In P. Mussen & M. Rosenzweig (Eds.), *Annual review of psychology.* Vol. 23. Palo Alto, Calif.: Annual Reviews, Inc., 1972. Pp. 375–412.

Stein, A. The effects of sex-role standards for achievement and sex-role preference on three determinants of achievement motivation. *Developmental Psychology,* 1971, *4,* 219–231.

Super, D. The critical ninth grade: Vocational choice or vocational exploration. *Personnel and Guidance Journal,* 1960, *39,* 106–109.

Super, D. Consistency and wisdom of vocational preference as indices of vocational maturity in the ninth grade. *Journal of Educational Psychology,* 1961, *52,* 35–43. Reprinted in I. J. Gordon (Ed.), *Human development: Readings in research.* Glenview, Ill.: Scott, Foresman, 1965.

Taborn, J. Some reflections on meeting the needs of youth: Implications for staff awareness. *University of Minnesota Center for Youth Development and Research Quarterly Focus,* 1972, *1,* 2–6.

Taschuk, W. An analysis of the self-concept of grade nine students. *Alberta Journal of Educational Research,* 1957, *3,* 94–103.

Thompson, A. Developmental stage and developmental needs at the junior high school level. *Personnel and Guidance Journal,* 1960, *39,* 116–118. Copyright 1960 American Personnel and Guidance Association. Reprinted with permission.

Trowbridge, N., Trowbridge, L., & Trowbridge, L. Self concept and socioeconomic status. *Child Study Journal,* 1972, *2,* 123–143.

Tuma, E., & Livson, N. Family socioeconomic status and adolescent attitudes to authority. *Child Development,* 1960, *31,* 387–399.

Turiel, E. Stage transition in moral development. In R. M. W. Travers (Ed.), *Second handbook of research on teaching.* Chicago: Rand McNally, 1973. Pp. 732–758.

Turiel, E., & Rothman, G. The influence of reasoning on behavioral choices at different stages of moral development. *Child Development,* 1972, *43,* 741–756.

Tyler, F. T. Stability of intra-individual patterning of measures of adjustment during adolescence. *Journal of Educational Psychology,* 1957, *48,* 217–226.

Vernon, P. E. Sex differences in personality structure at age 14. *Canadian Journal of Behavioral Science,* 1972, *4,* 283–297.

Ward, J. The saga of Butch and Slim. *British Journal of Educational Psychology,* 1972, *42,* 267–289.

Weir, M. Developmental changes in problem solving strategies. *Psychological Review,* 1964, *71,* 473–490.

Wickens, A. Reading interests: Grades seven through nine. In J. Seidman (Ed.), *The adolescent.* (Rev. ed.) New York: Holt, Rinehart & Winston, 1960. Pp. 504–510.

Yeatts, P. Developmental changes in the self-concept of children grades 3–12. *Florida Educational Research and Development Council, Research Bulletin,* 1967, *3(2).*

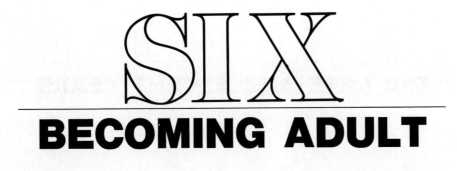

SIX
BECOMING ADULT

CHAPTER 17
THE LATE ADOLESCENT YEARS

Let us now in youth rejoice,
None can justly blame us.
For when golden youth has fled
And in age our joys are dead
*Then the dust doth claim us.**

THE ESTABLISHMENT OF
PHYSICAL STABILITY

Perhaps the most important aspect of physical development in late adolescence is the establishment of stability. By and large, the years from 15
to about 20 are ones in which the body reestablishes its equilibrium.

The rapid growth spurt is over for most children, and final heights are
essentially reached by the end of high school. Of course, some boys are
still not at their ultimate height, but only a very few are still in early adolescence in terms of physical development by the time they reach 18.

The erratic pattern of peaks of great activity and valleys of lethargy
diminish for both boys and girls, and in addition, for girls the normal menstrual cycle becomes established at about 28 days. Both sexes arrive,
physiologically, at a more even keel by the end of the late adolescence.

Part of the acceptance of the body by the adolescent involves the
acceptance of difference both from others and from one's ideal. When
youngsters reach their final height, two individuals may be mature but may
still differ by as much as 10 to 12 inches. To some degree, previous differences may have been due to differential rates of maturity. Now, these
differences will remain.

The boy who dreamed that he'd "catch up" is faced with the task of
acceptance of his final height; others who thought that such differences

* Medieval student song.

would disappear with age also have to face the facts. Acceptance of individuality is still a problem to the late adolescent. The interaction of rate of maturity and acceptance of self carries over from the early adolescent period. The concept of one's body is influenced not only by rate of maturity but also by one's total view of self. For example, Weatherley found that late-maturing males tend to be less dominant than early maturers and see themselves as more autonomous from both parents and peers. (Weatherley, 1964) Fisher (1964) asked boys to estimate their own height and found overestimation was related to needs to be superior to the female. In this age of tall basketball players in high school, height is certainly a significant variable in the boy's acceptance of self.

The following discussion of the significance of physical stability is a theoretical account of its meaning to the adolescent and not a description based upon empirical data. In order to test these ideas, a series of hypotheses would need to be deduced from them and then data collected and analyzed. Such data could be gathered through self-reporting techniques, projective devices, interviews, and compositions. Our purpose here is to raise ideas, with the understanding that our knowledge is incomplete.

With regularization of function, some of the adolescent's concerns over his own body are alleviated; the awkwardness of the gangling early adolescent, which was caused by both physical and social factors, gives way to the grace of maturity. The adolescent's assurance and confidence in his own body returns, and he handles himself more efficiently. By the end of adolescence, the youngster feels he can count on his body to perform in certain ways. He perceives himself as possessed of unlimited energy. He has an optimistic view of the limits to which he can test his body resources. He demands much of his body, and it meets his demands. If there is ever a time in life in which it seems as though the candle can be burned at both ends, it is now. Sleep seems unnecessary; partying and thrill seeking are highly valued.

Testing bodily limits becomes a sport in high school. For example, Moore (1972) found that Canadian boys saw accepting challenges that involved physical risk as a normal part of their lives. Adolescents don't believe their bodies can wear out or fail to respond. They see experimentation as exciting and reject both moralistic and futuristic warnings about the dangers of alcohol, drugs, tobacco, and sex. This is not just thrill seeking. The adolescent has just passed through a period in which he could not count on his body. Now he seeks to find out all he can about what his body will take. This is a part of the process of establishing stability; it is a part of his learning to accept and use his changing body.

The problem of the use of drugs is of increasing concern in the early 1970s. There has obviously been an increase in the use of marijuana, in trying out "acid" (LSD), and in the use of narcotics by teenagers, not only to explore their bodily limits but also to test some societal standards. The whole drug scene, reaching into the upper elementary grades, is incomprehensible to many adults and, as discussed later in this chapter, is a basic element of a large subculture in the peer society. No area is as surrounded by fear and emotion on the part of adults, yet facts on drug use and abuse are difficult to attain. What seems true is that usage is a function of the interaction of various attitudes as well as of situational factors, only one of which is acceptance of one's body and its limits. Difficult problems are posed for parents and schools in their attempt to teach children to deny themselves an experience simply because the adult world either says it should be delayed or it is no good for them. The problem is compounded when teenagers look at adult behavior and see very few attempts to delay gratification. After all, from their viewpoint, what is the difference between an adult getting "bombed" on alcohol and a youngster getting "stoned" on pot.

THE INTERPERSONAL WORLD
OF THE LATE ADOLESCENT
The Family

The late adolescent years see the continuation of the struggle between dependence and independence. The struggle occurs not only between parents and child but also within the individual child. He both identifies with and is in conflict with his parents. This drive toward independence occurs in the family setting, so the total emotional climate of the home influences both the process and the outcome.

Climate of Feeling. Much has been made over the need of the infant for TLC—tender, loving care. Does TLC still make a difference to the adolescent?

The importance of "Pop" as a significant person in the development of his children has often been as slighted as the role of "Mom" has been emphasized. Several studies have reemphasized the importance of the father. The studies described in Chapter 15 illustrated that a disruption of the father-son relationship in early childhood and a sustained break in communication was closely related to aggressive, antisocial behavior in adolescent boys. Both Biller (1971) and Hetherington (1972) examined the impact of fathers on daughters. Biller's review led him to conclude that there was a positive relationship between heterosexual satisfaction and positive relationships with fathers. Hetherington investigated the impact of father absence due to divorce or death on girls 13 to 17 years old and found that early separation was more disruptive than later and that separation affected heterosexual relationships.

TLC has been defined to include support and nurturance. Two studies illustrate how these variables continue to influence adolescents. Gecas (1971) used the semantic differential as a measure of self-evaluation and related it to parental behavior. The significant parental behavior that influenced adolescents' self-evaluation of their power and worth was parental support. In his study of psychopaths and nonpsychopathic delinquent boys, Fodor (1973) used the Kohlberg moral-development scales and a self-report by these boys of parental child-rearing practices. The psychopaths saw their fathers as less nurturant and praising; the nonpsychopaths saw their mothers as more achievement-oriented.

The top 30 percent on intelligence tests of all tenth- and twelfth-grade pupils in the Quincy, Illinois, public schools in 1957–1958 served as subjects of an intensive study of achievement motivation. High-achieving boys and girls saw the father as more important in their lives than did low achievers of equal intelligence. Mothers of high-achieving boys differed from those of low achievers in being less strict, less intrusive, less suppressive of sex, less authoritarian, more approving of activity, and more communicative. On the other hand, mothers of high-achieving girls were more strict. (Pierce and Bowman, 1960)

Boys and girls seem to attach different meanings to achievement; differing maternal attitudes toward each influence their needs to achieve. This conclusion emerges not only from the longitudinal work of Kagan and Moss (1962) but also from the study by Shaw and Dutton (1962) of parental attitudes of bright, underachieving youngsters. The middle class boy from the democratic home is more achievement-oriented, whereas achievement orientation for the middle class girl seems to come from a more restrictive home environment. Further, achievement is desirable for boys in our society, and may not yet be so for girls. ". . . boys, even at the preschool level, are more pressed for achievement by their parents than are girls, from whom less is expected and from whom less is acceptable." (Block, 1973, p. 518) Whether such findings are still sound in the mid 1970s is unclear; we really do not know the effects of changing life styles, women's liberation, and social expectations.

We all are well aware of sex differences, yet we sometimes tend to hunt for commonalities between boys and girls when they do not exist on all dimensions. The important thing to consider is the personal meaning of behavior or attitude. These meanings may be very much dependent on sex. But when we single out any one variable, such as achievement, and compare by sex, we may lose the concept that each attitude, or pattern of behavior, is imbedded in a total organization—the self—and may take on different meanings depending upon that organization. The way the adolescent views his sex role, social class position, and family values is a unique combination of variables, and no one part of it explains it all.

What Can We Conclude? The family as an interpersonal field, providing a climate in which concepts of self are cultivated, continues to play its role throughout the growing-up years. The continuing impact of the family throughout the adolescent period serves to strengthen the original concepts formed in earlier periods. It is within this setting that all other family issues and problems occur, and solutions are dependent upon the climate of feeling.

Cultural Expectations. As we would expect, cultural variables are interwoven with emotional factors in their influence upon the adolescent. The Quincy researchers concluded: "Parents of high achievers were better educated (based on highest grade completed) than parents of low achievers. . . . High achievers' mothers held higher educational aspirations for them. . . . Small families produced proportionately more high achievers than did large families." (Pierce and Bowman, 1960, p. 65)

Another study of achievement motivation showed that middle class high school seniors, when material rewards were removed, continued to strive because they saw satisfaction as its own reward. Their lower class classmates, however, were more motivated by material reward than by success itself, and quit when the reward was withdrawn. (Douvan, 1956)

But life is not simple, and there are no perfect relationships between any one set of variables, such as class or education, and another set, such as achievement or attitude. We know that some youngsters from so-called disadvantaged homes make it, whereas some from advantaged homes do not. Harrison (1968) explored this phenomenon in relation to high school achievement. He studied the views of four groups (advantaged-successful, advantaged-nonsuccessful, disadvantaged-successful and disadvantaged-nonsuccessful) on control over the environment, attitude toward education, and the school group's and peer group's attitude toward education. He found that successful students, regardless of background, shared common attitudes, but this meant that the disadvantaged-successful adolescents broke away from their peer group's view of education. Social class was obviously not a useful single predictor. What leads the disadvantaged-successful to hold optimistic views of education and their own future, to differ from their peers? Much more needs to be known.

Tuma and Livson (1960) analyzed the children in the Berkeley Growth Study Group. These youngsters had been studied from their second year of life up until age 18. Although they were adolescents during World War II, the general findings still hold. They found that the late-maturing boy from a lower social class was the most conforming to both peer and school, whereas the boy from the higher socioeconomic class was the most unconventional in his behavior. Social class did not seem to matter in attitudes toward authority in the girls. If we extend Tuma and Livson's findings to observations of college students' behavior as they reacted to the Vietnam War, as they participated in becoming members of the "beat generation," and as they saw themselves as flower children, the picture seems to hold up. The more affluent were also probably the more openly rebellious.

Leaders in high school affairs, as judged by teachers, peers, and counselors, differed in home conditions from those not so identified. Whether the mother worked did not matter, but the presence of the father in the evening was related positively to leadership for girls. Other cultural and emotional factors favoring the leaders were ample work assignments in and out of the home, the use of praise and reasoning, adequate recreation facilities, participation in family planning, and freedom of choice on moral issues. (Barr and Hoover, 1957) Another way in which the emotional climate and cultural expectations are interwoven into the self of the adolescent is through the continuing process of identification.

Identification.   The key to the satisfactory emergence of the adolescent into independence may lie in the degree to which he has been successful in his identification with the parent of the same sex. We saw that the identification process began during infancy. With sexual maturity, a new understanding of oneself as male or female has to be accomplished. Indeed, sexual identification has been seen by Kagan and Moss (1962) as the central governor of behavior.

We know that the child's initial attempts at identifying succeed or fail upon the basis of his perception of their reception by the significant adult. If he receives feedback indicating that his father enjoys and fosters his attempts at identifying, if he perceives love as accompanying his efforts, then he probably makes a satisfactory identification. How well does this seem to survive in adolescence?

The evidence from clinics, juvenile courts, and the guidance counselors in high schools seems to support the importance of father-son identification as a significant variable in the self-concept and behavior of the adolescent boy. Research evidence (Bandura and Walters, 1959; and Mussen, 1961) strengthens the hypothesis that identification is both important to adolescent boys and has its roots in the early childhood relationship. The adolescent's present perception of his father is highly related to identification. The boy who identifies with his father is also, on the average, the boy who perceives of his father as a highly rewarding, affectionate person and of the parent-child relationship as warm and rewarding. Medinnus (1965) found that for both boys and girls high self-acceptance was related to the perception of parents as loving and nonrejecting. This seems to be more true for boys than for girls. In his study, in contrast to the ones above, the role of the mother seemed more critical than that of the father.

Identification in adolescence is not equivalent to copying the behav-

ior of parents, nor is it equivalent to absorption of the parental image *in
toto.* It seems to be a selective process in which the boy or girl evaluates
various aspects of parental behavior, feelings, and values and chooses
those particular life patterns that harmonize with his total self-structure.
For instance, college freshmen women rated a series of ideas for themselves and as they thought their mothers would rate them. What seemed
to emerge was that the daughters' subjective appraisal or perception of
the mothers' similarity to her was more important in identification than any
real similarity. (Dignan, 1965) The survey research by Douvan and Adelson (1966) indicated that feminine girls accepted their inner conflicts and
revealed a high degree of self-organization. They seemed more able than
the nonfeminine to identify with some particular adult or group of adults,
to name more sources of self-esteem, to be more open to looking at their
future, and more involved in social activities. These researchers seem to
agree that girls seek their models from a wide variety of sources, rather
than just the mother. Girls seem more oriented toward interpersonal adequacy, whereas boys are more oriented toward occupational achievement.

The potency of sex-role identification and its effects on other attitudes and behavior is illustrated in Baruch's (1972) finding that a college
woman's devaluation of professional competence was a function of a
standard learned from a nonworking mother. Block's (1973) analysis of
sex-role stereotypes held by university students in five European countries
and the United States demonstrated cross-national agreements that men
were practical, shrewd, assertive, dominating, competitive, and self-controlled; women were loving, affectionate, impulsive, sympathetic, and
generous. According to Block, who based her theory on her interpretation of Bakan's (1966) dichotomy of behavior into agency and communion,
men are reared to favor the agency aspects, women the communion. The
above variables found to differentiate in the cross-national study reflect
these two modes. That is, agency is more active, aggressive, and indi-
vidualistic; communion is more empathic, affective, and communal. From
her viewpoint, "personal maturity is associated with greater integration of
agency and communion." (Block, 1973, p. 520)

How is this related to identification within the family? Block and her
colleagues analyzed data from the California longitudinal studies to seek
antecedents. They were able to categorize adolescents into four groups
on the basis of scores on the California Psychological Inventory femininity
and socialization scales: high on sex-role identity and socialization, low
on both, and two groups of high on one and low on the other. Those
adolescents who were high on sex-role appropriateness and socialization
or low on sex-role and high on socialization came from homes where
parents were psychologically healthy. In the former case, "both parents
were available to the child, both physically and psychologically, through
adolescence, and the like-sex parent appeared to be the more salient

figure for identification." (p. 523) In the latter case, the "parents offered more complex, less traditional sex-role differentiations as a model . . . [and] had established emotionally satisfying and value-inculcating homes for their children." (Block, 1973, p. 524) In the case of low-socialized adolescents, family patterns were unhealthy. Block concludes that socialization has a freeing effect for men but a restricting one for women.

Another example of identification with stereotyped roles is the study by Williamson and Seevard (1971) of Chilean adolescents. Boys perceived men as braver, stronger, wiser, more competent, and with higher leadership than women; girls saw women as more sensitive, less excitable, and more passive than men. The picture is not much different from the cross-national one.

Conflict. The cause of conflict is not a result only of the adolescent years; its roots lie in the total family situation and history. However, because of the particular demands of this age group, conflict becomes a focal factor in the parent-adolescent relationship.

There seems to be a degree of universality in parent-adolescent conflict in technological societies. We find it reported not only in American, Japanese, and West European research publications; it also seems to exist in Communist states. A Polish psychologist, using self-reporting techniques, found that adolescents living in small towns near Warsaw perceived that the conflict stemmed from restrictions placed upon them, differences of opinion with adults, and adult character traits. Only 3 percent were not bothered by such conflicts, and one-third reported that conflict was frequent. (Skorijpska, 1958) It is interesting to note the projection of blame onto the adults!

Why is conflict so visible, and perhaps universal, at this time? Ausubel claims, "The most important single cause of parent-youth conflict is the perseveration of parents' attitudes that interfere with the adolescent's greatly expanded need for volitional independence." (Ausubel, 1954, p. 226) This is true particularly when the youngster possesses a car and holds a part-time job, the manifestation of a modicum of economic independence. Previously, parents could be resisted only to a point, and even then much of the resistance had to be covert. The late adolescent can no longer easily accept many of the restrictions that continue to be placed upon him.

The adolescent boy is perhaps in a more favorable position than his sister. Even though his parents worry about his "hotrodding" or joyriding, his choice of friends, his late hours, they somehow recognize the cultural axiom that "boys will be boys."

Girls, however, even in homes that tend to be permissive, find their activities much more curtailed. The attitude of parents becomes more, rather than less, authoritarian. Both parents are haunted by the specter that their daughter might get "in trouble." They tend to doubt the impact of whatever moral training they themselves have imparted and try to clamp down. Of course, the adolescent being what she is, clamping often has the reverse effect. Girls often report that their parents don't trust them and rationalize their own behavior on this account. The threat of pregnancy looms much larger to the parent than it does to the girl.

Unfortunately, parents' fears are reinforced by statistics that show not only an increase in the number of illegitimate births but also a decrease in the average age of the unwed mother. Although these girls represent all social classes in our society, the statistics are biased by the ability of the upper middle and upper classes to resort to abortion or to arrange adoption. Although the overt manifestation of the conflict may be the time of homecoming or the choice of friends, the latent issue is often sex and, seen concomitantly by parents, drugs.

Cottle (1971), in reflecting as an adult on adult reactions to adolescents, expresses it most lyrically:

> Another part of socialization is the onset of the battle of battles, that war against oppression and imperialism fought out first in the hideaway tree houses and alleys of childhood. It is the battle against those by whose loins our existence owes its permanence. . . .
> In the end, however, we come to recognize the well-delineated stress points of independence and dependence. For despite our protestations, it is essential that we believe that our place of origin, our home base, will not budge one millimeter under the impact of our energies, our shoving off, or our first steps and later stampeding in space. [Cottle, 1971, pp. 327, 331]

Perhaps the movement toward early marriage or living together represents youth's search for the solution to the conflict. Youth wants independence but cannot fully achieve it in the home; youth wants a mature sex relationship and recognizes that clandestine or promiscuous relationships are unsatisfactory; youth wants to be adult in a society that requires that longer and longer years be devoted to education. Although older generations may deplore the trend, it may actually be a better solution to youth's problems than continued frustration of the urge toward growth and maturity. Whether the new patterns of living create other problems remains to be seen.

Some conflict will most likely occur in all families. However, we can infer from the data that the family that has involved the child in decision making, that accepts the growth urge, and that provides him with a supportive but liberating emotional climate most likely will enable the adolescent to develop a value system and a sense of personal worth and dignity. An adequate and secure concept of himself may enable him to resolve the dependence-independence quandary successfully.

The Community

A fundamental change in the relationship between the youngster and the adult world occurs during the adolescent period. Although it would be difficult to say exactly when this occurs, it becomes quite marked during the high school years. This change is the emergence of the adolescent as a market.

The adolescent as a consumer is big business. The mass media are turned to not only for stories but for market trends in clothes, records, tapes, cosmetics, and entertainment. The place of the adolescent in the large community as a purchaser of services has led to youth consumer surveys, the popularity of the disc jockey, the creation of special-appeal magazines such as *Mad, Seventeen,* and *Hot Rod,* the establishment of teenage credit card systems, and the lowering of the age of majority to 18. Most American teenagers buy their own records and sports equipment and their own clothes. They seem to have the pocket money to spend on electronic equipment—cassette recorders, stereos, tapes, etc. The late adolescent is a force in shaping his community. Because he is the consumer, movies feature his rock stars, unknowns sell records by the million, TV ads cater to his taste, TV programs include his music groups.

The record industry is an excellent example of the effect of the teenager on the adult world. Records purchased by teenagers or played on the radio provide spectacular profits for record companies. It is impossible to listen to the radio for any length of time without becoming aware of the broadcaster's concept of his most important audience. In a very real sense, teenage taste dictates what adults hear and see in the entertainment field. The size and importance of the market is indicated also by the periodic scandals about payoffs (cash, drugs, sex) to disc jockeys to push certain records. To know what teenagers think or believe, listen to any "top 40" station. But don't let the words alone divert you—the sound is also essential for an understanding of the values and concepts of the adolescent peer culture. Buying and judging are serious affairs. One's status may well rest upon the ability to consume wisely. Consumption is a key societal value, and although what is consumed may be related to the age group, the elevation of consumption to its prime position was accomplished originally by adult training. The late adolescent is thus demonstrating that he has met a major qualification for admission to the adult American world: he spends money.

Generally, the late adolescent plays a more significant role than younger age groups in influencing the adult world. This influence is brought to bear through the actions of his peers as a group, rather than by his behavior as an individual. He even brings his group into family situations to help him persuade his parents to allow him to behave in certain ways. He influences both the economy and the political situation of adult society. Although he is still denied adult status (until 18 in elections), he makes his presence felt. Just look back on the 1960s (and even through the 1972 election) to note the effect of youngsters both on the conscience of society (the civil rights movement and the Vietnam War) and on its political and moral scandals (Watergate being explained by officials as part of a reaction to youth antiwar attitudes and behavior).

The School

The adolescent's role as a molder of society is not limited to the transactional fields of entertainment, politics, and the home. The effect of peer group life on the high school and the attempts of the high school faculty to understand and use peer group dynamics are realities beneath the academic surface.

The process by which what were once extracurricular activities became first "cocurricular" and then "curriculum" is an excellent example of adolescent influence on the school program. Baton twirling, formerly a stunt, is now taught in many schools as a part of physical education. Clubs and societies, formerly limited to after-school time, now meet during the school day.

But the high school of the 1970s is in trouble. In the early 1970s (1969–1972 at least), the normal structure of organized clubs, student government, and planned activities decayed rapidly. Youth just did not want it. It may be being reassembled now, but the formerly placid scene is gone. Part of this may be due to drugs, but part is due to the increasing awareness of youth that the high school, as presently constituted, is, in their words, "a bad scene." At best it is irrelevant in its curriculum and organization for many; at worst it resembles a prison. "A large part of the high school population . . . finds itself enmeshed in an institution that has little relevance to present and future needs." (Handlin, 1969, p. 353)

In Chapter 8 we saw that the schools become what the powerful elements in the community wish them to be. If football and basketball are more important than academic work, the fault lies neither with the faculty nor with the philosophy of education but with the people who would rather build a stadium than a library and who pay the coach more than the principal. The adult community, wanting its bread and circuses, its parades and football games, not only sanctions but encourages such situations. The school, under such circumstances, is exploited by both the adult and adolescent communities.

Schools do influence their students, although not always in the way that teachers or society planned. The school as a total culture, including the socioeconomic makeup of its student body, serves as a force. Elder (1968) indicates that lower class youngsters are more vulnerable to school pressures. He further suggests, however, that we need many more careful studies that pay more attention to subgroups (such as bright students from lower social class families) in our analyses of information. Kleinfeld (1972) found that black high school girls were more influenced by teachers' evaluations of their academic ability than were white girls. Boyle (1966) surveyed Canadian adolescents and reported that these students' college aspirations were related to the status of the high school they attended. This may be due in part, he said, to the academic programs, but it also seemed to be due to the influence of the peer group.

Just how do faculties view their responsibilities toward adolescents? How does teacher behavior affect pupil self-development? High school faculties are fundamentally concerned with subject matter. They see the high school as a place for intellectual training. They set academic standards and enforce them. But many also recognize the importance of social and personal development and see the school as having some responsibility in this area.

The high school culture is a fusion of teacher and adult cultural forces and peer cultural forces. The student is influenced by both and uses the peer society to aid him in finding his way through the adult-imposed patterns. Let us take a look at how this works out in practice. First, we will examine the impact of the adult pattern on the pupil; then we will study the high school peer group.

Academic expectations are made known to students in a variety of ways: grading, grouping, reprimanding, warning slips, and parent conferences. Behavioral standards are enforced by suspensions, dismissals and assignments to special adjustment schools.

In many schools dress regulations are in force—mostly dealing with the length of boys' hair and the shortness of girls' skirts. Subject-matter requirements are still in Carnegie units—so much history, English, math. Attendance and conduct are regulated. Track systems separate the academic from the nonacademic students. Separate high schools teach vocational subjects. There are a variety of ways by which the schools establish status positions for students based on achievement, social class, race, sex, age.

But, it would be dangerous to see the high school as homogeneous. Many are trying varieties of approaches—individual learning, time modular units, open campuses, community involvement. Students respond to their own school climate, from their own frameworks, rather than *all* high schoolers responding to *all* high schools. For example, Ptaschnik used a Q-sort approach to see what students saw as relevant and irrelevant in three city schools—one predominantly black, one white and one integrated. There were common elements; students saw schools as preparing them for more schooling, as helping them learn about degree-type job opportunities, and as helping them learn about other people. Academic subjects, however, were not seen as relevant. In particular, business and secretarial skills, history, science, and learning about sex were irrelevant. There were differences across schools that seemed to be functions of the school's unique climate. One of the reasons for student classifications seemed to be the discrepancy between what was going on and what students wanted—in both directions. That is, schools might be stressing something students thought they already knew or didn't need to know; or schools might not be teaching what students wanted.

In either case, school and students are out of phase. Many schools are now going to implement preparenthood programs based on the concept that there are parenting attitudes and skills. For example, there is the program for the Educational Development Corporation funded by the U.S. Office of Education and the Office of Child Development "to help teenagers prepare for effective parenthood through working with young children and learning about child development and the role of parents." (HEW, 1973, EDC, 1972) Will students see this as relevant, or will it be out of phase, too, as they struggle with their own identities and find little energy or ambition left over to care for day-care center children? Adult expectations are thus differentially perceived by students, and the degree to which they are fulfilled seems to be a function of teacher behavior and pupil perception of self and teacher.

How important to the high school pupil is the acceptance of adult expectation? C. W. Gordon's intensive sociological study of a midwestern high school led him to conclude: "The behavior of the adolescent was found to be associated with his generalized status . . . the dominant orientation to action was to accept those roles which would establish a prestige position in the informal [peer] organization. Grade achievement was least significantly related to general status; achievement in student activities was most significantly related to a favorable social position." (Gordon, 1957, p. 22) Coleman (1965) came to a similar finding.

It may be said that the high school, as constituted today, presents the students with a dual image: a formal, adult-controlled, and supervised program of instruction and an informal, peer-controlled program. Both attempt to manipulate the other, both copy techniques from the other; but the peer culture is dominant in the perception of the student.

THE PEER CULTURE

The role of the peer culture as an aspect of higher education has long been recognized by college personnel workers and researchers. Perhaps Freedman's comments on the entering American college student, vintage 1959, are relevant to an understanding of the high school junior and senior and the school culture as a setting for peer culture. He says of the peer culture:

> *We contend in fact that this culture is the prime educational force at work in the college, for as we shall see, assimilation into the student society is the foremost concern of most new students. Suffice it to*

say now that in our opinion the scholastic and academic aims and processes of the college are in large measure transmitted to incoming students or mediated for them by the predominant student culture. . . .

The students' culture provides order and comfort. It teaches students how to behave in various social situations, what to think about all manner of issues, how to deal with common problems and troublesome external influences. It offers instruction in how to keep the faculty at a distance, how to bring pressure that will insure that the faculty behave in expected and therefore manageable ways. . . .

There are students who have been unable to develop internal agencies of control, who consequently have depended for a long time upon the direction of their peers. Separation from the peer group would put them under a very severe strain. This is a source of that rigid adherence to peer values which we sometimes see in individual students. It is also a factor making for resistance to change in the culture itself. [*Freedman, 1960, pp. 4–5*]

Indeed, Sanford suggests that one of the main functions of the peer culture is to allow some college students to avoid any real involvement with adults and to maintain their stereotypic views of adults. (Sanford, 1962) Coleman's (1965) study of a number of midwestern schools leads to similar conclusions. Status was a function of athletics and activities far more than of scholarship. However, in the minds of the parents, being a brilliant student was more important than either being popular or an athletic or activity leader.

Functions of the Peer Group

Gordon defines the four functions fulfilled by the high school cliques in his study:

1. *As collective prestige units which defined the individual's status.*
2. *As a means for cooperative competition for preferred objects such as dates, school offices, gossip, home work assignments, clothing knowledge, and transportation.*
3. *To provide the individual with a sense of adequacy in grade achievement competition. The capacity of the grading system to threaten the personal security of the individual was greatly reduced by the protection the clique afforded.*
4. *As arbiters of approved behavior and raters of persons in such a way as to operate the "rules of the game" by demanding conformity of both clique and nonclique members to approved standards of conduct* [*Gordon, 1957, pp. 105–106*]

Belonging to a clique is deemed vital by adolescents. It is through such group membership that dates are arranged, experimentation in liquor, sex, and smoking provided and discussed, consumption styles in clothes set, and moral reputations made and broken. In the small, face-to-face group, the communications network that permeates adolescent culture begins and ends.

The clique, or peer group, thus functions as the arbiter of social behavior, the protector from adult pressure, and the provider of experience and status. If one belongs to the "right" group and behaves in the "right" way, he's "got it made." To arrive at this enviable position takes time, effort, and money, but the satisfactions, as perceived by the adolescent, are generally worth the cost.

Organization

There is a definite hierarchical pattern both among and between peer groups in high school. Groups are known as "wheels," "brains," and by various other nicknames that convey their status position. The athletic crowd may be called "the jocks"; the drinking group, "the beer boys." There are the "potheads," and the "squares," and so on. Each group member knows this status system, even though he may express resentment about his place in the pecking order. Within the group, status is related to reputation and behavior. The more closely one approximates the values of his group, the more secure is his position and the higher his status. Since adolescent groups tend to value the doer, the roles of the "go-getter," "the popularity kid," and the "athlete" are accorded high status. To become a leader in the eyes of one's peers requires performance. The "brain" (the obvious academic scholar) is not valued, except within his own clique of "brains," who are usually low in the general social order.

A Canadian study of eleventh-grade boys serves as an example of the status system within the group. A sociometric, a social-reputation test, and a variety of personality test data were collected and analyzed. The only widely acknowledged leader of this particular group of boys was an active, carefree, optimistic, cheerful youngster, who actually lived up to his group's expectation that he would take an active lead. The followers in this group were less active and tended to be less emotionally stable and more subdued. "The reasons for isolation by the group appeared to be a lack of conformity to group standards and undue criticism of the group." (Munro, 1957, p. 159) In microcosm, this group might be said to be fairly typical of the adolescent peer culture.

Social class membership also acts as a variable in determining one's role, reputation, and behavior in the peer culture and the peer group. Where clothes are a sign of belonging, the lower class youngster often cannot compete. The values of leisure time, record collections, electronic gear, and a car as prestige symbols also discriminate against the lower class high school student. He belongs to his own peer groups, but they tend to have low status in the overall high school picture.

With desegregation of schools, ethnicity has become an increasingly important factor in the peer culture. The high school status system is influenced by the percentage of mixture as well as by prevailing attitudes. (Lundberg and Dickson, 1952) Ethnic groups within the high school differ on how they see leadership (Maas, 1954, Mastroianni and Khatena, 1972), on government, and on whether neighborhoods, clubs, and friends should be on a segregated basis. (Mastroianni and Khatena, 1972) Interracial relationships are exacerbated by militant whites who see other whites as "nigger lovers" and by militant blacks who see other blacks as "Toms" or "Oreos."

Peer groups are nonegalitarian in their organizational framework. Status is a function of approved behavior, which, in turn, is influenced by social class and caste membership and by personality variables.

How do adolescents perceive this pecking order? Coleman (1965) asked, "What does it take to get into the leading crowd in this school?" There were, as we would expect, differences for boys and girls, as well as differences depending upon whether the school was urban or rural or middle or lower class. For the girls, personality, good looks, good clothes, and a good reputation were the major criteria. For the boys, achievement, particularly athletic achievement, was a prime path to acceptance. Having a car was more significant in many of these schools than good grades. The leading crowd in these schools seemed to be defined mostly in terms of social success.

Activities

Perhaps the most significant activity, both from an adult and an adolescent point of view, is *dating*. Going steady becomes an important pattern for social behavior in the high school, although the pressures begin in junior high. Originally, dates are sought because of the pressure of the peer culture rather than the presence of a real, intrinsic interest in a particular person of the opposite sex.

Dating becomes a device by which one has a partner to be with when the gang goes someplace. Going steady seems to be an extension of this arrangement rather than a precursor of marriage. It provides one with security, status, and reduced competition. Although going steady may be perceived as a highly useful practice by teenagers, "Adolescents often found it difficult to make adjustments to the expectations and intimate associations. . . . The desire for security and predictability of social activity and the expectations of peers often made it very difficult to dissolve the relationships." (Crist, 1953, p. 26)

For boys, sexual desire reaches its peak between the ages of 14 and

18. Both boys and girls realize that boys see dating as providing opportunities for the boy to "go as far as he can." Christensen's study of the opinions of 2500 high school youths shows that boys are seen as more thoughtless, natural, and sex-driven and that girls are categorized as more inhibited, touchy, and money-minded. (Christensen, 1952)

Unfortunately, much of the research on dating is dated or outdated. It may even be that, for many youngsters, the concept of dating as known in literature through the early 1960s is no longer relevant to their lives. New forms of boy-girl relationships, some even without overt sexual overtones, may be emerging. However, dating and sexual behavior are not equivalent terms; there may be one without the other. Blaine (1967) analyzed the problems on both the high school and college campus and concluded, "There seems to be no thoroughly satisfactory answer to the problems presented by our instinctual sex drive. Perhaps this is why the story of the eating of the apple in the Garden of Eden is so deeply appealing." (p. 1975)

Offer (1971) conducted a longitudinal study of a group of suburban, middle class adolescents from their entry into high school until three years after graduation. His youth had entered high school about 1963 and were unaffected by the impact of the last decade. He found girls dated earlier than boys and were more preoccupied with sexuality. Ten percent of his group had intercourse before the end of the junior year. He later studied a large sample of youth in the United States and Australia and reported little change in attitude between 1962 and 1970. He didn't see a sexual revolution. (Offer, 1972) On the other hand, Robinson, King, and Balswick (1972) saw signs of such a revolution for college girls between 1965 and 1970 in both attitudes and behavior. In the case of Marty (Chapter 16), we saw her confusion about sex and the expectations concerning it in her group. It is now even more complicated, because it is somewhat interwoven with the drug scene:

> *Although the language remains unchanged, actions of "procuring" and "scoring" today refer to drugs. The prophylactic, its slick package dirtied by months in the seams of an old wallet, has been replaced by the nickel bag: "Always be prepared." A funny reversal, furthermore, concerns sex role functions in a new economic market, as girls now solicit funds to pay for their boyfriends' stuff. I was stopped by one of these girls in the street on a beautiful October afternoon: "Excuse me, sir," she began her proposal, "how about a quarter for a cup of God knows what?" . . . The subject, however, is close to the conversational surface. It is as intimate as it ever was, but seemingly beginning to be freed of its irrational ties to some mysterious and primordial secrecy. As with much of their behavior, many of the young merely make overt what their elders do covertly.*
> [Cottle, 1971, p. 84]

At best, we can say that much of what is reported in the media may be more myth than fact; real data are hard to come by, and we lack a true perspective on the current high school rating and dating scene. Although there seems to be much more openness, some say this began after World War I, and we are merely seeing the covert become overt. For instance, a generation ago Farnham said, "any society which gives drivers' licenses and automobiles to boys of seventeen and allows them to take girls of the same age out in those cars is clearly in no position to police the situation. That is exactly what is going on." (Farnham, 1952, p. 124)

Sexual behavior is a central problem for the high school youth. As Early (1973) reports, adolescents are ill-informed about sex, and its possible consequences (VD and pregnancy), and how to prevent them; and state laws and administrative procedures prevent them from gaining access to information. Adolescents do not seem to be concerned about the possibilities (or probabilities) of getting VD, although college youngsters are concerned about the risk of pregnancy. The irony is that it is often the very parents who are unable to communicate about sex to their own children (Sorenson [1973] indicates that over 70 percent of adolescents say they cannot talk freely with their parents about sex) who have been most adamant in their resistance to sex education in the schools.

It is clear, then, why the peer group attains such great significance. The adolescent spends much peer-group time talking about sex; he reads helpful hints in newspaper columns and magazines; he reports this as a major concern on problem checklists and opinion polls. We can understand this anxiety when we view dating and partying as the activity in which the youngster comes to grips with the conflicts between his sex-role identification, physical urges, religious and social class mores, peer pressure, and the value system he has internalized up to this time. It is no wonder that so much time and effort are expended in the reflective bull sessions or hen parties that occur after and between dates or parties.

THE DRUG SCENE

The one phenomenon that is perhaps different in this generation of adolescents is the drug scene. Drugs have been with us for centuries and have been used by sophisticates or subcultures without much uproar. Cole Porter's song of the 1930s, "I Get a Kick Out of You" originally had as its first line, "I get no kick from cocaine"; the last word was changed for radio to *champagne*.

The differences seen in today's society seem to be (1) the widespread use of marijuana as well as psychedelic, barbiturate, and narcotic drugs; (2) the much lower age level involved; (3) the use by middle and upper middle class youth; and (4) the relationship that has been assumed between drug use and a counter culture tied into the politics of the last two presidential elections and the struggle against the Vietnam War. However, teenage drug use seems to be worldwide (we lack data from such countries as the Soviet Union and China), at least in industrial societies.

As in the case of sexual behavior, much has been written and sensationalized, but hard data, unlike hard drugs, is difficult to procure. What is the percentage of use? When does use become abuse? How harmful is pot? Who really becomes addicted? Aren't cigarette smoking and alcohol consumption both more prevalent and more dangerous? The answers are not in, but considerable research of all kinds is being conducted. It seems clear that alcohol is a more serious national and personal problem than drugs; that cigarettes may kill more people (and are being smoked more heavily by adolescents [Tamerin, 1973]); and that the verdict on marijuana is not in. Hard drugs, barbituates, and LSD are definitely harmful. The current (1973) fad of quaaludes, made in chemistry labs on college campuses, is dangerous. The phenomenon of seeing smoking and drug and alcohol use used as a common category, with the assumption, therefore, of some common causation and perhaps common effects, is found, for example, in *Psychological Abstracts,* which uses the three terms together as a classification for research reports.

What little do we know? Tec (1971) indicated that high school youngsters were aware that some of their friends used marijuana but that most had not tried it themselves; they accepted that others had without rejecting them and saw other drugs as harmful. Various studies on college campuses indicate both the casual acceptance and heavy use of marijuana by students in all fields. Indeed, peer rumors float that medical students are not only into pot but know how to make the best synthetic drugs, such as quaaludes.

Winick states that there are "between 16 and 17 million young drug dependents . . . glue sniffing peaks from eleven to thirteen, marijuana use is common from fourteen to eighteen, amphetamine use is most common from seventeen to nineteen, and barbituates and LSD tend to be used by young adults in their 20s." (Winick, 1973, p. 433) He suggests ten reasons for the increase in drug use since 1945: affluence, changing sex roles, need for rituals, Vietnam, rock music, television, nonrationality, competition, reward for illness, and risk-taking behavior (pp. 434–435). This view that many of the causes are social rather than personal may mean that our usual academic approach—drug education—will prove useless. There are already indications that this is so. It seems fairly clear that drug use is related to involvement in a subculture (Gay and Gay, 1971; Garritano, 1972; Whitehead, Smart and Laforest, 1972; Cohen, 1972; David, 1972; and Goode, 1972), which means that any approach to both understanding and treatment (for abuse) requires that we go beyond the individual and beyond moralistic and legalistic approaches. This does not mean that there are not personality and family variables associated with abuse. Streit and Oliver (1972), for example, demonstrated a high relationship between drug abuse and perceived lack of family closeness. It means that both personal and societal factors, working in a transactional fashion, influence who will be an abuser and the degree of drug use and abuse in the population.

It may be that personality and family variables are the key to who *does not* become a user in the midst of widespread use. The report of the House Select Committee on Crime, as quoted by Gailey in the *St. Petersburg Times* on June 30, 1973, stated: "Drug abuse in our schools has become so extensive and pervasive that it is only the uniquely gifted and self-possessed child who is capable of avoiding involvement with some form of drug abuse." (Gailey, 1973, p. 19A)

It should not be inferred that sex and drugs are the sole activity of high school youth. They are active in games and sports; they watch TV and listen to the radio and records; they have hobbies of all sorts. About a third of the high school youngsters spent three or more hours a week working on a hobby or on other special interests. (Purdue, 1967) Although the poll showed that television viewing had dropped off since 1960, the average youngster still watched between one and four hours a day. Radio listening seemed to be related to social class, sex, and age. Girls from high-income groups and older students listened more to radio. Boys, younger students, and students from low-income families were more likely to watch television.

Peer-Adult Interaction

The previous discussion makes any lengthy discussion here unnecessary. We can say that the nature of the adult-adolescent interaction is essentially limited by hostility at one end and dependence-submission at the other, with most contact being essentially analogous to an armed truce, at least in Western society. The adolescent peer culture continues to exist because it offers that certain something to the youngster that the adult world denies—status. Although individual adults may be respected and even idolized, the adult world as a whole is viewed with suspicion. Although adult values permeate the peer group and the peer culture influences the adult world, the relationship is not a peaceful one.

The Peer Group and the Individual

The demands for conformity during the high school years are great. To belong, the boy or girl is expected to accept the group's values, conduct, dress, and speech. Although this may be seen as essential by group members in helping them accomplish whatever purposes they may have, it raises the problem of the loss of individuality. Must one surrender to belong?

The answer lies within the self of the individual adolescent. Certainly, most adolescents seek to participate actively in the peer culture. We know they are highly aware of the hierarchical structure. Some need so desperately to belong to prestige groups that they seem to be willing to go to any length. Others draw the line at different points and join groups more compatible with their own goals.

Social psychological research on resistance to pressure seems to indicate that it is very difficult for most youngsters to be the lone holdout against group judgment. The presence of others who disagree or the existence of other peer groups one can join make it easier for the adolescent to maintain his position. If he is caught in a situation in which he perceives that "everyone is doing it," the going gets rough.

McDavid's study (1959) seems to indicate that the ability of adolescent boys to withstand group pressure may depend upon whether they are task-oriented or person-oriented. One hundred and sixty-five boys between 16 and 18 were placed in situations in which it appeared that they were alone in arriving at a particular conclusion (number of clicks heard over a "radio"). The evidence suggests that those who yielded and changed their count were boys who were motivated to conform by the desire not to be different. They were person-oriented. Those who resisted were message-oriented or task-oriented. They maintained a relatively firm perceptual view and shaped the interpretation to conform to this view; they chose not to change.

In view of the popularity of the claim that we are becoming more and more a person-oriented or "other-directed" society, we may wonder how many adolescents would be able to maintain their views. Maybe, at home, in the culture at large, and in school, we are training them to be more person-oriented, thus defeating our professed concern for the integrity of the individual.

In any event, to the individual adolescent, insofar as he perceives it to be crucial to him to belong, the peer group will be a shaper and molder of his values and behavior. His total self-concept and the situations in which he finds himself will determine the roles he will play in his peer culture.

SUMMARY

In this chapter we have considered both the physical and social forces at work upon the self of the late adolescent. We have seen both the continuation of earlier patterns of self-environment transactions and the emergence of new meanings and behavior. We have noted the increasing power of the late adolescent not only to cope with but also to modify his social situation. Not only is he physically mature by the end of the late adolescent period; he is also ready to absorb adult ways of relating to the world.

In Chapter 18 we will explore the concomitant changes in his private world and self-concept as he moves toward adulthood.

REFERENCES AND ADDITIONAL READINGS

Ausubel, D. *Theory and problems of adolescent development.* New York: Grune & Stratton, 1954.

Bakan, D. *The duality of human existence.* Chicago: Rand McNally, 1966.

Bandura, A., & Walters, R. *Adolescent aggression.* New York: Ronald Press, 1959.

Barr, J., & Hoover, K. Home conditions and influences associated with the development of high school leaders. *Educational Administration and Supervision,* 1957, *43,* 271–279.

Baruch, G. K. Maternal influences upon college women's attitudes toward women and work. *Developmental Psychology,* 1972, *6,* 32–37.

Biller, H. Fathering and female sexual development. *Medical Aspects of Human Sexuality,* 1971, *5,* 126–138.

Blaine, G. B., Jr. Sex and the adolescent. *New York Journal of Medicine,* 1967, *67,* 1967–1975.

Block, J. Conceptions of sex role, some cross-cultural and longitudinal perspectives. *American Psychologist,* 1973, *28,* 512–526.

Boyle, R. The effect of high school on students' aspirations. *The American Journal of Sociology,* 1966, *71,* 628–639.

Christensen, H. Dating behavior as evaluated by high school students. *The American Journal of Sociology,* 1952, *57,* 580–586.

Cohen, H. Multiple drug use considered in the light of the stepping-stone hypothesis. *International Journal of the Addictions,* 1972, *7,* 27–55.

Coleman, J. S. The adolescent culture. *Social Climates in High Schools.* Cooperative Research Monograph No. 4. Washington, D.C.: U.S. Department of Health, Education, and Welfare, 1965. Pp. 9–29. Reprinted in I. J. Gordon (Ed.), *Human development: Readings in research.* Glenview, Ill.: Scott, Foresman, 1965.

Cottle, T. J. *Time's children: Impressions of youth.* Boston: Little, Brown, 1971.

Crist, J. R. High school dating as a behavior system. *Marriage and Family Living,* 1953, *15(1),* 23–28.

David, H. P. Drugs and the adolescent: A WHO report. *Journal of Psychiatrict Nursing & Mental Health Services,* 1972, *10(1),* 30–32.

Dignan, M. H., Sr. Ego identity and maternal gratification. *Journal of Personal and Social Psychology,* 1965, *1,* 476–483.

Douvan, E. Social status and success strivings. *Journal of Abnormal and Social Psychology,* 1956, *52,* 219–225.

Douvan, E., & Adelson, J. *The adolescent experience.* New York: Wiley, 1966.

Early, G. Adolescent sexual attitudes and behavior. *Sharing,* 1973, 12–15. Washington, D.C.: Consortium on Early Childbearing and Childrearing.

Educational Development Center. *Exploring childhood.* Cambridge, Mass.: EDC, 1972.

Elder, G., Jr. *Adolescent socialization and personality development.* Chicago: Rand McNally, 1968.

Farnham, M. *The adolescent.* New York: Harper & Row, 1952.

Fejer, D., & Smart, R. G. Drug use, anxiety and psychological problems among adolescents. *Ontario Psychologist,* 1972, *4(1),* 10–21.

Fisher, S. Power orientation and concept of self height in men: Preliminary note. *Perceptual and Motor Skills*, 1964, *18*, 732.

Fodor, E. Moral development and parent behavior antecedents in adolescent psychopaths. *The Journal of Genetic Psychology*, 1973, *122*, 37–43.

Freedman, M. Some observations of students as they relate to orientation procedures in colleges and universities. *The Journal of College Student Personnel*, 1960, *2*,2–10.

Gailey, P. Drug "crisis" seen in schools. *St. Petersburg Times*, June 30, 1973, p. 19A.

Garitano, W. W. Youth and drugs. *Drug Forum*, 1972, *1*(2), 195–199.

Gay, A. C., & Gay, G. R. Haight-Ashbury: Evolution of a drug culture in a decade of mendacity. *Journal of Psychedelic Drugs*, 1971, *4*(1), 81–90.

Gecas, V. Parental behavior and dimensions of adolescent self-evaluation. *Sociometry*, 1971, *34*(4), 466–482.

Goode, E. Cigarette smoking and drug use on a college campus. *International Journal of the Addictions*, 1972, *7*(1), 133–140.

Gordon, C. W. *The social system of the high school.* New York: Free Press, 1957.

Handlin, O. Live students and dead education. In J. Stone & F. Schneider (Eds.), *Readings in the foundations of education.* New York: Crowell, 1969. Pp. 351–362.

Harrison, I. Relationship between home background, school success, and adolescent attitudes. *Merrill-Palmer Quarterly*, 1968, *14*, 331–344.

Hetherington, E. M. Effects of father absence on personality development in adolescent daughters. *Developmental Psychology*, 1972, *7*, 313–326.

Jimerson, P. How selected classifications of pupils in two city high schools perceive various dimensions of the school environment. *Psychological Abstracts*, 1971, *32*, 5106A.

Kagan, J., & Moss, H. *Birth to maturity.* New York: Wiley, 1962.

Kleinfeld, J. The relative importance of teachers and parents in the formation of Negro and white students' academic self-concept. *Journal of Educational Research*, 1972, *65*, 211–212.

Lundberg, G., & Dickson, L. Inter-ethnic relations in a high-school population. *The American Journal of Sociology*, 1952, *58*, 1–10.

McDavid, J. Personality and situational determinants of conformity. *Journal of Abnormal and Social Psychology*, 1959, *58*, 241–246.

Maas, H. The role of member in the clubs of lower-class and middle-class adolescents. *Child Development*, 1954, *25*, 241–251.

Mastroianni, M., & Khatena, J. The attitudes of black and white high school seniors toward integration. *Sociology and Social Research*, 1972, *56*, 221–227.

Medinnus, G. R. Adolescents' self-acceptance and perceptions of their parents. *Journal of Consulting Psychology*, 1965, *29*, 15–154.

Moore, R. Canadian adolescents and the challenge to demonstrate competence at personal physical risk: I. *Adolescence*, 1972, *7*, 245–264.

Munro, B. The structure and motivation of an adolescent peer group. *Alberta Journal of Educational Research*, 1957, *3*, 149–161.

Mussen, P. Some antecedents and consequents of masculine sex-typing in adolescent boys. *Psychological Monographs*, 1961, *75* (2, Whole No. 506).

Offer, D. Sexual behavior of a group of normal adolescents. *Medical Aspects of Human Sexuality*, 1971, *5*, 40–49.

Offer, D. Attitudes toward sexuality in a group of 1500 middle class teen-agers. *Journal of Youth and Adolescence*, 1972, *1*, 81–90.

Pierce, J., & Bowman, P. Motivation patterns of superior high school students. In *The gifted student,* Cooperative Research Monograph No. 2, Washington, D.C.: U.S. Department of Health, Education, and Welfare, Office of Education, 1960. Pp. 33–66.

Ptaschnik, J. A comparison of the relevance of education in three city high schools: Black, white and integrated. Paper presented at AERA convention, February 1973.

Purdue Opinion Panel. High school students' leisure time activities and attitudes toward network television. Lafayette, Ind.: Purdue University, February 1967.

Razavieh, A. A., & Hosseini, A. A. Family, peer, and academic orientation of Iranian adolescents. *Journal of Psychology,* 1972, *80(2),* 337–344.

Robinson, I. E., Ing. K., & Balswick, J. O. The premarital sexual revolution among college females. *Family Coordinator,* 1972, *21(2),* 189–194.

Sanford, N. Developmental status of the entering freshman. In N. Sanford (Ed.), *The American college.* New York: Wiley, 1962. Pp. 253–282.

Shaw, M. C., & Dutton, B. E. The use of the parent attitude research inventory with the parents of bright academic underachievers. *Journal of Educational Psychology,* 1962, *53,* 203–208. Reprinted in I. J. Gordon (Ed.), *Human development: Readings in research.* Glenview, Ill.: Scott, Foresman, 1965.

Skorijpska, J. Konflikty mlodziezy djorzewajacej z osobami doroslymi w opinii samej mlodziezy (Conflicts between adolescents and adults as viewed by young people). *Psychology Wychowaucza,* 1958, *1,* 206–227.

Sorenson, R. *Adolescent sexuality in contemporary America.* New York: World, 1973.

Spencer, C. P. Selective secondary education, social class and the development of adolescent subcultures. *British Journal of Educational Psychology,* 1972, *42,* 1–13.

Streit, F., & Oliver, H. The child's perception of his family and its relationship to drug use. *Drug Forum,* 1972, *1,* 283–289.

Tamerin, J. Recent increase in adolescent cigarette smoking: A disquieting phenomenon examined. *Archives of General Psychiatry,* 1973, *28,* 116–119.

Tec, N. Drugs among suburban teenagers: Basic findings. *Social Science & Medicine,* 1971, *5,* 77–84.

Tuma, E., & Livson, N. Family socioeconomic status and adolescent attitudes to authority. *Child Development,* 1960, *31,* 387–399. Reprinted in I. J. Gordon (Ed.), *Human development: Readings in research.* Glenview, Ill.: Scott, Foresman, 1965.

Weatherley, D. Self-perceived rate of physical maturation and personality in late adolescence. *Child Development,* 1964, *35,* 1197–1210.

Whitehead, P., Smart, R., & Laforest, L. Multiple drug use in Eastern Canada. *International Journal of the Addictions,* 1972, *7,* 179–190.

Williamson, R., & Seevard, G. Concepts of social sex roles among children and adolescents. *Human Development,* 1971, *14,* 184–194.

Winick, C. Some reasons for the increase in drug dependence among middle class youths. In H. Silverstein (Ed.), *The sociology of youth, evolution and revolution.* New York: Macmillan, 1973. Pp. 433–436.

Zellermayer, J., & Marcus, J. Kibbutz adolescence: Relevance to personality development theory. *Journal of Youth & Adolescence,* 1972, *1,* 143–153.

CHAPTER 18

SELFHOOD IN LATE ADOLESCENCE

You'll drink a farewell drink
And I'll take a farewell take
We'll talk about our times
And crack a few worn jokes.
Then I'll board the trackbound train
And you'll board the airborne plane
And we'll never see each other again.

You've got to live a little on the inside
But you've got to live mostly on the outside.
You've got to live a little on the underside
But you've got to live mostly on the topside.

I'm gonna miss you when the jokes have all been told.
I'm gonna miss you when our young times all grow old.
But I know you'll keep on livin', even when I'm gone.
And though I've sorta stopped, I'll start livin' 'fore too long.
And we'll smile about our times
And we'll laugh at well-worn jokes
And we'll always see each other, again.

Gary D. Gordon

CONCEPTUAL DEVELOPMENT
Attitudes and Values

In late adolescence, each youngster organizes his values according to the patterned ways of life he sees around him. He adopts certain beliefs from his culture but modifies them within his own self. He is more able to recognize the various origins of the demands made upon him for behavior. In the terms of moral development used in preceding chapters, he should be able to function at Piaget's mature level and Kohlberg's stages 3, 4, and 5.

There is much evidence of the similarity of late-adolescent and adult views of life. This does not mean that adult behavior and late-adolescent behavior are identical but that they share a common system of values. Friesen (1972), for example, found little evidence of a generation gap in values, but rather cultural continuity. Conger (1972) states that on such values as competition, private property, control of one's fate, and the need for legal authority, most adolescents agree with their parents. There seem to be some differences between adolescents and adults, however. Youth seem more intense and tend to display their values a little more openly and fully. They tend to move more toward the poles rather than toward the middle. However, as Figure 18.1 so vividly illustrates, the outward signs of morality were reversed between 1972 and 1973 in the White House. Those who looked fully Establishment in age, demeanor, appearance, and education engaged in various crimes that a few years before (and even then) would have been attributed to militant youth and minority groups.

The analysis of adolescent values in 1973 is a tricky business, because it is not at all clear what these values are and how rapidly they will change. The world situation is changing, and the goals and values of adolescence seem to be making corresponding shifts. Wright and Cox (1971) replicated in 1970 a study of English adolescents' attitudes that had first been done in 1963. There was movement toward more permissive attitudes toward sex, gambling, and acceptance of others across racial lines. Changes in moral belief were independent of religious commitment. Conger (1972) suggests that adolescents are more tolerant of behavior, but he also points up what may be an essential difference between the generations: The current generation "appear less knowledgeable about the past and less convinced that there are lessons they can learn from it." (Conger, 1972, p. 207) Further, from their view of their own past (childhood), they infer that impersonality, war, and rapid change are the normal conditions, whereas their parents view these as unusual. It may be that part of the cry for "relevance" from students who are asked to study anything that occurred before they were born stems from their ahistorical and apocalyptic view of the world.

Although Sherif and Sherif (1965) indicated that the immediate interests of adolescents, at least in the southwestern part of the United States, were still material (that is, cars, appliances, home), their behavior seems to reflect a growing concern for the nature of the American society and the direction in which it seems to be moving. Mixed in with the "cool" attitude of many is an orientation toward social action, which exists in the university and high school student in other lands. This trend is not confined to ghetto youth who protest the indignities that surround them. The 1968 and 1972 presidential campaigns revealed the high level of activity of middle class college students in working both in and out of the normal political

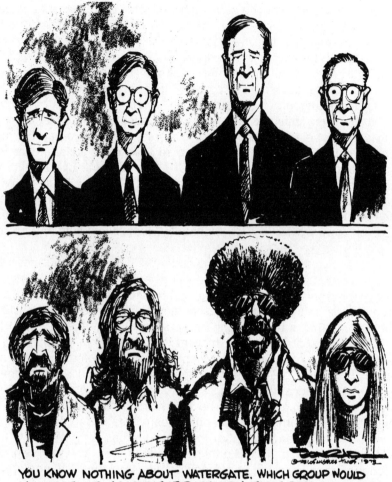

YOU KNOW NOTHING ABOUT WATERGATE. WHICH GROUP WOULD
YOU MOST LIKELY SUSPECT OF BURGLARY, THEFT, BREAKING AND
ENTERING, WIRETAPPING, ELECTION LAW VIOLATIONS AND CONSPIRACY?

FIGURE 18.1
From an editorial cartoon by Paul Conrad, Copyright *Los Angeles Times,* 1973.
Reprinted by permission.

process to influence events. The spread of university sit-ins in the spring
of 1968 and the campus upheavals in the fall and winter of 1968–1969, the
Kent State and Jackson State killings, related both to antiwar demonstrations following the brief incursion into Cambodia and civil rights in 1970
which led to demonstrations, are other examples. The campuses turned
"cool" in late 1972, with no mass upheavals as the bombing continued
in spite of Congressional efforts. But this, one may guess, was not due to

any change of value but to a recognition of the futility of the approach. It may also relate to the escape into drugs and apathy.

Similarly, the evolution of the hippie movement suggested to many that this group of youngsters was seeking to drop out from the normally materialistic and success-oriented American society. The hippie movement as such has passed from the scene, as have the movements of previous generations (such as the beat generation of the 1950s), but it has left behind a widespread belief among youth that getting and spending is not the only, nor the right, way of life.

Research by Block, Hann, and Smith (1968) seems to indicate that the student activist comes from the privileged class and that his attitudes often resemble those of his parents. According to Block et al., "Rejection of major *societal* values does not necessarily imply rebellion against *parental* attitudes. Although placing themselves squarely in opposition to many of the prevailing views and practices of the culture, the activists have identified with and accepted many of their parents' values." (1968, p. 15) They may have moved further than their parents (Pugh, 1971), but in the same direction. Another indication of the link between the family and boy adolescents' values can be found in the University of Michigan's survey of a large sample of these boys. (Bachman, 1970) The only background variable related to social values (honesty, kindness, reciprocity, self-control, social responsibility, social skills) was the boy's relationship with his family. Further, these students seemed to be concerned with integrity and humanity rather than with the material things of life.

Although political activities, both within and without the traditional political and economic structure, are highly visible, it may be that the great majority of youth still resemble those reported by Sherif and Sherif. Gottlieb (1971), for example, found that poor black youth wanted white-collar jobs, a steady income, middle class standing; it was the white youth who were more alienated. The paradox of this period may be that it was the children of the affluent, with the education and the leisure, who were in the forefront of the anti-Establishment struggle, while the children of the poor were struggling to enter the Establishment, even though on their own terms.

Perhaps the best that can be said is that adolescent values reflect the adult world. The flux and confusion of their values is but an indication of the moral dilemmas that face the society at large. Along with their own personal anxieties about their place in the scheme of things, adolescents felt deeply the impact of the Vietnam War and the struggle of blacks, Chicanos, and women for first-class citizenship. This does not mean that those who are seeking and finding ways to participate are all on the same side of the issue. The adolescent seems to pride himself on being able to scoff and ridicule the adult world. The emergence of satire magazines

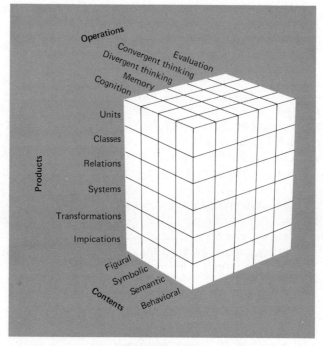

FIGURE 18.2

A cubical model representing the structure of intellect. Reprinted from J. P. Guilford, The three faces of intellect. *American Psychologist,* 1959, **14,** 469–479. Copyright 1959 by the American Psychological Association. Reprinted by permission.

such as *Mad* and *Lampoon* represent an effort by youth to show that they want to face a "real" world, not one hidden behind sham and hypocrisy.

Intellectual Development

In this book we have consistently described intelligence, or intelligent behavior, as reflecting learned patterns and the self of the growing person, rather than as stated quantity or a "given" native ability, fixed and unchanging.

Current views of intellectual growth recognize the concept of differentiation-integration; intelligence is seen as a many-faceted process. As the person develops, there is movement toward complexity and toward differentiation of the many factors that combine to make up intellect.

Guilford's three-dimensional model may serve to illustrate one scheme for deciding what "intelligence" is. This scheme, Figure 18.2, enables us to recognize that there is no such simple entity as intelligence, but rather that there are a number of operations in which the person engages, a number of kinds of material (contents) he uses in these operations, and a number of results (products) that emerge from intelligent behavior. "Each cell in the model calls for a certain kind of ability that can be described in terms of operation, content and product, for each cell is at the intersection of a unique combination of kinds of operation, content and product." (Guilford, 1959, p. 471) For example, many high school tests of the objective type rely heavily on the cells that are labeled "memory" and "semantic." All the pupil has to do is recall the right phrase or recognize the right word.

In an up-date of this model, Guilford (1971) points out that 10 of his 15 categories relate to information, illustrating its great importance and leading to the idea of the person as an information processor. He further indicates that the six products bear a resemblance to Piaget's logical operations in that they may be the results of such operations. In addition, Guilford ties in his structure of intellect model with a new view of problem solving that stresses the interrelationships among operations, contents, and products. This is a dynamic, active view of intelligence; it is the intelligent behavior of the person in the solution of problems. As such, it moves us away from static definitions of intelligence as a fixed quantity of a single something. His scheme stresses a nonunitary, nonimmutable view of intelligence. Such a scheme does not apply solely to the late adolescent. However, the development of some of the abilities represented by cells in Guilford's model probably do not occur until adolescence.

One way to see scores on intelligence tests as reflective of life experiences and as composed of many of Guilford's cells is to examine the research on patterns of performance. For instance, as the children in the primary grades illustrated, the pattern of performance on intellectual tests seems to be a function of ethnic membership. Japanese, Chinese, Caucasian, Filipino, and Hawaiian students were assessed state-wide in Hawaii in the tenth and twelfth grades. Analysis of a sample of 20 percent of these youngsters revealed that their scores on the School and College Test (SCAT) and on two subtests in mathematics of the California Achievement Test were functions of their backgrounds. The Japanese and Chinese ranked above all other groups. The Hawaiian subjects were consistently on the bottom with the Filipinos just above them. The Japanese girls were superior on verbal measures in both the tenth and twelfth grades. The boys' quantitative scores on the SCAT exceeded their verbal scores in all populations except Caucasian in both the tenth and twelfth grades. (Stewart, 1967)

Backman (1972) analyzed the scores of a large sample of youngsters who had been measured on verbal knowledge (VKN), English language (ENG), Math (MAT), visual reasoning (VIS), perceptual speed and accuracy (PSA), and short-term memory (MEM) as part of project TALENT, a large-scale survey made in 1960. The adolescents were Jewish whites, non-Jewish whites, blacks, and Orientals. She found sex more important than ethnicity or social class; girls were higher on ENG, PSA, and MEM; boys, on VKN, MAT, and VIS. Within ethnic groups, Jews did better on VKN and MAT than they did on PSA and MEM. The non-Jewish whites had little variation. Backman indicates the latter was probably true because the tests had been standardized on this group.

These results, Guilford's work on conceptualizing intelligence, the findings in the Michigan study (Bachman, 1970), and the creativity material presented below all point up the difficulty of using the single label "intelligence" to describe the complex organization of intellectual abilities within the person and the importance of cultural impacts (sex-role expectations, racial prejudice, cultural values) upon the intellectual performance of the person.

Creativity

The concept of divergent thinking, or creativity, in high school youths has been studied with most interesting and thought-provoking results. How the person performs on an intelligence test is not only related to how he perceives himself, but is also a function of how he perceives his world and the way he sees the particular stimulus of the test item. Those who score high on the traditional type of intelligence test tend to engage in "convergent thinking"; that is, they zero in on the task, focus on the problem, analyze it, and produce the conventional or "right" answer.

The divergent thinker, who may fail to show up as highly intelligent on the standardized test, uses the stimulus as a tickler for his imagination and soars off from the cue. Although researchers use labels such as "high intelligence" and "high creativity" (Getzels and Jackson, 1960; Yamamoto, 1964), they may be describing two aspects of intelligent perception and behavior: convergent and divergent thinking.

An example from Getzels and Jackson illustrates the different kinds of perception. They studied two groups of students drawn from a larger group of 500 adolescents at a private school. One group of 26, labeled the high creativity group, scored in the top 20 percent on creativity tests. (A sample test item: Give as many uses as you can for a brick.) But they were not in the top 20 percent on the standard IQ tests. The second group was composed of those in the top 20 percent on IQ tests, but they were not in the top creativity bracket. One of the tasks presented to these youngsters was to look at a picture and write a story.

> One picture-stimulus was perceived most often as a man in an airplane reclining seat returning from a business trip or conference. A high-IQ subject gave the following story: "Mr. Smith is on his way home from a successful business trip. He is very happy and he is thinking about his wonderful family and how glad he will be to see them again. He can picture it, about an hour from now, his plane landing at the airport and Mrs. Smith and their three children all there

welcoming him home again." A high-creative subject wrote this story: "This man is flying back from Reno where he has just won a divorce from his wife. He couldn't stand to live with her anymore, he told the judge, because she wore so much cold cream on her face at night that her head would skid across the pillow and hit him in the head. He is now contemplating a new skid-proof face cream." [Getzels and Jackson, 1960, p. 9]

These two groups of youngsters did not differ in scholastic achievement or need for achievement, although the "intelligent" group averaged 23 IQ points higher. Interestingly, the teachers preferred the convergent to the divergent thinkers!

Torrance (1960) reports partial substantiation of the Getzels and Jackson study in elementary, high school, and university groups. He found in all situations a significant difference between the mean intelligence scores of the two groups. Torrance also found that, if a "gifted" group were being selected for special work, "about 70 percent of the most creative would have been eliminated . . . on the basis of the intelligence test or Miller Analogies." (Torrance, 1960, p. 7) Many a creative high school youth, on the basis of IQ and teacher choice, would thus be overlooked.

From their research, Wallach and Kogan (1965) formulated four categories of children:

[1] *High creativity–high intelligence: These children can exercise within themselves both control and freedom, both adult-like and child-like kinds of behavior.*

[2] *High creativity–low intelligence: These children are in angry conflict with themselves and with their school environment and are beset by feelings of unworthiness and inadequacy. In a stress-free context, however, they can blossom forth cognitively.*

[3] *Low creativity–high intelligence: These children can be described as "addicted" to school achievement. Academic failure would be perceived by them as catastrophic, so that they must continually strive for academic excellence in order to avoid the possibility of pain.*

[4] *Low creativity–low intelligence: Basically bewildered, these children engage in various defensive maneuvers ranging from useful adaptations such as intensive social activity to regressions such as passivity or psychosomatic symptoms. [Wallach and Kogan, 1965, pp. 367–368]*

As in the case of performance on the more traditional, convergent measures discussed earlier in this chapter, such variables as sex and social class influence scores on measures of divergent thinking. Kogan and Pankove (1972) retested at tenth grade the middle class children

Wallach and Kogan had studied five years before (see classification above). They found that creativity and IQ became positively related for the boys, but not for the girls. In addition, they found long-term stability over the five years on their measures of creativity. Olive (1972a) found, in her study of youngsters from three eastern high schools, that there was a considerable relationship between IQ (as measured by the Otis) and divergent thinking (as measured by several Guilford scales). However, IQ was more highly related to social class and scholastic achievement than was divergent thinking. She also reports (Olive, 1972b) that although there were no sex differences on IQ, girls outperformed the boys on five of the seven divergent thinking measures she used.

By late adolescence, intellectual functioning is an extremely complex system of behavior. The boy or girl manifests many types of intelligent behavior, some of which are perceived by adults as more "intelligent" than others. Not only their total score on tests but also, and of more fundamental importance, the way in which they approach and solve their problems will be influenced by the nature of the experiences they have had and the way they perceive them.

Interests

The main differences between the interest patterns of early and late adolescents can be seen in terms of quantity and variability. School demands more and more time, so leisure pursuits must decrease. The importance of heterosexual interests increases, so time spent in sports and other physical pursuits decreases. The trend is away from participating in play and toward becoming a spectator, notably of varsity athletics.

Interest patterns, including vocational interests, tend toward more stability during the late adolescent period. With the decrease in absolute number of interests comes the concentration of effort on fewer activities. If a boy or girl is interested in collecting, he or she moves from collecting everything to collecting stamps, coins, girls or boys, or some particular class of objects. Accompanying this specializing process is the trend to higher levels of complexity. This can be seen not only in an organized sport such as football with its variety of formations, plays, and options but also in hobbies. For example, when a youngster owns a hot rod, he learns a whole new language and engages in complicated operations to modify engine and chassis in order to produce a "new" car.

Vocational Interests and the Self. The idiosyncratic, personal, and "self" nature of interests becomes even more visible in late adolescence than in earlier periods of life. Choice of particular interests, degree of variability, and depth or breadth of interests reflect the adolescent's self-image as well as peer situation.

For example, stability of vocational interest choices were examined by Schmidt and Rothney (1955) who found that only one-fifth of the youth they studied expressed the same choice throughout high school and during the follow-up after graduation. Approximately one-half were consistent in their last two years, one-third for three years. Though we can identify the trend toward increasing consistency, we need to recognize that, for the individual adolescent, maturation is only one factor. Who constituted those who were highly consistent and stable? What were their choices? What led them to consistency? We don't know. Holland (1966) proposed that stability was related to overall self-integration flowing from the interaction of person and environment. Although this fits in with the overall thesis of this book, we still need considerably more information.

Several additional clues as to the relationship between self and interest patterns may be found in the Marks (1957) study and the previously mentioned work by Getzels and Jackson (1960). Marks used the Adolescent Growth Study material to explore the interaction between interests and clique leadership. He found, on an interest questionnaire, that those who are identified as leaders by their peers "do not follow the norms of the group to the extent of being conformists and may actually be more deviant in their interest behavior than are followers." (Marks, 1957, p. 172) Since his test was verbal, there may be a discrepancy between interests checked and those actually pursued, but this study may indicate a relationship between peer status and diversity of interests. It is impossible to assign the causes of such a relationship at this time with the little we know. It may be that once a youngster has status in his adolescent peer group, he becomes free to deviate. It may be, though more unlikely, that those who deviate somewhat, at least verbally, are accorded status.

The Getzels and Jackson study included work in the area of occupational choice. The "creative" (divergent thinkers) and the "intelligent" (convergent thinkers) were given sentence-completion and other personality tests. They found that the high-creatives not only mentioned more choices but also more unusual fields, choosing such careers as adventurer, writer, and inventor rather than doctor, lawyer, and professor. They feel that convergent youth may prefer safe fields; divergent youth may prefer the challenge of growth. In either case, occupational choice was a function of the interaction of cognitive and personal-social variables.

Warren (1961) studied college students' choices of major and shifts of field and found that there was not always a relationship between choice of role and self-concept as measured by self-report. Majors were still unstable. Almost half the subjects changed majors by the end of the sophomore year.

Reality of Vocational Choice. We have noted the unreality of vocational choice in younger age groups. Although many high school seniors and college students are unsettled or unrealistic about vocational aspirations, there seems to be a movement toward more realism. Girls seem to view work choice as related to the enhancement of the feminine role. Almost half of them chose noncareer types of jobs. Douvan and Adelson (1966) found that almost all the girls' job choices fell into four categories: personal aide, social aide, traditional white-collar work, and glamour-type jobs.

However, this picture is obviously changing. The notion of sex-related jobs is diminishing and is being replaced by the recognition that interests and competence need not be seen as functions of gender. For example, Cole's (1973) analysis of four common vocational interest inventories (Strong Vocational Interest Blank, Kuder Occupational Interest Survey, Holland's Vocational Preference Inventory and The American College Test Vocational Interest Profile) revealed that there is a difference in the interests of men and women, but these do not override across-sex common occupational or vocational interest patterns. Vocational choice might rest more on the common element of interest than on the sex-related elements.

In setting vocational goals, late adolescents show an awareness of competition, training, and societal needs. For example, in a study of both immediate and long-range goals, the immediate goals perceived were graduation, good health, and acceptance into college. Longer-range goals were family- and job-oriented. There were intelligence and social class differences that also indicated a greater awareness of reality. For instance, brighter youngsters perceived college as immediate and viewed competition, hard work, and lack of confidence as obstacles; less bright youngsters saw entry into the labor force or armed services as immediate and lack of ability, being drafted, and a poor educational background as obstacles. (Crowley, 1959)

The interrelationship of job choice and social and personal factors can be seen, for instance, in two studies. Romanian (Dragan, 1972) high school students perceive little relationship between intellectual interests and occupational choice, make inconsistent choices, but show a high degree of relationship between personal preference (subject matter) and occupational choice. American high school boys' (Bachman, 1970) job attitudes and occupational goals were related to family relations, religion, race, and socioeconomic status, as well as to intellectual ability.

In general, adolescents' interests reflect the movement toward a more integrated self-picture. Interest patterns include a clearer understanding of the future and the world at large; they are less dependent on particular situations and more stable. By the end of late adolescence, the adolescents' interests and aspirations resemble those of adults. The transition from the less complex, more open, variable interests of the child to the more complex, specialized, relatively fixed adult pattern is being completed.

THE SELF-CONCEPT
Self-definition

Sex-Role Identification.   We have seen throughout this book that identification is a key process in self-development. In these last chapters on adolescence, we have recognized that the establishment of identity and integration are closely related to acceptance of one's biocultural sex role. We know that adolescents, viewed externally, are working on their sex role through dating and other peer group activities, through vocational and recreational patterns, and through family transactions.

As a way of gathering data, we may ask youth how they look at sex roles. We know that concepts of sex-appropriate behavior are changing in the American culture. How are these changes reflected in the self-concepts of late adolescents? Unfortunately, we do not have completely up-to-date research. McKee and Sherriffs (1959) used an adjective checklist with California college freshmen men and women. These students were asked to check for ideal self, real self, ideal member of opposite sex, and beliefs (what they think others expect of them). Their findings clearly indicate that these college youngsters were aware of changing social patterns. The man included in his evaluation of his real self the formerly female characteristics of warmth, human feelings, and concern for interpersonal relations. He recognized that women want these characteristics in him, and he accepted them as part of his real self, although he did not fully accept them into his ideal self. The woman, on the other hand, did not incorporate such male attributes as aggressive, rugged and daring behavior into her ideal self.

In contrast to our earlier discussion (see chapters on preadolescence) of constriction of the male role, these college students see the female role as more sex-typed and the male role as less rigid. In agreement with our hypotheses of the girl's self-concept, the woman's real self in this study is seen as more unfavorable than the man's. Both sexes are aware of the changing culture, but boys seem to feel more positively about themselves and their roles than do their female college classmates. We should emphasize that this study and several other studies we will cite in this section were on college students in the 1950s and 1960s. We have no guarantee that college youngsters are typical late adolescents, and we know the picture is changing. We need current studies of the McKee type on both college and noncollege youth.

The split between what may be called feminine role behavior and attitudes toward female personality traits in college girls was examined by Kammeyer (1964). A girl may engage in "modern" role behavior while holding "traditional" views about basic differences between men and women. A traditional statement of role behavior would be, "In marriage, the major responsibility of the wife is to keep her husband and children happy." A traditional attitude would be embodied in an item such as,

"Women are more emotional than men." Kammeyer found that girls who had interaction with others in college as well as many contacts with parents were more likely to have consistent views than were girls who had few friends and dated rarely. Most girls were consistent in their role behavior and attitudes, which may indicate that they had worked out their identifications pretty well and were not particularly suffering from role confusion.

Central to the self-concept of the late adolescent is his identification with and acceptance of his sex role. Although the cultural shifts in what behaviors may be considered appropriate continue, each youngster will continue to hold himself against some standard and measure his adequacy against it.

Personal Attributes.   When late adolescents define themselves, what do they consider good personal attributes?

A comprehensive assessment covering college freshmen in 21 institutions was conducted by Richards (1966). Students rated themselves on 31 traits, which Richards factor analyzed by sex. He found no factor unique to one sex and seven factors common to both. These are listed below:

(1) *Physical well-being* (athletic ability, physical energy, and physical health);
(2) Scholarship (mathematical ability, scholarship, scientific ability, and self-confidence-intellectual);
(3) *Estheticism* (originality, artistic ability, speaking ability, writing ability, expressiveness, and acting ability);
(4) *Pragmatism* (self-control, independence, conservatism, practical mindedness, and perseverance);
(5) *Technical-scientific ability* (mechanical ability, artistic ability, scientific ability, and research ability);
(6) *Sociability* (leadership, popularity with opposite sex, sociability, aggressiveness, cheerfulness, self-confidence, popularity);
(7) *Sensitivity to others* (understanding of others, sensitivity to the needs of others, cheerfulness, and sense of humor).

The How I See Myself Scale (Gordon, 1968) yielded factors for both boys and girls in high school that may be compared to Richards' findings. The physical adequacy factor relates to physical well-being in that it includes energy, athletics, and health. The academic adequacy factor relates to scholarship; autonomy, to estheticism in that it contains items on art, speaking, music, individual projects; emotions, to pragmatism; and interpersonal adequacy, to sociability.

Of course, all factors on self-rating scales are functions of the original items placed on such scales. Nevertheless, the degree of overlap between the high school factors and the college freshmen factors suggests a considerable degree of organization and stability between the late high school years and the early college years in the dimensions adolescents see as making up their images of themselves.

Ekehammar (1972) reviewed the literature on sex differences in reported anxiety and found that girls reported higher levels than boys; she also studied Swedish adolescents' self-reports. She used a 5-point scale (very much to not at all) on such personal items as hands shaking, mouth dry, and restlessness and on situational items such as dentist, new job, and fire at home. Girls consistently reported more anxiety, which she interprets from both a cultural and physiological framework.

Locus of Control. Another dimension along which people can define themselves is that of locus of control. (Rotter, 1966) How much does an adolescent feel he is a victim of circumstances (external), and how much does he think his own behavior influences what happens to him (internal)? How one views himself along this dimension has been related to a variety of cultural background factors such as family, nationality, class and race (Sarason and Smith, 1971: DuCette and Wolk, 1972) as well as to behavioral variables such as performance in school (Coleman, 1966) and intellectual factors. (Bachman, 1970) DuCette and Wolk (1972) studied juniors and seniors from three high schools representing different social backgrounds. They conclude that how the youngster sees locus of control is related to his orientation toward reality; the more internal adolescent responds to the environment more accurately than does the external youngster. They suggest that an "internal person" does not simply perceive that the environment can be controlled; instead, he accurately perceives whether the environment can be controlled and then responds to this perception with appropriate behavior. (DuCette and Wolk, 1972, p. 502) It is an interesting hypothesis. It may help to explain (1) shifts in adolescent behavior in spite of the steady trend by college students, for example, toward alienation (Schneider, 1971); (2) differential behaviors toward school and life by people who come from diverse backgrounds but react similarly on measure of locus of control such as Rotter's I-E scale; (3) why campuses are quiet in 1973 when they were noisy in 1970. Their hypothesis also illustrates the continuing difficulty encountered from a simple view of life that expects high relationships between a self-perception and behavior without taking into account both the place of that perception in the person's total organization of self-concepts and the situations in which he finds himself. The meaning of a personal attribute is highly individual; prediction of behavior must take into account the totality of the person-situation transaction.

Another way of looking at locus of control is the degree to which the person solves the problem of individuality and group living. The college freshman still looks to his social group for self-definition and is highly vulnerable to the evaluations others make of him. As Sanford indicates, "Over the long pull he must, if he is to become highly developed, build up an internal base for self-evaluation. . . . He must evolve a self-conception that includes as much as possible of his real self, his abilities, inclinations . . ." (1962, pp. 265–266) The balancing of external to internal orientation is thus a major task in adolescence, even though it obviously has its roots much earlier in time. Resolving the inner and outer self and other conflicts is not completed by late adolescence; it continues throughout life. However, the pressures to submerge one's self in one's peers are probably highest during the adolescent period.

Self-acceptance

In Chapter 16 we examined the evidence concerning the stability of the early adolescent's self-concept. Those studies also included data on late adolescence. In general, there seems to be a movement toward both increased stability and more positive self-report in late adolescence. We can hypothesize that this is in keeping with what is known about development. We would expect that the 18-year-old will be closer to finding himself than the 13-year-old. He is more able to differentiate various aspects of himself and to see the world more realistically.

The degree of distortion of perception of self and world is probably related to both the stability and reality of the self-concept in adolescence. The youngster who feels adequate can afford to see self and world for what they are. He has established his anchorage points, including himself as one. He is more open to the meaning of his experience, to his own feelings, and to self-evaluations than is the youngster who is either seeking to find himself or who has defined himself in negative fashion.

But, as we have encountered throughout this book, the problem of the locus of evaluation remains when one attempts to understand the inner feelings of another. Who determines what is "the real world" of another? One way to do this has been to study the youngster's own stated view of what his ideal self would be against his stated report on his real self. Katz and Zigler (1971) used an adaptation of the Coopersmith scale and an adjective checklist with middle class suburban adolescents. They found that self-ideal discrepancy *increases* with age and is also positively related to IQ. We can interpret that to mean that the older adolescent is more aware (or at least more willing to admit) that he's not all he would like to be. This is a sign of maturity and lowered defenses toward both himself and the outside world.

On the other hand, delinquent youngsters who were interviewed about their images of self and others define themselves in terms of "What I am, others are too." (Rosenberg and Silverstein, 1973, p. 174) For example, a young Washington girl who has had many illicit sexual relationships and regards herself as both good and bad, when asked what a good girl is, says, "I don't think there are any good girls." The interview proceeds:

> [*You don't think there are any?*]
> *I don't know of any. All the girls I thought were good and pure and never had anything to do with boys, I found out they weren't doing anything but fooling the public.*
> [*Just like everybody else?*]
> *Yeah. They just kept everything secret. But sooner or later people find out.* [*Rosenberg and Silverstein, 1973, p. 174*]

To them, "goodness" and "badness" are pragmatic terms; if you are caught, you are bad. Smoking pot is worse than mugging because the sentence is stiffer if you are caught.

We can tie these two versions of self-acceptance (Katz and Zigler versus Rosenberg and Silverstein) together by referring to the egocentrism-decentering process developed by Piaget. Youngsters who recognized the self-ideal gap might be seen as decentered. They could stand off from themselves and accept themselves. The delinquents mentioned above are still egocentric; they cannot separate self from other. Further, they are operating at a low stage of moral development on both the Piaget and Kohlberg schemes. One should not infer that *all* suburbanites or *all* delinquents are as described above. The point here is that there are several ways to look at self-acceptance and that the internal frame of reference has to be placed in its social and developmental context. Bachman (1970) also measured adolescent self-esteem and found that the tenth-grade boys surveyed reported a fairly high level of self-acceptance and that self-esteem was related to reported good relationships with parents.

The impact of the early adolescent growth experience on the self of the late adolescent and adult seems to be long-lasting. Jones (1957) followed up the early- and late-maturing boys who were studied at 17 when they were 33. She found that, on personality tests, the psychological differences between these groups had persisted, although, of course, the physical differences had disappeared. Another longitudinal study to examine stability of values was conducted by Himmelweit and Smith (1971). They collected follow-up data on Englishmen age 24 to 25 who had been previously measured on their attitudes eleven years earlier. They were primarily concerned with authoritarianism and its relationships to other psychological and social variables. They did not find a high direct relationship between family relations and authoritarianism in early adolescence as might have been predicted. However, they found that attitudes of powerlessness, fear of venturing, and acceptance of one's place at age 24–25 were positively related to feelings of lack of parental warmth at age 13–14. To a degree, their measure of powerlessness corresponds to externality on the internal-external dimension discussed above. Further, they indicate that attitudes such as authoritarianism can best be studied in relationship to cognitive, personal, and social factors. Any attitude can only be understood in such a context.

If one generalizes from these longitudinal efforts, it seems that there is stability of attitudes, which would include self-regarding attitudes. However, one's concepts of self are in constant transaction with the social environment, and stability does not mean complete lack of change. Self-definition continues throughout life, but the view one holds as an adolescent will act as a predisposing factor to maintain itself.

Self-concept and Behavior

Our basic assumption throughout this book is that behavior and self-concept are reciprocally related. In the late adolescent period, we can examine this relationship in respect to school, peers, and goal-setting behavior.

School Achievement.   Why some bright youngsters do poorly in school is a question of great concern because of our desire to enable each child to achieve his maximum development. What makes a gifted adolescent an "underachiever"? Counselors who have engaged in research on this question seem to agree that gifted underachieving adolescents perceive themselves differently than do their peers. These youngsters, as seen by observers, are hostile, unsociable, indifferent to their responsibilities, and hard to reach. In addition—or perhaps at the root of the problem—most of them question their giftedness. (Broedel et al., 1959) When asked to rate themselves by means of an adjective checklist, the results show "male underachievers seem to have more negative feelings about themselves than do male achievers. Female underachievers tend to be ambivalent with regard to their feelings toward themselves." (Shaw et al., 1960, p. 195) They just don't believe they are good, and resist the pressures and demands for performance that are placed upon them by parents and teachers.

We would expect that high achievers value themselves and their ability and see themselves as able to learn. In spite of the differences in their approach to problems, both the convergent and divergent thinkers we described earlier in this chapter achieved highly and did not differ on their needs for achievement. They shared a common concept of self as "able."

The Quincy study of achievement yields similar results. High-achieving boys seem to possess strong needs for achievement and to view school as a favorable environment and self as industrious and imaginative. They also express high educational motivation. The girls follow this pattern, except on need for achievement, and score even higher than the boys on seeing self as active and industrious and school as positive. (Pierce and Bowman, 1960) Taylor (1964) reviewed 30 years of research on achievement and found that, among other traits, overachievers had higher self-esteem (variously measured), good peer relationships, and controlled, as opposed to free floating, anxiety. Since we are faced with a relationship, it is not possible to talk in terms of cause and effect. One might speculate as to what role the school itself has in stigmatizing pupils as slow learners or underachievers and how that categorization affects both performance and self-concept.

One way to see the direction of influence is to measure self-concept at one point in time (such as entry into junior college) and relate it to academic performance later on (grade point average at the end of the first year or graduation at the end of the second). The How I See Myself Scale was part of a battery of predictions used at St. Petersburg Junior College in Florida. It was found to be an important predictor of grade point average (Clarke, 1968) and graduation. (Ammons, 1971)

The pattern of the relationship between self-concept and achievement seems clear. There is a relationship between positive self-concept and high achievement and negative self-concept and underachievement. Although self-concept predicted performance in the junior college studies, the long-term relationships are more complex. Chances are we can see a circular pattern beginning earlier with perception of experiences as "successes" or "failures" leading to development of a concept of self, which in turn, influences both the selection and evaluation of subsequent experiences.

Self and Others.   Does the adolescent's self-concept influence his acceptance of and by his peers? Is acceptance of self related to acceptance of others? Most of the research on the latter question, unfortunately, has been done either on older age groups or on clinical cases. We may summarize it by saying that the relationship is present, and the problems of demonstrating it seem to be more a matter of technique than theory. A big stumbling block has been the inability to agree on what constitutes self-acceptance and how it should be measured. Several approaches have been used to answer this question with respect to high school youngsters. Combinations of Q-sort, sociometric techniques, and self-rating techniques have been used.

Morval and Morval (1972) used a self-report approach with French-speaking Canadian girls of average intelligence. They report a positive relationship between self-esteem and a need to be included in groups and a negative relationship between self-esteem and the need to control others. Wilk (1957) found that Girl Scout leaders elected by their peers saw themselves as more able to supply leadership than did nonleaders. Catholic senior high school girls who saw self and others as accepting were seen by peers as having better interpersonal relationships than those who were not accepting. (Kennedy, 1958)

The above suggests that there are some relationships between concept of self and peers and peer status. The data on peer life and the adolescent value system would certainly suggest a high relationship. We still lack sufficient evidence approaching the problem from a self, transactional point of view. Theoretically, we may assume that the way one sees self and peers is a crucial concept; research, however, lags behind the theory.

Self and Social Mobility. Does the way the adolescent sees himself relate to mobility? Does the youngster who drops out of high school and settles for a lower class position do so in relation to his view of self? Does the lower class adolescent who makes the effort to go to college see himself differently than his peers?

Two studies seem to be related to these questions. We may assume that one tool for upward social mobility is increased education. Douvan and Adelson studied high school boys for the characteristics of upward- and downward-mobile youth. The upward-mobile boys are not only more energetic, active, and independent of their parents; they also see themselves differently:

> *Upward mobile boys show a high degree of self-acceptance, and a confidence in social situations . . . we find signs of self-rejection and demoralization in the downward mobile boys' answers to the questions, "What would you like to change about yourself if you could about your looks, or your life or your personality?" They more often desire changes so gross or so central as to indicate alienation from the self; and they more often wish for changes that are unlikely to occur. The upward mobile boy more often refers to changes he has the power to effect himself. He is more realistically critical of himself, and less self-rejecting. [Douvan and Adelson, 1958, pp. 39–40]*

In their study of girls, Douvan and Adelson (1966) reported that girls almost always see themselves as upwardly social mobile. However, this upward mobility does not seem to be related to achievement motivation. What seems to matter for the girls who seek to move upward into college is the collegiate climate rather than the end goal of degree or occupation. Most girls, they suggest, hope to accomplish their mobility through the men they marry rather than through their own achievements. Whether this is still so is questionable.

Beilin's research into the upward-mobile boy of the lower class indicated that this boy is independent of his family and sees self as able to achieve more than the family has (with their blessings). He has high energy, and had shifted his identification to include school personnel and upward-mobile peers. He has taken over the school values as a part of his self. (Beilin, 1956)

These studies suggest a clear relationship between self-acceptance, the accomplishment of self-identification and independence, high energy, and upward mobility.

The elimination of the draft, as well as changing economic and social conditions, may influence many in their decision of whether to go to college, or take time out, or even drop out of the academic life in ways that dispute a simple high self-concept = stay-in-school equation. We indicated earlier the dissatisfaction of youth with the high school. This is equally true of higher education. It may be that youngsters with positive self-concepts and with high degrees of feeling of internal control and divergent thinking patterns are exhibiting autonomy and maturity by leaving school. We need more and better research on this type of dropout.

SUMMARY

Late adolescence is a period of both increasing complexity of behavior and the integration of the self. The adolescent becomes more "adult" in his attitudes and values and in his clearer view of his self. Within the self-system, his personal organization becomes stable.

He has not yet reached the point of self-definition, however, in which he accepts his own uniqueness as desirable and worthwhile. Even though he differs from his peers in many ways, he still seeks their acceptance. He has a somewhat narrow perspective and still lacks a broad view of man. He is more peer-group oriented than self-oriented and is subject to many demands for conformity.

Intellectually, he is capable of highly complex, abstract thought. He can engage in both logical operations and imaginative endeavors, and he can use problem-solving approaches to complex problems. The extent to which he uses a variety of the intellectual factors of which he is capable seems to be highly related to learning and experience. If he has been taught to think in creative ways and experiences have encouraged him to apply thought processes to a variety of issues, the late adolescent is able to utilize these skills.

Those who think creatively, or divergently, rather than convergently, seem to perceive self and world in different fashions. Some are able to do both, and this would seem to be highly desirable.

The late adolescent, on the whole, has identified successfully with the appropriate sex role. His concepts of the behavior that accompany playing the role still fluctuate somewhat with cultural change, but generally, he knows who he is.

His behavior in school and with his peers and family seems to be more a function of his self-concept than his general ability. The use to which he puts his self-system seems to be determined not only by specific concepts of self in relation to life situations but also, and more fundamentally, in relation to the core of his self, his concept of his own adequacy and security. Success or failure in academic achievement, work, and human relationships are all tied into his view of self.

Since late adolescence is an integrating period, the view of self he holds becomes less open to easy modification by environmental forces. Although the self is always an open system, the defenses of the person become less permeable with age. As new experiences in adulthood—marriage, career, and children—occur, certain aspects of self will continue to develop and become more elaborated. The degree of self-consistency, already developed as youth enters adulthood, is high, and the direction of self-development is fairly well set.

We may expect comparatively little fundamental change in basic orientation toward self and life during the early adult period. The values and self-concepts held by the late adolescent will essentially continue to be the values and self-concept held during the next period of development.

A FINAL WORD

What are some of the implications of these conclusions? It is beyond the scope of this book to present a list of specific "oughts" to parents, teachers, and other professionals who work with children and youth. To do so, considering the point of view maintained throughout this book, would be presumptuous on the part of the author. If, however, we accept the challenge of individuality and the goal of self-development for youth, several generalizations suggest themselves. They are presented not as solutions or cookbook gimmicks but only as guideposts for further study and thought. They fall into two categories: research and application.

Research Needed

We have seen that we still know very little about the private world of children and youth. If we accept the importance of the self as a main governor of behavior, we then need to develop research methods to learn more about (1) concept formation, including self-concept formation; (2) the relationships between self-concept, behavior, and experience; (3) the impact of others, especially family, peer, and school, on the developing self of the child; (4) techniques for securing valid pictures of self-concept, whether through the interpretation of behavior, projective techniques, or self-report; (5) self-in-situation relationships, which means both a more complex definition of self beyond self-esteem and a more careful study of the role of the situation in the transaction between the two (Gecas, 1972); and (6) the integration of cognitive and self-concept development.

We are still a long way from integrating the inner and the outer worlds of humans. We have a good start in the area of moral development and such concepts as egocentrism-decentering, but much remains to be learned.

All these research efforts, however, should fall within a value framework based upon respect for the integrity and individuality of the person. We have no right to violate the child's private world to use the data against him. How can we learn more about the person and still leave him free? The implications for research and application in connection with social values are serious, and we can only suggest their existence here.

Application

The importance of family relationships as an important force in positive identification and the development of secure and adequate concepts of self comes through clearly. This raises a number of significant questions about the continued role of the family, the effect of changing life styles, the high divorce rate, and the perpetuation of the nuclear family. It also raises issues of education for family living and a restructuring of the relationships between the family and other social agencies. If family relationships seem so crucial, how can we maintain the institution or learn to provide, by other means, whatever it is the family does that makes the difference? Or is the family indispensable? At the moment, we have no answers, but this author's value system argues for the strong resurgence of the family as the primary learning environment.

The importance of body image to the self of the adolescent suggests that some agency, either the home or school, needs to concern itself more with preparing youth for adolescent body changes, the meaning of these changes, and the chances that a particular boy or girl will be temporarily out-of-step with his peers. With the pressure to be like others and the odds that one won't be what he'd like to be physically, it is important that adults assist youngsters in accepting themselves. The effects of nonacceptance seem to linger for a long time, and it may be that they can be diminished if assistance is given as early as preadolescence.

The role of the school is not fully understood, but the data seem to indicate quite clearly a relationship between self-concept and achievement. A task of the school, then, is to develop in youth concepts of adequacy, self-respect, and self-confidence. Since these concepts depend upon experience in being evaluated in these ways and being treated as worthy, the implications for school practice are many. As only one example, can we really demonstrate trust in youth when we allow them virtually no choice? If we perceive guidance, for example, as testing and steering, how can the adolescent learn to value his own decisions? If we persist in having de facto segregated schools, unequal in facilities, space and resources, how can the child in less well-financed and maintained schools come to value himself? If we organize high schools in ladder or track systems and categorize youngsters according to some external means removed from their own needs and perceptions, how can they come to see themselves as adequate? If we see skill learning in a vacuum removed from all its emotional components, how can an adolescent come to know himself? If we assign youngsters to classes on the basis of standardized intelligence tests, how can the creative youngster experience his worth? How can the youngster with high motivation but less than 120 or 130 IQ demanded see himself as adequate? Especially when we know that motivation contributes as much as ability to success, how can we continue to justify exclusion on the basis of ability alone?

The question remains: How can we organize the school and teaching to demonstrate our belief in individuality and in the validity of the youngster's self-concept? How can we make the educational experience in high school less constrictive and more broadening? This works both ways: We need to allow the youngster who perhaps does not fit the definition of "giftedness" to try the advanced math course if he so desires and to allow the youngster who fits the definition to take typing if he sees this as important to him.

Who can judge for the person? It is his life and his right to choose. We hope he will not waste it, but which would be better—a career choice in which he is happy and profitably engaged and at peace with self and world, or one in which he goes through the motions because he ought to but feels little satisfaction?

We need equally to concern ourselves with the high school dropout or the youngster who graduates with no salable skill. We have, perhaps, made a shibboleth of academic education. Entrance requirements to jobs are often at a far higher level than really are needed for performance. We need to move rapidly into career-development patterns for youth in order to make them not only productive in the society but also productive for themselves. The variety of programs needed amply indicates that it may take a heavy investment of time and money, but these youngsters can learn and function with dignity.

We need to find ways in which youth can use their talents fully, but which allow them wide opportunities for exploration, even if this means the postponement of decision making until after high school graduation or even, for the college-bound, until after the first two years of college.

The evidence points up the narrow view of the adolescent about other groups of people outside his immediate circle of family and peers. He knows little about other cultures, even other culture groups in his own country. He tends to see different customs or religious beliefs as somehow inferior to his own. He has distorted perceptions of other class and ethnic groups within the broad American culture. Even within the consolidated, comprehensive high school, he has little contact with others in ways that modify his perceptions.

One of the greatest challenges of the transactional view of adolescence rests in the area of modification of concepts of those who differ from oneself. All we can do is pinpoint the issue: Schools and youth-serving agencies need to develop techniques for broadening the individual adolescent's experiences with other culture groups. Of course, those situations in which the individual develops more self-acceptance must be provided as an accompaniment. We know there is a relationship between acceptance of self and acceptance of others. We probably cannot expect the adolescent to learn to accept others if he lacks self-acceptance. Ways need to be found in which both goals are accomplished.

Knowledge of how adolescents conceive of self and other and knowledge of how this influences behavior leads to a host of implications with regard to the role of adults in assisting them to find and develop themselves. We can only hope that such knowledge will be used within the democratic ethos. The goal of all development, as we said in the first chapter, is to maximize and use one's capacities to the fullest. With this goal in mind, those of us who work with youth can find many ways to help them move toward healthy adulthood.

REFERENCES AND ADDITIONAL READINGS

Ammons, R. M. Academic persistence of some students at St. Petersburg Junior College. ERIC 063929, Office of Testing Services, St. Petersburg Junior College, May 1971.

Ausubel, D., & Schiff, H. Some intrapersonal and interpersonal determinants of individual differences in socioempathic ability among adolescents. *Journal of Social Psychology*, 1955, *41*, 39–56.

Bachman, J. *Youth in transition, Vol. II. The impact of family background and intelligence on tenth-grade boys.* Ann Arbor, Mich.: Institute for Social Research, University of Michigan, 1970.

Backman, M. Patterns of mental abilities: Ethnic, socioeconomic, and sex differences. *American Educational Research Journal*, 1972, *9*, 1–12.

Beilin, H. The pattern of postponability and its relation to social class mobility. *Journal of Social Psychology*, 1956, *44*, 33–48.

Block, J., Haan, N., & Smith, M. B. Activism and apathy in contemporary adolescents. In J. Adams (Ed.), *Understanding adolescence.* Boston: Allyn & Bacon, 1968. Pp. 198–231.

Block, J., Haan, N., & Smith, M. Socialization correlates of student activism. *Journal of Social Issues*, 1969, *25*, 143–177.

Boshier, R. The effect of academic failure on self-concept and maladjustment indices. *Journal of Educational Research*, 1972, *65*, 347–351.

Bradway, K. P., & Thompson, C. W. Intelligence at adulthood: A twenty-five year follow-up. *Journal of Educational Psychology*, 1962, *53*, 1–14. Reprinted in I. J. Gordon (Ed.), *Human development: Readings in research.* Glenview, Ill.: Scott, Foresman, 1965.

Broedel, J., Ohlsen, M., Proff, F., & Southard, C. The effects of group counseling on gifted underachieving adolescents. (Mimeo) University of Illinois, 1959.

Clark, J. et al. "Identification of disadvantaged junior college students and diagnosis of their disabilities." St. Petersburg Junior College, St. Petersburg, Florida, 1967.

Cole, N. On measuring the vocational interests of women. *Journal of Consulting Psychology,* 1973, *20,* 105–112.

Coleman, J. et al. *Equality of educational opportunity.* Washington, D.C.: U.S. Office of Education, 1966.

Combs, A., & Gordon, I. J. Attitudes and behavior of biological science curriculum study special materials classes in two Florida counties, 1965–66. A final report to the Biological Science Curriculum Study Director, Boulder, Colorado, March 1967.

Conger, J. A world they never knew. In J. Kagan and R. Coles (Eds.), *Twelve to sixteen: Early adolescence.* New York: Norton, 1972.

Crowley, F. The goals of male high school seniors. *Personnel and Guidance Journal,* 1959, *37,* 488–492.

Douvan, E., & Adelson, J. The psychodynamics of social mobility in adolescent boys. *Journal of Abnormal and Social Psychology,* 1958, *56,* 31–44.

Douvan, E., & Adelson, J. *The adolescent experience.* New York: Wiley, 1966.

Dragan, I. Les intérêts intellectuels, prémisses de l'orientation scolaire et professionnelle. *Bulletin de Psychologie Scolaire d'Orientation,* 1972, *21,* 11–14.

DuCette, J., & Wolk, S. Locus of control and extreme behavior. *Journal of Consulting and Clinical Psychology,* 1972a, *39,* 253–258.

DuCette, J., & Wolk, S. Locus of control and levels of aspiration in Black and white children. *Review of Educational Research,* 1972b, *42,* 493–504.

Ekehammar, B. Sex differences in self-reported anxiety for different situations and modes of response. *Reports from the Psychological Laboratories, #363.* The University of Stockholm, Sweden, 1972. 11 pp.

Elder, G. *Adolescent socialization and personality development.* Chicago: Rand McNally, 1968.

Feldman, K. Some theoretical approaches to the study of change and stability of college students. *Review of Educational Research,* 1972, *42,* 1–26.

Flacks, R. The liberated generation: An exploration of the roots of student protest. In I. J. Gordon (Ed.), *Readings in research in developmental psychology.* Glenview, Ill.: Scott, Foresman, 1971. Pp. 341–351.

Freedman, M. Some observations of students as they relate to orientation procedures in colleges and universities. *Journal of College Student Personnel,* 1960, *2,* 2–10.

Friesen, D. Value orientations of modern youth: A comparative study. *Adolescence,* 1972, *7,* 265–275.

Getzels, J., & Jackson, P. The study of giftedness: A multidimensional approach. In *The gifted student,* Cooperative Research Monograph No. 2, Washington, D.C.: U.S. Department of Health, Education, and Welfare, Office of Education, 1960.

Gordon, I. J. A test manual for the How I See Myself scale. Gainesville, Fla.: Florida Educational Research and Development Council, 1968.

Gordon, I. J., & Combs, A. W. The learner: Self and perception. *Review of Educational Research,* 1958, *28,* 433–444.

Gottlieb, D. Poor youth: A study in alienation. In I. J. Gordon (Ed.), *Readings in research in developmental psychology.* Glenview, Ill.: Scott, Foresman, 1971. Pp. 312–326.

Guilford, J. Three faces of intellect. *The American Psychologist,* 1959, *14,* 469–479.

Guilford, J. Three faces of intellect. In I. J. Gordon (Ed.), *Readings in research in developmental psychology.* Glenview, Ill.: Scott, Foresman, 1971. Pp. 10–23.

Gurin, G., Veroff, J., & Feld, S. *Americans view their mental health.* New York: Basic Books, 1960.

Harris, D. Sex differences in the life problems and interests of adolescents, 1935 and 1957. *Child Development,* 1959, *30,* 453–459.

Himmelweit, H., & Swift, B. Adolescent and adult authoritarianism reexamined: Its organization and stability overtime. *European Journal of Social Psychology,* 1971, *1,* 357–384.

Holland, J. *Psychology of vocational choice.* Waltham, Mass.: Blaisdell, 1966.

Hollender, J. Self-esteem and parental identification. *The Journal of Genetic Psychology,* 1973, *122,* 3–7.

Hollingsworth, H. *Psychology and ethics.* New York: Ronald Press, 1949.

Hunt, D. Adolescence: Cultural deprivation, poverty and the drop-out. *Review of Educational Research,* 1966, *36,* 463–473.

Jackson, P., Getzels, J., & Xydis, G. Psychological health and cognitive functioning in adolescence: A multivariate analysis. *Child Development,* 1960, *31,* 285–298. Reprinted in I. J. Gordon (Ed.), *Human development: Readings in research.* Glenview, Ill.: Scott, Foresman, 1965.

Jones, M. The later careers of boys who were early- or late-maturing. *Child Development,* 1957, *28,* 113–128.

Kammayer, K. The feminine role: An analysis of attitude consistency. *Journal of Marriage and the Family,* 1964, *26,* 295–305.

Katz, P., & Zigler, E. Self-image disparity: A developmental approach. In I. J. Gordon (Ed.), *Readings in research in developmental psychology.* Glenview, Ill.: Scott, Foresman, 1971. Pp. 341–351.

Kennedy, P. *Acceptance of self and acceptance of others as interdependent variables in interpersonal relations.* Washington, D.C.: Catholic University of America Press, 1958.

Kibrick, A. K., & Tiedeman, D. V. Conceptions of self and perception of role in schools of nursing. *Journal of Counseling Psychology,* 1961, *8,* 62–69.

Kipnis, D. M. Changes in self concepts in relation to perceptions of others. *Journal of Personality,* 1961, *29,* 449–465. Reprinted in I. J. Gordon (Ed.), *Human development: Readings in research.* Glenview, Ill.: Scott, Foresman, 1965.

Kogan, N., & Pankove, E. Creative ability over a five-year span. *Child Development,* 1972, *43,* 427–442.

Lent, A. A survey of the problems of adolescent high school girls. *Alberta Journal of Educational Research,* 1957, *3,* 127–137.

MacDonald, K., & Gynther, M. Relationship of self and ideal-self description with sex, race and class in southern adolescents. *Journal of Personal and Social Psychology,* 1965, *1,* 85–88.

McKee, J., & Sherriffs, A. Men's and women's beliefs, ideals and self-concepts. *American Journal of Sociology,* 1959, *44,* 356–363.

Marks, J. B. Interests and leadership among adolescents. *Journal of Genetic Psychology,* 1957, *91,* 163–172.

Maslow, A. *Motivation and personality.* New York: Harper & Row, 1955.

Matteson, R. Self-estimates of college freshmen. *Personnel and Guidance Journal,* 1956, *34,* 280–284.

Mead, M., & Metraux, R. Image of the scientist among high school students. *Science,* 1957, *216,* 384–390.

Moore, B., & Holtzman, W. *Tomorrow's parents: A study of youth and their families.* Austin, Texas: University of Texas Press, 1965.

Morval, J., & Morval, M. Self-esteem and interpersonal needs in girls between 15 and 18. *Revue de Psychologic Applique,* 1972, *22,* 67–75.

Okaji, J. Studies on characteristics of adolescents' attitudes toward life. *Japanese Journal of Educational Psychology,* 1958, *6,* 7–13.

Olive, H. The relationship of divergent thinking to intelligence, social class, and achievement in high-school students. *Journal of Genetic Psychology,* 1972a, *121,* 179–186.

Olive, H. A note on sex differences in adolescents' divergent thinking. *Journal of Psychology,* 1972b, *82,* 39–42.

Ostlund, L. Environment-personality relationships. *Rural Sociology,* 1957, *22,* 31–39.

Piaget, J. Intellectual evolution from adolescence to adulthood. *Human Development,* 1972, *15,* 1–12.

Pierce, J., & Bowman, P. Motivation patterns of superior high school students. In *The gifted student,* Cooperative Research Monograph No. 2, Washington, D.C.: U.S. Department of Health, Education, and Welfare, Office of Education, 1960. Pp. 33–66.

Pugh, M., Perry, J., Snyder, E., & Spreitzer, E. Participation in anti-war demonstrations: A test of the parental continuity hypothesis. *Sociology and Social Research,* 1971, *56,* 19–28.

Purdue Opinion Panel. High school students' leisure time activities and attitudes toward network television. Lafayette, Ind.: Purdue University, 1967.

Remmers, H., & Radler, D. Teenage attitudes. In J. Seidman (Ed.), *The adolescent.* (Rev. ed.) New York: Holt, Rinehart & Winston, 1960. Pp. 579–605.

Richards, J. M., Jr. A factor analytic study of the self-ratings of college freshman. *Educational and Psychological Measurement,* 1966, *26,* 861–870.

Rogers, C. The concept of the fully functioning person. (Mimeo) 1958.

Rosen, E. Self-appraisal and perceived desirability of MMPI personality traits. *Journal of Counseling Psychology,* 1956, *3,* 44–51.

Rosenberg, M. Society and the adolescent self-image. Princeton, N.J.: Princeton University Press, 1965.

Rosenberg, B., & Silverstein, H. Moral socialization and moral anomie. In H. Silverstein (Ed.), *The sociology of youth, evolution and revolution.* New York: Macmillan, 1973. Pp. 166–184.

Rotter, J. Generalized expectancies for internal versus external control of reinforcement. *Psychological Monographs,* 1966, *80* (Whole no. 609).

Ryckman, R. M., Martens, J. L., Rodda, W. C., & Sherman, M. F. Locus control and attitudes toward Women's Liberation in a college population. *Journal of Social Psychology,* 1972, *87,* 157–158.

Sanford, N. Developmental status of the entering freshman. In N. Sanford (Ed.), *The American college.* New York: Wiley, 1962.

Sarason, J., & Smith, R. Personality. In P. Mussen & M. Rosenzweig (Eds.), *An-*

nual review of psychology. Vol. 22. Palo Alto, Calif.: Annual Reviews, Inc., 1971. Pp. 393–446.

Saugstad, P., & Raaheim, K. Problem-solving past experience, and availability of functions. *British Journal of Psychology,* 1960, *51,* 97–104. Reprinted in I. J. Gordon (Ed.), *Human development: Readings in research.* Glenview, Ill.: Scott, Foresman, 1965.

Schmidt, J., & Rothney, J. Variability of vocational choices of high school students. *Personnel and Guidance Journal,* 1955, *34,* 142–146.

Schneider, J. M. College students' belief in personal control, 1966–1970. *Journal of Individual Psychology,* 1971, *27(2),* 188.

Shaw, M., Edson, K., & Bell, H. The self-concept of bright under-achieving high school students as revealed by an adjective check list. *Personnel and Guidance Journal,* 1960, *39,* 193–196.

Sherif, M., & Sherif, C. W. *Reference groups.* New York: Harper & Row, 1964.

Silber, E. et al. Adaptive behavior in competent adolescents: Coping with the anticipation of college. *Archives of General Psychiatry,* 1961, *5,* 354–365. Reprinted in I. J. Gordon (Ed.), *Human development: Readings in research.* Glenview, Ill.: Scott, Foresman, 1965.

Singer, J., & Singer, D. Personality. In P. Mussen & M. Rosenzweig (Eds.), *Annual review of psychology.* Vol. 23. Palo Alto, Calif.: Annual Reviews, Inc., 1972. Pp. 375–412.

Stewart, L. H. Cultural differences in abilities during high school. *American Educational Research Journal,* 1967, *4,* 19–30.

Strunk, O. Relationship between self-reports and adolescent religiosity. *Psychological Reports,* 1958, *4,* 683–686.

Taba, H. The moral beliefs of sixteen-year-olds. In J. Seidman (Ed.), *The adolescent.* New York: Dryden Press, 1953. Pp. 314–318.

Taylor, R. Personality traits and discrepant achievement: A review. *Journal of Counseling Psychology,* 1964, *11,* 76–81.

Torrance, E. P. Educational achievement of the highly intelligent and the highly creative. Minneapolis: Bureau of Educational Research, University of Minnesota (Research Memorandum BER–60–18), 1960.

Wallach, M. A., & Kogan, N. A new look at the creativity-intelligence distinction. *Journal of Personality,* 1965, *33(3),* 348–369.

Warren, J. R. Self concept, occupational role expectation, and change in college major. *Journal of Counseling Psychology,* 1961, *8,* 164–196.

Wilk, R. E. The self perceptions and the perceptions of others of adolescent leaders elected by their peers. Doctoral dissertation, University of Minnesota, 1957.

Wright, D., & Cox, E. Changes in moral belief among sixth-form boys and girls over a seven year period in relation to religious belief, age and sex difference. *Journal of Social and Clinical Psychology,* 1971, *10,* 332–341.

Yamamoto, K. A further analysis of the role of creative thinking in high-school achievement. *Journal of Psychology,* 1964, *58,* 277–283.

Zuk, G. Sex-appropriate behavior in adolescence. *Journal of Genetic Psychology,* 1958, *93,* 15–32.

INDEX OF NAMES

406

INDEX OF SUBJECTS

415

Strong Vocational Interest Blank, 261–262, 327
Structure-function, 6, 9, 184
Sweden, breast feeding in, 46
children in, 271, 389

T

Tactile communication, 33, 63
Teachers, 154, 157–158. *See also* School
relations to students, 154, 162, 191–192, 206, 228–230, 242–244, 249–250, 271, 292, 310–311, 363–364
Television. *See* Mass media
Television for children, 134
Temperament, 28, 29
Tennessee Scale of Self-Concept, 344
Thematic Apperception Test, 274, 294–295, 302, 343
Thought, 63, 102–107, 196–198, 202, 239–241, 275, 320–321. *See also* Cognition; Conceptual development; Language; Meanings; Operations
Toilet-training, 45–46
Transactional viewpoint, 3–4, 45, 83, 93, 122, 206–207, 211, 286–287, 314, 372, 389, 392, 394–399
Transactions. *See* Interpersonal relations; Learning; Self-system; Development; Instruction; Parent-child relations; Transactional viewpoint
Turkey, children in, 248–249
Twins, study of, 27, 29–30

U

Uniqueness, 4, 13–17, 19, 37, 55. *See also.* Individual differences; Physical growth

V

Values, 70–72, 116, 133–134, 143–146, 152–154, 156, 160, 162–163, 177–180, 202–207, 230, 232–235, 248–251, 312–317, 328–332, 344, 360, 362, 376–380, 397. *See also* Moral development
Venereal disease, 31, 307, 369
Vietnam, children in, 263, 357, 362, 369–370, 379
Vocational aspirations, 258, 333–335, 384–386, 394–395

W

Warner Scale for Social Class, 51
Watergate, 362, 377–378
Women's liberation, 47, 257, 339, 355

75 76 77 7 6 5 4 3 2 1